Foreword

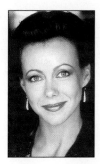

Over the last couple of decades the range and availability of natural health treatments, therapies and products has increased so dramatically. Now we can choose to use natural approaches that have been developed over hundreds and in some cases thousands of years, and yet have only reached the masses during our children's lifetimes. Other therapies are based on new, exciting principles and discoveries.

Natural Health Direct is the second in a series of directories celebrating the cosmopolitan community that has grown around natural health. Complementary medicine, integrated health care, holistic medicine, all come together and have a place in this publication. Looking after yourself is about making choices. If we choose to use natural medicines or therapies then the more informed we are the better, and the more options we have.

My son suffered with Colic for his first six months. Had I known of Cranio-sacral therapy at that time I am sure it would have helped him. Bowen Technique helps those with age related illnesses such as Parkinson's Disease, Physiotherapy techniques have been developed to help children with cerebral palsy. These are only sparse examples of the many ways in which natural health can add to our lives. Natural Health Direct gives access to the people, services and products that will enable and support informed choice.

While I do not feel that using natural medicines and therapies should in any way preclude the use of the more orthodox treatments, I do believe that they have often helped the healing process. My work with Ovacome, a support group for women suffering from ovarian cancer, has made me aware of remedies that have been used alongside some of the more toxic cancer drugs to good effect.

I have been helped by natural approaches to self-care in my career too. Acting requires energy and concentration, both of which have been improved for me by Yoga. I also enjoy the benefits of Aromatherapy, massage and Reflexology.

We live in a world of fast foods at a fast pace. Health should never be taken for granted. I think we need to be aware of the best ways to look after ourselves. I hope this directory will help you to find some extra ways to keep up with the pace in a healthy way.

Jenny Agutter

The Natural Health Directory

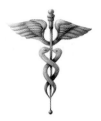

ISBN: 190336100-1

Published
by
Kingsley Media Ltd, Plymouth.
Tel: 01752 559999   E-mail: admin@naturalhealthdirect.com
Copyright: Kingsley Media Ltd
All rights reserved.

The purpose of this directory is to educate, inform and entertain. Its objective is to provide accurate and useful information to the consumer. Whilst every care is taken the publisher accepts no responsibility for any errors or misinformation contained in the articles or claims made by advertisers. The information included is not intended as advice for self-diagnosis; readers are advised to consult a medical practitioner prior to adopting dietary guidelines or any form of nutritional or medical treatments. The views expressed are those of the authors of the text and not necessarily those of the publisher or advertisers.

Kingsley Media Ltd wishes to thank the experts and health care professionals who have contributed their support and knowledge and the advertisers for their enthusiastic support. Without them this book would not have been possible.

Thanks are given to The Media Team and all at Kingsley Media for their invaluable assistance in bringing this book to you. We hope you find the book useful in pursuing a healthier lifestyle and sourcing a natural health professional for whatever therapy or service you may require.

Typeset by The Media Team, Plymouth, Devon.
01752 519736
www.media-team.co.uk
Printed and bound in the United Kingdom by
J.H. Haynes & Co. Ltd.

Concept by M.Willcocks. PhD. (Chairman)
Edited by Louise O,Neill

Contents

Continued overleaf

How to use this book

To find out more about a specific therapy and find relevant therapists or services, please refer to these Contents Pages. All information is provided in a simple A-Z format.

To fast track finding a therapist or service in your area please consult the directory section at the back of the book for a subject and locality index.

To locate organisations, societies and charities please go to Page 386

Alternative medicine should be available to all on the NHS

It has always been a subject close to his heart. Now PRINCE CHARLES is anxious to share his views on alternative medicine with as wide an audience as possible

For years, the NHS has found complementary medicine an uncomfortable bedfellow – at best regarded as 'fringe' and in some quarters as 'quack'; never viewed as a substitute for conventional medicine and rarely as a genuine partner in providing therapy. But at last there are signs of a genuine partnership developing as more and more NHS professionals and complementary therapists find themselves working alongside one another.

That patients are interested in complementary therapies is undeniable. A BBC poll revealed one in five Britons opts to use such therapies. Yet, we have a situation in which substantial numbers of people are looking beyond the NHS for healthcare; indeed are using complementary and alternative medicine in parallel with conventional provision, and – if continued demand is any indication – are presumably satisfied with the results. All well and good, perhaps, but if there are advantages in this approach, clearly they should not be limited to those who can pay.

This interest in non-conventional approaches is far from one-sided. According to a survey by Birmingham University in 1998, about half the family doctors who responded provided access to one or more complementary therapies, either by practising a non-conventional therapy themselves, or by suggesting their patients to go to a local complementary practitioner.

The response to the recent Guild of Health Writers' Award for Good Practice in Integrated Healthcare, held in association with the Foundation for Integrated Medicine, of which I am proud to be president, suggests that integrated medicine is more widespread than expected. To qualify for entry, the integrated healthcare team had to include at least one conventional health professional. The number of entries – 81 to be precise – far exceeded expectations and the sheer diversity, the quality of work and the real integration of disciplines was astonishing. Even more remarkably, the majority were operating within the NHS. Homeopaths, osteopaths, reflexologists, acupuncturists, T'ai chi instructors, art therapists, chiropractors, herbalists and aromatherapists; these practitioners are working alongside NHS colleagues in hospitals, on children's wards, in nursing homes and, in particular, in primary healthcare, in GP practices and health clinics up and down the country.

What the best demonstrate is that integrated medicine – the collaboration of two seemingly opposed disciplines for the benefit of patients – is not only possible, but actually works. There was little that was haphazard or ad hoc about these teams – they worked as professionals in teams of mutual respect. By dint of intensely hard work and innovation, many of the entrants also found ways to research and prove the effectiveness – and cost effectiveness – of complementary therapies.

The winner, Complementary Therapies within Cancer Services at the NHS

Hammersmith Hospitals Trust, was outstanding for the sheer depth of its integration in offering massage therapy, reflexology, aromatherapy, relaxation training and art therapy to cancer patients at Charing Cross and Hammersmith Hospital.

Records indicate that complementary therapies have significantly decreased palliative drug use among radiotherapy patients. Another example, this time in primary care. Glastonbury Health Centre, runner-up in the award, set out to develop a model of a fully integrated NHS primary care service that could be replicated in other NHS practices. Patients are offered courses of acupuncture, herbal medicine, homeopathy, massage therapy and osteopathy in the same way as orthodox practices offer physiotherapy or medication. No-one would deny that there are not considerable hurdles in assimilating systems that in many respects, notably language and philosophy, may seem diametrically opposed. Obviously, compromises must be made on both sides. But patients do benefit. Studies show that complementary therapies help patients' general vitality, social functioning, emotional and mental health, and are particularly effective in relieving pain and physical discomfort for patients with musculoskeletal problems.

As an NHS practice, how does Glastonbury Health Centre afford this service? A practice-based charitable trust enables patients to access the required therapies for the price of an NHS prescription, or free of charge if necessary. Although providing complementary therapies tends to be slightly more expensive, patients appear to reduce their usage of other health services such as GP time, prescriptions, X-rays and other tests.

This is tremendously important information for all of us who would like to see the NHS offering a broader kind of care for a greater number of people.

Complementary therapies afford enormous scope for self-care and their very popularity is often attributed to patients' desire to take more responsibility for their own well-being. One of the most appealing entrants in the Guild of Health Writers' Award involved a single intervention with enormous potential. A team at Queen Charlotte and Chelsea Hospital showed that teaching mothers with post-natal depression to massage their babies not only enhanced mother-child bonding, but relieved the depression. If one considers that post-natal depression afflicts ten per cent of the 70,000 women who give birth in the UK each year, it is clearly a major problem, affecting the mental health of the infants, who often grow up with behavioural problems, or with a reduced IQ. Set against this the sum of £30 – the estimated cost of five lessons in infant massage that, with appropriately trained therapists, could be provided in any baby health clinic or GP practice.

These are pragmatic examples, with easily quantifiable benefits, of the kind of future that integrated healthcare could provide in the NHS. Complementary therapies are not a woolly cul-de-sac, but a very real option with promising advantages for patient care and primary health group budgets. Communication is the very oxygen of innovation, but too often ground-breaking initiatives are not well publicised. With this in mind, the Foundation for Integrated Medicine is establishing an information database and resource centre for practitioners who want to develop integrated services.

It is not a question of hacking through unexplored jungle. The way is landmarked, the goals and prizes are visible. All that is needed is courage – and a little imagination.

The Regulation of Complementary and Alternative Medicine

By the Federation of Holistic Therapists

The House of Lords Select Committee recently issued a report into 'Complementary and Alternative Medicine'(CAM). This is partly in response to growing public concern regarding the safety of this largely unregulated industry. Recent programmes such as 'Tonight' with Trevor McDonald have highlighted the dangers of using unqualified practitioners who claimed to diagnose medical conditions.

The Federation of Holistic Therapists, the largest professional body for Complementary Therapists such as Aromatherapists and Reflexologists, has welcomed the impetus behind the Report to seek clarification of the scope of these fields and the protection of the public against unscrupulous or poorly qualified therapists.

Summary of Report

The report covers a wide range of therapy practice. The Committee has categorised complementary and alternative medicine (CAM) therapies into three groups:-

Group 1 includes the most organised professions in what may be called the principal disciplines. The group includes osteopathy; chiropractic; acupuncture; herbal medicine and homeopathy.

Group 2 contains those therapies that most clearly complement conventional medicine and do not purport to embrace diagnostic skills. It includes aromatherapy; the Alexander Technique; body work therapies, including massage; counselling, stress therapy; hypnotherapy; reflexology and probably shiatsu, meditation and healing.

Group 3 cannot be supported unless and until convincing research evidence of efficacy, based upon the results of well designed trials, can be produced. The third group favours a philosophical approach and are indifferent to the scientific principles of conventional medicine. Group 3a includes long-established and traditional systems of healthcare such as Ayurvedic medicine and Traditional Chinese medicine. Group 3b covers other alternative disciplines which lack any credible evidence base such as crystal therapy, iridology, radionics, dowsing and kinesiology.

The report recommends that the existing regulatory bodies in each of the healthcare professions should develop clear guidelines on competence and training in the CAM disciplines and on the position they take in relation to their members' activities in CAM. The report recommends, however, that only those CAM therapies which are statutorily regulated or have robust mechanisms of voluntary self-regulation should be available through the NHS.

Reasons for accessing CAM – survey data

The BBC Survey of CAM use in the United Kingdom shows the reasons for the public using CAM was firstly that it 'helps relieves injury/condition' (25 per cent). Other reasons include 'Just like it' (21 per cent); 'Find it relaxing' (19); 'Good health/well-being generally' (14); and 'Preventative measure' (12). These 'other reasons' add up to more than the 25 per cent of 'Helps or relieves injury/condition'. This demonstrates that many people go to complementary practitioners for reasons other than to cure them of an illness and the hidden health benefits attached to these reasons should not be underestimated.

The Government view regulation as important. In May 1998, the then Secretary of State for Health, Frank Dobson, addressed a conference at FIM at which he stated that the Government expected CAM professionals "to attain the same standards of professional self-regulation expected of other healthcare professionals". The Department of Health's evidence also explained their aims for regulations within healthcare: "In matters of regulation, it is the Government's intention to maintain freedom of choice while ensuring that appropriate safeguards are in place".

On the issue of the protection of title: "The Common Law right to practise medicine means that in the United Kingdom anyone can treat a sick person. The Common Law right to practise springs from the fundamental principle that everyone can choose the form of healthcare that they require. Thus, although statutory regulation can award a therapy protection of title, it cannot stop anyone utilising the methods of that therapy under a slightly different name." This is an important point.

Features of an effective regulatory system

The primary benefit of effective regulation is that it protects the public. This is done through five main features which the BMA outlined: "To provide a code of conduct, a disciplinary procedure, and a complaints procedure; to provide minimum standards of training and to supervise training courses and accreditation; to understand and advertise areas of competence, including limits of competence within each therapy; to keep an up-to-date register of qualified practitioners; and to provide and publicise information on CAM".

Which therapies would benefit from statutory regulation?

The Report opines that acupuncture and herbal medicines are two therapies which are at a stage where it would be of benefit to them and their patients if practitioners strive for statutory regulation under the Health Act 1999, and it is recommended that they should do so. Statutory regulation may also be appropriate eventually for the non-medical homeopaths. Other bodies must strive to come together under one voluntary self-regulating body and some may wish ultimately to aim to move towards regulation under the Health Act once they are unified with a single voice.

Jacqueline Palmer, Chief Executive of the Federation of Holistic Therapists said: "The FHT welcomes the Lords' attempt to tackle the complexities of this problem head on. Nobody wants the public to be exposed to unnecessary risk through incompetent or poorly trained therapists. However, we were disappointed to note that there was much reliance upon the information contained in the University of Exeter Report into Complementary Therapies which actually contained many inaccuracies which have already been pointed out to the Department of Health who commissioned it.

"It was interesting to note that the Select Committee did not feel that those therapies classed in Group 2 were ready to move towards state registration at present. Instead they were encouraged to bring therapists together to form a single body to work towards that end. The FHT supports progress in this area so long as the body concerned is a genuinely independent group made up of those with no commercial interests."

Acupuncture
By the British Acupuncture Council

Acupuncture is an ancient system of healing developed over thousands of years as part of the traditional medicine of China, Japan and other Eastern countries.

Optimal health, according to traditional Chinese philosophy, is dependent on the body's motivating energy – known as Qi – moving in a smooth and balanced way through a series of channels beneath the skin. Illness occurs when the flow of Qi is insufficient, unbalanced or interrupted.

Qi flow can be disturbed by a number of factors including poor nutrition, stress, infections, weather conditions, trauma, and emotional states such as grief, anger, fear or anxiety. In acupuncture, diagnosis and therapy are aimed at identifying any imbalances in the body and correcting them. Treatment usually involves having extremely fine needles inserted into appropriate points along the meridians or energy pathways in the body.

Its origins

The earliest record of acupuncture is found in the Huang Di Neijing or Yellow Emperor's Classic of Internal Medicine (300 BC). The practice of acupuncture is thought to have begun with the discovery that the stimulation of specific areas on the

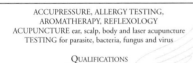

skin affecting the functioning of certain organs of the body. Since then, acupuncture has evolved into a system of medicine that is practised worldwide.

How it is used?

At your first consultation, the acupuncturist will need to assess your general state of health in order to identify the underlying pattern of disharmony and to give you the most effective treatment. You will be asked about your current symptoms and what treatment you have received so far, your medical history, your diet, digestive system, sleep patterns and emotional state. Your tongue and pulse will also be examined as these both give a good indication of your physical health. Based on the diagnosis, the appropriate acupuncture points will be selected. Once inserted, the needles may be manipulated or left still. The treatment may be supplemented with other methods of stimulation including, moxibustion or cupping to encourage the Qi to flow smoothly.

Conditions that acupuncture treats

Many people will visit an acupuncturist with specific symptoms or conditions, such as pain, anxiety or high blood pressure. While extensive practice and research has shown that acupuncture is effective in helping people with such conditions as well as with many others, it does more than simply relieve symptoms. The aim of traditional acupuncture is to improve the overall well being of the patient, rather than the isolated treatment of specific symptoms. Many people have acupuncture as a preventative treatment.

Some of the conditions acupuncture treats:

• respiratory tract infections and broncho-pulmonary disorders such as acute sinusitis, rhinitis, common cold, acute tonsillitis, hay fever, acute bronchitis and bronchial asthma

• dermatological disorders such as urticaria, eczema, and psoriasis

• gastro-intestinal problems including hiccough, indigestion, spastic colon, gastroptosis, acute and chronic gastritis, colitis, constipation, diarrhoea

• gynaecological disorders such as pre-menstrual tension, irregular menstruation, dysmennorhea,

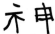

amenorrhea, uterine bleeding, leucorrhea, malposition of foetus, difficult labour, endometriosis, menopausal symptoms, impotence, infertility

• neurological and musculo-skeletal disorders such as headache, migraine, trigeminal neuralgia, facial paralysis, sciatica and lumbar pain, rheumatoid and osteo-arthritis, tennis elbow, 'frozen shoulder', intercostal neuralgia, Menier's Syndrome, cystitis, nocturia, peripheral neuropathies, sequelae of poliomyelitis (early stage)

• ear, eye and mouth disorders such as acute conjunctivitis, retinitis, myopia in children, cataract, tinnitis and toothache

• other conditions such as depression, anxiety, stress, hypertension, addictive disorders, ME and MS

Finding a practitioner

People often find practitioners through referrals from a friend or another medical professional, logging on to naturalhealthdirect.com, or by using this directory.

What to look for in a practitioner

Ensure the practitioner has completed training of at least three years in traditional acupuncture including biomedical sciences appropriate to the practice of acupuncture. Wherever treatment is offered it is important to check the qualifications of the practitioner and their registration with a reputable professional body.

Case history

A 55-year-old man suffered from chest pain on exercise. Apart from this, he had not many other symptoms at all, except for some lower backache and a cold feeling. However, his tongue and pulse clearly showed the presence of a definite pathology. His tongue had a normal colour but was purple on the sides in the chest area, his pulse was firm, especially on the right side and weak on both rear positions (kidneys).

The firm pulse is wiry but only at the deep level and it usually indicates blood stasis in the interior. The diagnosis was blood stasis in the heart occurring against a background of Kidney-Yang deficiency.

The treatment; Red Stirring, two tablets twice a day to treat the manifestation, i.e. blood stasis in the heart, and acupuncture for the root. After two months, the purple patches on his tongue had completely disappeared and no further chest pain was experienced.

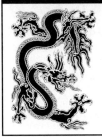

Aikido
By The British Aikido Association

Aikido can benefit everyone; male or female, young or old, of any ethnic or national origin. All can enjoy and improve their health and fitness by attending regular and well-run classes. The formal and more spiritual aspect of Aikido appeals to some, the physical side to others. Its full and natural body movement has aerobic benefits for all.

When practised regularly it will assist in developing a fitter, suppler and stronger body with improved flexibility, reflexes and reactions. Aikido is essentially non-violent, encourages harmony of mind, body and spirit and the avoidance of confrontation. Force is never opposed by force. Students learn how to improve self-awareness and also grow in self-confidence. In this Aikido teaches self-defence.

Aikido is today's fastest growing recreational activity with Japanese origins that go back many centuries. Aikido as practised today includes joint locking techniques and body movements from ancient fighting methods perfected by Samurai in feudal Japan. Aikido principles are based on exploiting the weaknesses of an opponent. Joints, posture, the mind can all be vulnerable areas when attacked or challenged. In essence Aikido is turning an opponents' power against themselves by using the exact degree of control required to neutralise their energy without inflicting undue harm.

The Aikido feeling

This is a simple illustration of aikido feeling which can be done by anyone. First, extend one arm away from the body with the palm facing the ceiling and the joint of the elbow also facing the ceiling. The arm should naturally bend upwards towards the body.

Now have someone attempt to bend the arm while you resist. Take care not to stress the arm unnaturally! The person should have superior leverage and be able to bend the arm at the elbow. Even if they do not succeed, by resisting, your arm will tire quickly.

Now try it again, but instead of resisting their attempts to bend your arm, extend your arm and think of it as a straight pole. Relax, pick an object which your arm is pointing towards and pretend that your arm is attached to this object. Do not try to resist the person bending your arm but instead concentrate on the attachment between your arm and the object; above all, relax. You will find that not only is your arm now unbendable but, more importantly, it requires far less energy to resist.

No special equipment is necessary for Aikido. There are Aikido coaches, known as Do-Jos, throughout the UK. For more information about Aikido or to locate a coach in your area, contact the British Aikido Association (see advertisement on this page).

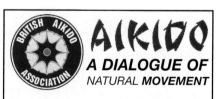

Alchemy

By Kate and Simon Kirkwood

Healing with Natural Incenses

The role of fragrant incenses in preparing the mind for healing and meditation has long been known by religions and cultures around the world, from the Catholic Church with the sweet heady aroma of the altar incense of frankincense, myrrh benzoin and storax, to the Plains Indians with their smudge-sticks of wild sage, copal, cedarwood and sweetgrass.

Many complementary therapists are also making the most of our sense of smell in creating a healing environment. Our sense of smell is one of our most subtle and powerful links to the deep levels of our psyche.

A particular smell can bring memories flooding back or provoke a strong emotion. To see a beautiful rose, our immediate reaction is to reach out to smell it, but if it is a rose that has been bred only for its bloom, we feel disappointed and walk away feeling let down. However if it smells as beautiful as it looks, for that moment our heart lifts and our mind is empty of everything except that wonderful perfume.

Incenses and fragrant oils can be used in this way to create a mental space for healing to occur, and can have a wide range of positive effects on physical and mental well-being, helping us to generate positive mental states and healing energy.

Incenses are now available to use in all aspects of healing. Blends containing lavender and rosemary, traditional cleansing herbs, can be used to clear a space before or after healing. Or specific incenses blended from herbs and fragrant tree resins specially chosen to stimulate the charkas, can be burnt while working on the specific energy centres of the body.

Using our sense of smell to bring a sense of well being to body and mind is a gentle complement to any healing tradition. As a tool for meditation it helps clear a special space for you to calm and centre in, and as a mood enhancing fragrance, different blends can be burnt to give an atmosphere of peace, or alternatively to fill yourself with energy.

Becoming aware of natures fragrances, and how they affect us, brings balance and harmony to mind body and spirit, and brings us into harmony with nature.

Allergy Therapy

An allergy is an inappropriate or exaggerated response of the body's defence system (the immune system) to something that in the majority of people causes no symptoms.

That which causes an allergic response is known as an allergen. Surprisingly, allergens are commonplace around the home. Among the most common are:

• The house dust mite and its droppings, found all around the home but especially in bedding and soft furnishings

• Animal dander – the tiny particles of skin, dried sweat and saliva found in the fur of cats and dogs

• Feathers in pillows, cushions and other soft furnishings

• The tiny spores released from mould and mildew

• Pollen from plants and flowers

• Certain household chemicals, such as formaldehyde, ammonia and phenol.

Allergens in the home can trigger or make worse a number of common conditions, such as allergic rhinitis, asthma or eczema.

Beds contain between 100,000 and 10,000,000 dust mites! To help make your bedroom as allergen-free as possible try barrier covers for your bedding. They are designed to prevent house dust mites and their tiny droppings escaping from your pillows, mattresses and duvets. You should be able to find this type of bedding in most department stores. Wash bedding at least once a week in a hot wash (at least 60°C)

Kill dust mites in soft toys, cushions and soft furnishings by putting each item in the freezer for 24 hours, then washing as recommended. Keep pets out of the bedroom.

To help create a less dusty living room, change carpets, curtains and cushions for wood, lino or hard floors and Venetian or roller blinds that are much easier to clean. Cushions and curtains also collect dust but if you prefer their look make sure you wash them frequently. Give rugs and mats a good beating outside regularly and dry-clean often. Don't use woollen blankets or anything that contains feathers. Leather, wood, metal or plastic furniture is less likely to capture dust. Buy furniture that's nailed rather than glued, as certain glues release irritant fumes into the atmosphere.

The kitchen is an active room for moulds and mildew, so when cleaning pay attention to the undersides of surfaces, around taps, doorknobs and under cupboard handles. Discard out of date food. Use an extractor fan or open a window when cooking to help reduce moisture and humidity.

The bathroom is another mould and mildew hot spot. Check behind the bath, around the basin and toilet and on shower curtains and use an extractor fan if you enjoy steamy baths or open a window to reduce humidity.

Try the following cleaning tips if allergies are a problem in your home:

• Use a high-filtration vacuum cleaner; ordinary cleaners stir up much of the dust they pick up and release it back into the air

• Wear a dust mask and gloves to reduce contact with potential allergens

• Dust with a damp cloth to 'soak up' dust, rather than flick it around

• Some of the worst irritants are found in cleaning fluids, such as formaldehyde, phenol and ammonia. Try 'natural' alternatives such as vinegar, soda crystals, lemon juice, water and good old elbow grease instead. Rather than spraying with man-made air fresheners, try placing a saucer of baking soda in a room to help neutralise smells

• Keep your home dry and well ventilated

• Open windows regularly and keep extractor vents open

• Open windows for at least half an hour a day. However, if you suffer from hay fever, keep windows closed as much as possible during the pollen season to keep out pollen

• A humidifier may help to reduce the symptoms of allergic rhinitis by softening the sensitive nasal membranes

• Dry clothes outside if possible, or indoors with windows open

• Humidity is a breeding ground for mould, mildew and dust mites. Dry the air with an air conditioning system or a dehumidifier if your house is humid

• Don't permit smoking. While smoking itself may not actually cause allergies, it can trigger asthma and, as an unhealthy habit, it may affect other allergies

• Think before you buy a pet. If you think you may be allergic to pets then it's best not to have one pet in the house. Alternatively, keep them outside or limit them to one room only, preferably one without carpet. The bedroom should be strictly out of bounds. Finally, try to bath them regularly.

To find out more about allergies and allergens, contact any of the advertisers in this section, who will be happy to help.

The Alexander Technique

By Joan Diamond

How does the Alexander Technique help you?

The Alexander Technique works differently than other bodywork techniques such as massage or osteopathy, in that you, the 'pupil', are required to become aware with the 'teacher' of the way you are thinking into your body. Together with the help of your Alexander teacher's hands and voice you learn to 're-think' the relationship between your mind and body according to Alexander's principles. Much like music lessons, this requires practice at home.

Under what conditions should the Alexander Technique be used?

Historically Alexander's work developed along parallel lines. One had to do with the voice, theatre, performing. So if you are an actor, a musician or an athlete, the Alexander technique can help to enhance your performance. The other line that Alexander's work developed along was that of ongoing chronic conditions mainly to do with the back. So if you have long term back troubles, frozen shoulders, recurring stiff necks and migraines, constricted breathing and asthma, the Alexander Technique can help you.

Dynamic Posture

When you start a series of Alexander lessons, you will begin to learn to stop the inappropriate patterns and allow the anti-gravity muscles to emerge with ease and do the job they were meant to. Your back muscles begin to support your trunk at the appropriate gentle level, while you release unnecessary tension. Posture is a dynamic process, an activity of mind, muscle and nerve.

We have two types of muscles: 'being' and 'doing' muscles. Some muscles are capable of 'being' and 'doing.' However, we know that the intrinsic muscles are made of non-fatigable material: they utilise oxygen. The extrinsic muscles fatigue faster because in using glucose they produce lactic acid, which fatigues muscle. If we slump when sitting, or need to lean on something when we stand, it shows that the intrinsic ('being') muscles have changed their state to fatigable.

The Alexander Technique is named after Alexander himself, an Australian actor who, at the turn of the last century, suffered from loss of voice. He discovered through seven years of self observation, with the help of three mirrors, a series of principles that affect the body and mind relationship.

The main principle is the relationship of the head to the neck to the back. Alexander discovered that if this head/neck/back relationship was in balance, the co-ordination of the rest of the body would follow. For example, breathing, digestion, reproduction, locomotion and speech. Alexander called this head/neck/back relationship the 'primary control'. He discovered that although he could not correct his voice problems directly, he could correct them indirectly through the restored good use of the primary control.

This work, which consisted of both verbal instruction and hands on experience, Alexander brought to London in 1905. He was considered the 'doctor' of the London Theatre and was much admired by Bernard Shaw, Aldous Huxley and Stafford Cripps.

Aloe Vera

By Dr. Peter Atherton

Aloe Vera or the 'true' aloe is the name that should be reserved exclusively for Aloe Barbadensis Miller, the most medicinally active of all the 300 or so types of aloe in the world. This plant, which has its origin in Africa, is a succulent related to the onion, garlic and asparagus.

Being an extremely successful plant it has now colonized many areas of the world, which provide a warm climate, and no frost – its main enemy.

One of the reasons it is so successful is that it can propagate itself sexually by producing seeds, arising from beautiful yellow tubular lily-like flowers arising from a tall central stem, or asexually by suckers or pups, which grow from the base of the mother plant.

Apart from possessing these two methods of reproduction it is also able to withstand long periods of drought and attack by animals, insects and microbes.

It is a perennial with a life span of about twelve years, reaching a maximum size in about four years when its leaves are about 60 cm in length and about 8-10 cm wide at the base. The leaves taper to a point and possess soft marginal spines.

When the outer leaves are cut and harvested this remarkable plant, like many xerophytes, is able to seal itself against water loss.

Within a few seconds of the wound being inflicted it films over and during the next few minutes a rubber-like protective coating stops further loss of sap so the main stem does not become desiccated and continues to live.

In a short time the wound heals completely so not surprisingly it is often referred to as 'the Wonder Plant' although its most common nickname is 'the Burn Plant'.

The word 'Aloe' probably stems from the Arabic word 'Alloeh', meaning 'shining bitter substance' obviously referring to the sap of the plant.

It was from the sap that bitter aloes were produced, either as a laxative or taken orally as a remedy for painting on children's nails to stop them biting them.

Today the sap is virtually excluded from modern aloe products, which use the leaf's

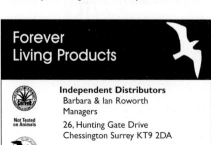
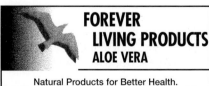

inner mucilage layer and parenchyma or gel to make tonic drinks or topical preparations.

Aloe Vera has a documented history going back over 4,000 years and was a popular remedy prescribed by many famous ancient physicians including Hippocrates, Dioscorides and Galen, the father of modern medicine.

They used both the sap of the plant as a laxative and a means of killing intestinal parasites as well as the inner gel as a wound-healing agent.

They knew that the application of the inner part of the plant to a wound would prevent infection, reduce pain and speed up healing.

It is said that Alexander the Great in 333BC was persuaded by his mentor Aristotle to capture the island of Socotra in the Indian Ocean on his return from Persia just to acquire its famed aloe supplies to treat his wounded soldiers.

An interesting feature associated with wounds treated with aloe is that they heal with minimal or no scarring.

The small amount of solid material (0.5-1.5%) of the plant contains over 75 different ingredients, which are balanced in such a way as to work in concert.

This synergistic action produces an effect far greater than the sum of the individual effects of the components.

Some facts about Aloe Vera

Aloe Vera originates in Africa, Asia and the southern Mediterranean. It has a long history of usage as a purgative and externally in the treatment of wounds and burns. Today, it is a common houseplant and adapts well to indoor living.

Aloe Vera is a member of the lily family. It grows to 40 to 50 cm long, 6-7cm wide at the base and forms a rosette of leaves.

These succulent like leaves are greenish/grey and have a slightly concave surface. They contain a greenish translucent juice. At their margins are small pale 'teeth' about two centimetres long. Its flowers range from greenish/orange to red to white and are borne on a slender stalk about 40 cm high. It should be noted that there are over 180 different Aloe species and not all contain the same healing characteristics.

ALOE VERA

THE ESSENTIAL ALOE VERA by Dr. Peter Atherton is probably the definitive book on this plant.

Cheques to the value of £6.50 per copy to incl. p&p made payable to:
Mill Enterprises,
The Mill House, Thornborough,
Buckingham. MK18 2ED

Alternative Dentistry

By Drs. G. & L. Munro-Hall

Alternative dentistry or holistic dentistry is a flexible term. Any dentist can call him or herself Alternative or Holistic but this is more than just hanging a crystal in the waiting room and not using mercury fillings.

A patient must use common sense when seeking alternative dentistry, must not be afraid to ask questions, ask to speak to other patients and demand the dentist give full explanations and results of all their treatment procedures.

A patient should enquire fully into any aspect of treatment because only by gathering full information can they make the appropriate decision to do what is right for themselves. The dentist advises the patient decides.

Alternative dentistry should be based on observation, experience and science. Always remember that no committee of experts can make a toxic material less toxic by saying so.

Alternative dentistry treats the mouth as the front end of the digestive system. It is not about the repair of teeth. It may involve the repair of teeth but only with due consideration of the whole body. Good dentistry takes the best from both the alternative and traditional camps.

Toxic materials associated with traditional dentistry should not be used and

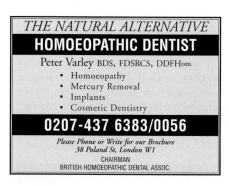
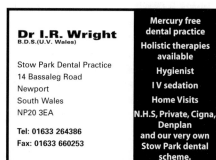
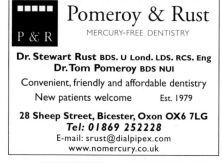
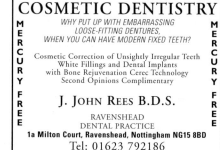

different diagnostic methods may be used from acupuncture to bio energy machines, Vega, Best etc. The alternative dentist will take time to know how to advise you. No metals should be used in the mouth.

Silver amalgam fillings are really 50 per cent mercury. This mercury comes off the fillings and is deposited all over the body especially the brain, heart and kidneys. Mercury is one of the most toxic metals on the planet. It is associated with Alzheimer's, Allergies, Depression, Autoimmune diseases and much more. Adults with four or more amalgam fillings have their health at risk.

Gold in dentistry is usually a mixture of five or more metals. These metals are also released into the body, but at a slower rate than mercury, and can depress immune systems and cause skin problems, especially palladium.

There are good non-metal alternatives, such as composites, polyceramics and ceramics. These materials require time and experience to be used successfully. Metal never has to be used.

You can be protected when removing metal fillings by the dentist fitting a rubber dam to seal the teeth, by breathing separate oxygen and taking supplements before treatment, especially Selenium at 200mcg and a teaspoonful of Vitamin C powder.

The normal local anaesthetic which numbs up teeth carries a cancer risk, it breaks down into aniline, but an alternative has just become available that is safer. Implants contain titanium. In some individuals titanium can be toxic. A blood test called Melisa can show whether you are sensitive to titanium or any other metal.

Root filling is needed if a tooth is dead or the nerve inside is damaged. The problem with root fillings is that even a small tooth has over a mile of tiny tubules coming off the main canal where the nerve was. These tubules contain bacteria, which remain even after the main canal is filled.

The toxins produced by the bacteria can be very toxic and effect any system of the body. If a tooth must be root filled all the tiny tubules must be filled too, at present only one material, Biocalex can do that. There is a test, the ALT test, which can show if a tooth is toxic or not. Best to avoid root fillings if possible.

Cavitations or NICOs are holes in the bone where the teeth have been extracted and are full of bacterial poisons. They can have a big impact on health and are hard to see with an X-ray. A CT scan can show them provided there are no metal fillings present to confuse the computer. Diagnosing and treating cavitations requires a lot of care and experience. They have to be opened and cleaned with military thoroughness.

To prevent cavitations, teeth must be extracted without causing trauma to the bone using the 'ogura' or similar methods and all infection under the tooth cleaned out.

Gum or Periodontal disease is a bacterial infection of the gums around the teeth. These bacteria can be the cause major health problems, heart disease, diabetes etc. The bacteria have to be destroyed. This is done with brushing, flossing and irrigation. The alternative dentist will use herbal means at first and use a microscope to see the effectiveness of the treatment.

Orthodontics is the straightening of the teeth with braces. Traditional dentistry extracts teeth and pulls the remaining teeth straight. However, the alternative of orthopaedic orthodontics develops the bone to allow the teeth to straighten, mostly without extractions. It is better functionally and aesthetically and can be done at any age.

Fluoride is classed as highly toxic. It is a nerve poison. It builds up in the body; half of what you take daily stays with you forever. There is evidence linking it firmly to reduced intelligence of children, osteoporosis with hip fractures and cancer, especially cancer in young men.

There is no valid double blind trial that shows it significantly reduces tooth decay.

Fluoride in the stomach reacts with the acid and turns into a very corrosive acid that can even dissolve glass. It is a toxic by-product of the fertiliser industry and is hard to dispose of. Best to avoid if you can.

Detoxification is used to remove poisons from the body. This can be done with chemical chelators like DMPS, DMSA, or by natural means such as vitamin C and other supplements.

Vitamin C is effective given intravenously and is far safer, but this should be left to experienced hands.

Chemical chelators should never be used, especially if amalgam fillings are present, as they will pull the mercury out of the fillings.

The only accurate method of testing your mercury level is the stool. Blood and urine tests are not reliable.

Amatsu

By Dennis Altram, Amatsu UK

Amatsu is an ancient form of Traditional Japanese natural medicine, which has been practised for thousands of years both as a therapy and self-maintenance programme.

Its traditional school was called the Hichi Buku Goshin Jutsu Ryu, which translates as the school of knowledge of the secret of the opening flower, the essence or Heart of Nature. Its curriculum includes medicine, philosophy, strategy, religion and martial skills.

Amatsu medicine has five basic levels of development under the traditional (Pre Edo Period) grades of:

1 Shoden **2** Chuden **3** Okuden **4** Menkyo **5** Kaiden

Shoden involves methods such as stretching and mobilisation of the soft tissues with massage techniques.

Chuden involves itself with the stimulation of kyushu (weakened areas or locked energy points) and gentle alignment adjustments of joints. This approach is known as seiti or body correction.

Okuden utilises spinal dynamics to re-establish neuro-muscular connections associated with natural movement. At Sekkotushi level – this is gentle adjustments to the ligaments and fascia soft tissue of the body and balancing the fluid systems of the

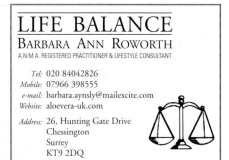
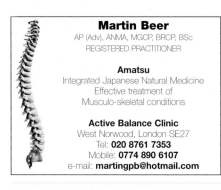
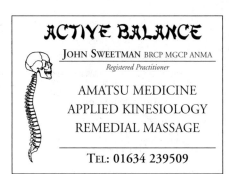

body promotes correction and well-being.

At Menkyo level – work is on the reciprocal cranial sacral reflex system and the functional levels of the problem or psychological and spiritual factors of the imbalance.

At Kaiden – level gentle touch to the body and kime or energy projection releasing deep archaic and emotional traumas to the body is employed.

The earliest records of this tradition exist some 2,000-2,500 years ago in Central Japan. Around this period in Japanese history a group of Malays (Tibetan, Chinese border people) fleeing from their own country, arrived in Japan.

Initially they were suspected of being an invasion force and consequently were attacked by local military personnel.

Fleeing through Japan, they were eventually captured and tried for treason, but later won a reprieve and were re-settled in central Japan. This group of people brought with them customs, practices, religion, Martial skills, writing and medical knowledge that were slowly integrated into Japanese society.

As such the Hichi Buko Goshin Jutsu Ryu could be said to have originated in Japan but from people of different lands.

The original scrolls are in a mixture of what appears to be Sanskrit mixed with old Chinese/Japanese Kana. In the early 1980s three people (Dennis Bartram, William Doolan and Chris Roworth) began studying the medical methods (Amatsu medicine) of the Hichi Buko Goshin Jutsu Ryu under Dr Hatsumi.

In 1995, these three received Kaiden (full mastery and teaching rights) in the Hichi Buko Goshin Jutsu Ryu. Since this time, Amatsu medicine has been registered with The Institute of Complementary Medicine as a Japanese natural medicine.

Japanese Gods and Goddesses

Japanese Gods

Aji-Suki-Taka-Hi-Kone ....god of thunder	Shina-Tsu-Hiko ....god of wind
Amatsu Mikaboshi ....god of evil	Taka-Okami ....god of rain
Bishamon ....god of happiness and war	Take-Mikazuchi ....god of thunder
Hiruko ....solar god	Tsuki-Yomi ....god of the moon
Ho-Masubi ....god of fire	
Inari ....god of rice	**Japanese Goddesses**
Izanagi ....creator god	Ama-No-Uzume ....fertility goddess
Kagu-Zuchi...........................god of fire	Amaterasu ....sun goddess
Kawa-no-Kami ....god of rivers	Benzaiten ....goddess of love
Kura-Okami ....god of rain	Izanami ....creator goddess
Nai-No-Kami ....god of earthquakes	Shina-To-Be ....goddess of wind
O-Kuni-Nushi ....god of sorcery and medicine	Sengen-Sama ....goddess of mount Fujiyama
O-Wata-Tsu-Mi ....god of the sea	Uke-Mochi-No-Kami ....goddess of food
Susa-No-Wo ....god of storms and thunder	Wakahiru-Me ....goddess of the dawn sun

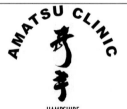

Animal Welfare

Respecting the Natural Lives of Animals
by Andrew Linzey

I n her Romanes Lectures delivered in Oxford during 1984-5, Miriam Rothschild said: "Looking back at the first half of my life as a zoologist, I am particularly impressed by one fact: none of the teachers, lecturers, or professors with whom I came into contact ... ever discussed with me, or each other in my presence, the ethics of zoology... no-one ever suggested that one should respect the lives of animals in the laboratory or that they, and not the experiments, however fascinating and instructive, were worthy of greater consideration." (Animals and Man, p50)

This honest admission should give us some pause. Especially so, when it is remembered that Rothschild is herself a distinguished scientist with a lifetime's experience in her subject, not least of all in practical laboratory work.

What is particularly striking in Rothschild's account is that her fellow scientists apparently felt no need to defend their work in ethical terms, even, to address the issue at all.

How is it, we may ask, that scientists who daily experimented on animals could conduct their research without even asking – at least notionally – questions about the morality of causing suffering to animals? To begin to answer this question, we need to recognise that scientists have not been alone in their apparent neglect of animal ethics.

For many centuries, despite periodic protests, humans have assumed that they have an automatic right to use animals, even in cruel ways.

"Animals are here for our use" is the familiar intellectual justification. It has been commonly accepted that our power over animals gives us rights to exploit

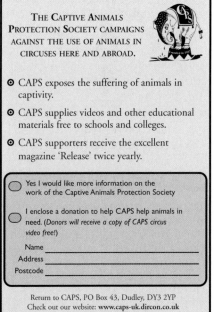

them. These justifications have a long religious and philosophical history. Alongside them has gone the moral marginalisation of animals as things without value in themselves. Historically, humans have regarded other animals as little less than things, objects, commodities, resources here for us.

Given this intellectual heritage, it is perhaps not surprising that scientists just didn't see the need to address the ethical issue. They have simply become accustomed, like most of us, to not thinking in moral terms about how we treat them.

For the most part, animals have simply not been on the moral agenda. When it comes to animal ethics, humans have been going through what can only be described as the 'Big Sleep'.

Since Rothschild spoke those words, however, animals have come to figure on the moral agenda – and increasingly so.

Nowadays no self-respecting scientist would want to be ignorant of the moral issues surrounding animal experimentation. And neither should anyone who is involved, directly or indirectly, in the use of animals – and that practically includes all of us.

What then is the challenge involved in thinking ethically about animals? Rothschild herself refers to two ideas that are at the heart of the debate.

The first concerns the 'worth' of animals. Rothschild rightly bemoans the fact that none of her colleagues dared to think that animals themselves might be worth more than the discoveries that might result from experimenting upon them. Historically, as we have seen, individual animals have counted for next to nothing.

But thinking ethically about animals requires that we regard individual sentient animals (that is, beings that can experience pain and suffering) not just as means to human ends but as ends in themselves.

Thinking ethically about animals means taking each individual animal – and their suffering – into account morally. It follows that it should be as inconceivable to deliberately inflict harm upon individual sentients as it would be in the case of individual human beings.

The second idea concerns 'respect'. Again, Rothschild expresses surprise that none of her colleagues ever suggested that the lives of animals 'should be respected'.

To respect something is to let it lead its own life and to desist from deliberately harming it. Here is the essence of the new ethical view of animals: we should not – in the words of Stephen Clark – be 'the cause of avoidable harm' to other sentient species.

Notice that the issue is not just about respecting animals as a species or as communities of life, but rather about respecting animals as individuals. Now it should be clear that this new ethical approach in turn challenges in a very practical way our contemporary use of animals. Let me take three examples:

The first concerns our keeping of animals as 'pets' or companions. Domestication has been a mixed blessing for animals. While some animals are well cared for, others

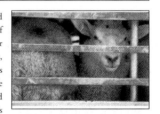
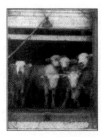

are kept in unsuitable environments or are subject to neglect, abandonment, or cruelty.

In fact, recorded complaints of cruelty against animals are at an all time high. In addition, companion animals are still exploited through puppy farms and pet shops where they are often viewed as little more than consumer items for sale.

Over-breeding inevitably results in the wanton destruction of animals. It has been estimated that the RSPCA and veterinary surgeons have to destroy up to a 1,000 unwanted dogs every week. Neutering programmes are essential to prevent yet more generations of unwanted animals.

The plight of exotic animals, like snakes, parrots, and lizards, merits special attention. These animals are seldom kept in suitable environments and much suffering is caused through ignorance or neglect of their basic behavioural needs.

Treating animals ethically requires that we care for every aspect of the lives of the animals under our control. No-one should keep an animal unless they can adequately provide for the range of needs, both emotional and environmental, that are essential for its wellbeing.

We need a new generation of concerned vets who will lead the way in fostering ethical attitudes towards animals.

The second area concerns the use of animals in sports and amusements, and specifically those held in captivity. It goes without saying that it is impossible to morally justify the infliction of suffering upon animals for sport and entertainment.

Although bear-baiting and cockfighting are illegal in Britain, it is still legal to hunt foxes, deer, mink, and hare, and also to exhibit wild animals in circuses.

Unquestionably, all these practices inflict stress or suffering on animals. In the case of circuses, animals have to suffer frequent transport in cramped, inappropriate accommodation, commonly known as 'beast wagons', in addition to the indignity of having to perform 'tricks' for public amusement.

It is important to recognise that animals suffer not only through the infliction of direct, physical harm but also through environmental deprivation.

When animals are denied the opportunity to live their natural lives – for example – to follow their innate behavioural patterns, to socialise freely, to groom themselves, and to interact creatively with their environment, suffering and stress are the inevitable result.

The moral principle here is that no animal should be held captive unless it is directly for its own individual benefit. To deprive wild animals of their ability to be wild is to deny them something fundamental to their own nature.

The third area concerns the exploitation of animals in modern farming, especially intensive farming.

Since we do not need to eat meat in order to have a healthy diet, there is an overwhelming case for treating farm animals with more generosity than we do today. Intensive farming compromises the welfare of animals.

While it is true that veal crates and sow stalls are now things of the past – at least in the United Kingdom – we have yet to successfully phase out the practice of keeping hens in battery cages.

Moreover, contemporary farming still involves a range of practices that are particularly objectionable, especially the non-veterinary mutilation of animals involved in tail docking, de-beaking, and castration.

While in theory it is possible to kill animals humanely, in practice farm animals suffer through genetic manipulation, poor welfare conditions, long periods of travel especially overseas, as well as through insensitive handling and inexpert killing in markets and abbatoirs.

The use of genetic science in relation to farm animals raises particular ethical problems since such developments frequently straddle the limits of the animal's physiological adaptability. We now have the ugly phenomenon of turkeys programmed to grow so fast that they can hardly stand their own body weight.

In these three areas – and many others – we have still to live out the challenge which thinking ethically about animals confronts us with. The issue, simply put, is how we respect the natural lives of animals. We need to acknowledge their right to live their own lives which means in practice that we have to find ways of living free of exploitation.

A Guide to Further Reading

Mark Bekoff and Caron Meaney (eds), Encyclopedia of Animal Rights and Animal Welfare (Greenwood Press, 1998). An indispensable guide to the new ethical thinking about animals.

Priscilla Cohn (eds), Ethics and Wildlife (Edwin Mellen Press, 1999). An important new collection of essays devoted to various aspects of our treatment of wildlife.

Hilda Kean, Animal Rights: Political and Social Changes in Britain since 1800 (Reaktion Books, 1998). A new history of the animal rights movement.

Andrew Linzey, Animal Theology (SCM Press, 1994). A systematic, ethical and theological critique of our treatment of animals.

Andrew Linzey and Dorothy Yamamoto (eds), Animals on the Agenda (SCM Press, 1998). A new collection of essays examining the intellectual and religious history of our abuse of animals.

Andrew Linzey, Animal Gospel (Hodder and Stoughton, 1998). A Christian case for treating animals with respect.

Danny Penman, The Price of Meat (Gollancz, 1996). Exposes the suffering to animals involved in the modern meat industry.

Tom Regan, The Case for Animal Rights (Routledge, 1983). A philosophical defence of the rights of animals.

Miriam Rothschild, Animals and Man, The Romanes Lectures 1984-5 (The Clarendon Press, 1986). A zoologist's approach to animal welfare.

Bernard E. Rollin, The Frankenstein Syndrome: Ethical and Social Issues in the Genetic Engineering of Animals (Cambridge University Press, 1995). A welcome critique of the genetic manipulation of animals.

Kate Solisti-Mattelon and Patrice Mattelon, The Holistic Animal Handbook (Beyond Words Publishing, 2000). A guide for those who want a holistic dimension to keeping animals as companions.

Yi-Fu Tuan, Dominance and Affection: The Making of Pets (Yale University Press, 1984). An important critique of the modern pet industry.

Some Useful Addresses

Animal Aid, The Old Chapel, Bradford Street, Tonbridge TN9 1AW.

Anglican Society for the Welfare of Animals, The Old Toll Gate, Hound Green, Hook, Hampshire RG27 8LQ. Tel: 0118 932 6586.

Captive Animals Protection Society, 171 Cherry Tree Road, Blackpool FY4 4PQ. Tel: 012553 765072.

Care for the Wild, 1 Ashfold, Horsham Road, Rusper, Horsham, West Sussex RH12 4QX. Tel: 01293 871596.

Compassion in World Farming, 5a Charles Street, Petersfield, Hampshire GU32 3EH. Tel: 01730 264208.

International Association Against Painful Experiments on Animals, 29 College Place, St Albans, Hertforshire AL3 4PU. Tel: 01727 835386.

International Fund for Animal Welfare, Warren Court, Park Road, Crowborough, East Sussex TN6 2GA. Tel: 01892 601900.

League Against Cruel Sports, 83-7 Union Street, London SE1 1SG. Tel: 020 7403 6155.

National Equine Defence League, Oaktree Farm, Wetherall Shields, Wetherall, Carlisle CA4 8JA. Tel: 01228 560082.

RSPCA, The Caseway, Horsham, West Sussex RH2 1HG. Tel: 01403 264181.

Respect for Animals, PO Box 500, Nottingham NG1 3AS. Tel: 0115 952 5440.

Vegetarian Society, Parkdale, Durham Road, Altrincham, Cheshire WA14 8QG. Tel: 0161 928 0793.

Educational Materials

A full range of educational materials for use in schools is published by the Education Department of the RSPCA. Visit their website on www.rspca.co.uk for details of current programmes.

The Animal World Directory

If you have enjoyed reading this piece by Professor Andrew Linzey watch out in your local book shop for THE ANIMAL WORLD directory, available in the autumn of 2001, price £7.95.

For more details please contact Kingsley Media Ltd, Kingsley House, College Road, Keyham, Plymouth PL2 1NT. Email: animal@naturalhealthdirect.com. Or see overleaf.

Aromatherapy

By M Willcocks PhD

Aromatherapy combines the soothing, healing touch of massage with the therapeutic properties of Essential Oils. Aromatherapy is an holistic treatment which can have a profound effect on the mind, body and emotions.

Many of the oils used in Aromatherapy have a long history of therapeutic use. Aromatherapy is one of the fastest growing canons in the 'new age' and 'holistic' repertoire. Critics once lumped it in with other energy healing practices and laughed it off as magical thinking about fragrances and feelings.

But Aromatherapy is gaining popularity and being accepted by the public. It is an increasing part of standard medical practice throughout Europe, where its modern-day rediscovery occurred. The Eastern world has always embraced the medicinal value of aromatics. They are a staple ingredient in India's Ayurvedic medicine and in China, aromatics, like herbs, are listed with modern medicine in the pharmacopoeia.

The myth to dispel is that aromatherapy is for the use of fragrance and its mood altering effects. While scent is directly related to our emotional and physical state, not every fragrance in the world is aromatherapy. Many manufacturers of air fresheners, perfume oils, magical oils, and other fragrance elements would like us to think so, but that is simply not the case. Unfortunately, the prodigious use of the term 'aromatherapy' to market every scented product known to man is only adding to

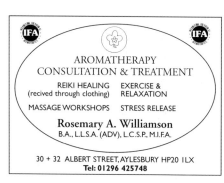
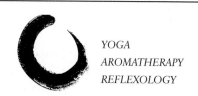

confusion about its true medicinal value. Aromatherapy can be defined as the responsible use of essential oils for physical, mental, and spiritual well-being. Essential oils are highly concentrated and volatile, meaning they evaporate quickly and are highly flammable, plant extracts. They are extracted from aromatic trees, resins, citrus fruits, flowers, plants, leaves, seeds, barks, and roots. True essential oils are extracted by steam distillation. In the case of citrus fruits, the essence is expressed from the rind in a process called scarification. Anything else you come across, no matter how lovely the scent, is not an essential oil.

A guideline to selecting quality essential oils is price. Prices on different oils 'should' vary greatly. This is because, different plant materials produce differing amounts of extractable essence. Some oils, like orange, grapefruit, eucalyptus, and peppermint, can realistically be in the neighbourhood of £2.50. to £5 for a half ounce bottle. Oils like Melissa, Neroli, and the ever-popular rose, should never be less than £30 to £40 for a tiny 2 ml. bottle. They could be much more, but if they are much less than that you can rest assured they are synthetic.

Jasmine is another expensive oil and is not, in fact, an essential oil. Its fragile petals cannot withstand distillation and the essence can only be extracted by solvent extraction or a process called effleurage. The resulting product is called an absolute or absolute of effleurage. 'Jasmine essential oil' is a misnomer and is another warning sign of fraud.

Another frequent mistitling marketing misnomer with potentially hazardous results is what often accounts for 'rosewater'. Read the label; if it says it's rose oil and water, it's not. There is an all-too-common practice of suspending synthetic rose oil in water and calling it rosewater. True rosewater, or *hydrosol of rose* is, in fact, the water

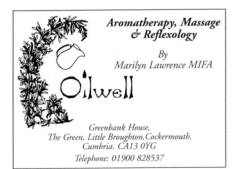
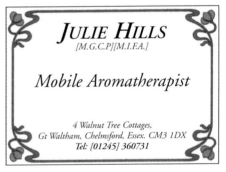
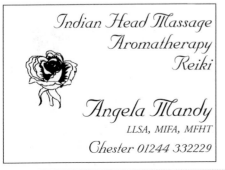
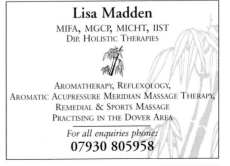

by-product of rose essential distillation. It is a glorious healing tool and an affordable substitute for rose Otto when the scent of real rose is desired. True aromatherapy uses essential oils because of their profound healing benefits, not because they smell good. Some of them do smell good, especially in synergistic blends. Other very effective oils, such as tea-tree, are not exactly perfumery.

I recommend that you have your hype detector with you when shopping for aromatherapy products and do not buy when it rings.

Essential oils are the most concentrated form of herbal energy available. They are actually the hormones of the plant. They work on the body in two different, but related capacities. Not surprisingly, the first is scent. The second is application to the skin. The molecules of essential oils are so small that they can actually be absorbed through the skin and into the blood stream. They can also penetrate the olfactory epithelium in the nose which filters out virtually all other substances and enter the bloodstream that way.

Our sense of smell is 10,000 times more sensitive than any other sense. It is our first and most primal sense. We interpret smell in the limbic or old brain, also called the rhinencephalon. Our neo-cortex grew on top of the old brain out of a piece of olfactory tissue but smell is not interpreted there.

Our sense of smell is one nerve synapse away from our limbic brain. All our other senses go through the neo-cortex first. That is why we have no adjectives that directly describe scent. Our reactions to scent are emotional, not intellectual. The limbic brain also regulates our autonomic systems, so scent also directly affects our physical responses. An example of this is sandalwood, which slows the breathing rate, and has

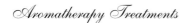

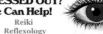

been used for centuries as a meditation aid. The benefits of dermal application of essential oils are many. Many oils aid in detoxification, lymphatic drainage, hormonal and menstrual balance, respiration, immunity, cellular regeneration, and much more. There simply isn't room in this article to list the benefits associated with a vast array of essential oils. It seems that information about the constructive use of these oils abounds. I have decided instead, to focus here on some of the precautions as they are not as well publicised and they are important to the safe usage of this remarkable healing tool.

First and foremost, do not apply essential oils directly to the skin or 'neat'. Essential oils are very strong and should be diluted in some type of carrier. Vegetable oils, such as canola, almond, grape seed, and jojoba work very nicely. For full body massage, essential oils should not comprise more than two-three per cent of your blend. The highest concentration you would ever use would be in the form of perfume oil, which can be up to 50 per cent of your blend, because you are only dabbing them onto pulse points. Even when properly blended, some oils have toxic properties and should be avoided by people with certain health conditions, or, in some cases, all-together. You may encounter some well-meaning individuals who have suggested that 'pure' or "organic" oils cannot be toxic. Nothing could be further from the truth. In the case of toxic oils, the greater the purity, the greater the concentration of toxic elements.

These oils should never be used by anyone as they could cause organ damage, neurological damage, spontaneous abortion, and even death: DWARF PINE – MUGWORT – PENNYROYAL RUE – TANSY – THUJA –WORMWOOD.

These oils should be AVOIDED, and only used by knowledgeable Aromatherapists as they have been associated with things like liver and neurological damage: ANISEED

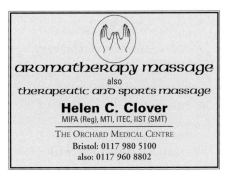

– *Camphor – Hyssop – Origanum – Parsley – Sage.*

These oils should not be used by EPILEPTICS as they can provoke seizures: *Eucalyptus – Fennel -Hyssop – Rosemary – Sage.*

These oils should be avoided during PREGNANCY. Many of them are menstrual regulators and, while that's usually a good thing, they can cause miscarriage: *Angelica – Arnica – Basil Bay – Camomile (first three months) – Carrot Seed – Cassia – Cedar Wood – Cinnamon leaf and bark – Clary – Sage – Cypress – Fennel – Geranium – Jasmine Juniper – Lavender (first three months) -Lavender Spike – Melissa – Marjoram – Myrrh – Peppermint (also contra-indicated during nursing) – Rose (first three months) Rosemary – Spearmint -Thyme.*

These oils cause PHOTOSENSITIVITY and should not be applied to the skin before being in the sun: *Angelica – Bergamot – Cumin – Lemon – Lime – Orange – Verbena.*

The above however does not cover everything you need to know. I recommend that you look at a few good books before delving into 'at home' aromatherapy. Using aromatherapy safely and to its fullest advantage requires a little dedication, but the benefits to health, skin care, hair care, and mental/emotional balance make it more than worth the effort.

A well-trained Aromatherapist should be knowledgeable about a wide variety of essential oils, including what they may be used for, how much to dilute them for various purposes, which other essential oils they may combined with, how to apply them and what safety precautions should be taken. The practitioner should have formal training in these areas plus in-depth experience treating a variety of people and ailments.

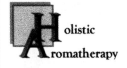

Some aromatherapists also are trained in other health practices, from massage to nursing. You will find many therapists in this directory who practice more than one therapy. If you are uncertain ask the aromatherapist about his or her training and experience.

Warning

Remember the following is a guide and you are advised to consult an aromatherapist for proper use of oils, and if you are using prescribed medicines tell your doctor what you wish to use before doing so. Most oils, should not be used on the skin without first diluting with a suitable carrier oil. This directory contains a number of qualified aromatherapists and oil suppliers who will be pleased to offer you a consultation.

The most effective method of using the oils involves combining their properties with the therapeutic power of touch. The oils should not be used undiluted, but should be diluted with an odourless carrier oil, such as rapeseed, sweet almond or peach kernel. A dilution of three per cent essential oil to carrier oil is a recommended starting point. (Less if using on sensitive skin such as babies). This is approximately one drop essential oil to two millilitres of carrier oil (six drops in two teaspoonfuls). But in all cases less can be definitely more!

Contrary to some popular beliefs, essential oils are not absorbed through the skin. Saying that oils go through the skin is a myth that needs to be exposed. Just because some books have said that oils go through the skin does not make it so.

There is no scientific evidence that oils are absorbed through the skin and then into the bloodstream. Dermatologists who have done experiments also show that oils do

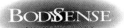

not go through the skin. Some chemicals in EOs do show up in the blood in very small amounts but is not proven that the amount is of therapeutic value. The skin is the largest organ of the body and is designed to keep out contaminants not let them in. Medical patches use specially designed synthetic compounds to go through the skin. It has been shown that those oils that do have penetrative affects are also those that are likely to be sensitisers or irritants thereby showing that the skin is working in stopping contaminants getting through the skin.

Baths

Using oils in baths is a simple, effective and pleasant way to relax and receive the therapeutic effects. Water itself has therapeutic value which enhances the powers of the oils. To use, add six to ten drops of essential oil (or a blend), to the surface of the water which has already been run, add no other substances, e.g. foam or bath oil, then immerse yourself for about 20 minutes, whilst you inhale the vapour. Again reduce the amount of oils used in baths for babies. Take care with plastic baths as some oils may stain.

Compresses

Add five to ten drops of essential oil to 100ml of warm water then soak a piece of clean cotton in the water, wring out the excess and place the cloth on the affected part.

Inhalations

Add five to ten drops of essential oil into a bowl of steaming water, then place a towel over your head and the bowl and inhale the vapour for a few minutes.

Vaporisation

All essential oils are antiseptic and evaporate easily, so they make very good air-

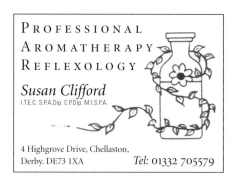
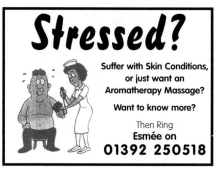
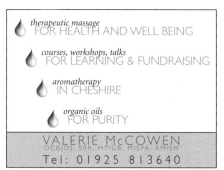

fresheners. Different oils create different atmospheres, so experiment! For example, relaxing Sandalwood or Clary Sage is good for parties; or Peppermint clears your mind when you need to work. There are many vaporisers on the market, from the simple bowl of water on the radiator with a few drops of oil on the surface, to vaporiser light bulb rings and specially made vaporiser bowls which sit above candle holders.

Perfumes

Make your own distinctive natural perfume by blending different oils. Many commercial perfumes use synthetic concoctions for their scent. Try experimenting with different combinations, which can be mixed with a carrier oil or non-fragrant alcohol.

Storing essential oils

Because essential oils are affected by sunlight they should be sold and stored in dark glass bottles, with stopper caps. Make sure that the cap is on securely and the bottle stored up-right in a cool dark place. The oils should be stored out of sight and the touch of children. Remember that children, especially small ones, are very inquisitive. Never store essential oils in plastic bottles. Good Essential oils should keep for several years if properly stored, though the oils of orange, lemon and lime will not keep as long. Patchouli is at the other extreme and actually gets better as it ages.

Mixing essential oils

It is strongly recommended that you use a dropper so that you can measure the actual number of drops easily. Use a different dropper for each oil to avoid cross contamination.

The 'droppers' supplied in bottles should be in different sizes according to the viscosity of the different oils. Good internal droppers have a grove on one side. With the grove uppermost you will get a 'slow drip', with the grove downward you will get a 'fast drip'.

The following oils may assist you. This list is not comprehensive, consult your local Aromatherapist for more advice on which oils to use, he/she will be able to obtain these oils for you.

ANGELICA: Herb Seeds Roots. Cough, Cold, Fever, Flatulence Indigestion.

ANISEED: Herb Seed Pod. Indigestion, Coughs, Bronchitis, Catarrh.

APRICOT KERNEL OIL: From the kernel. Premature skin aging, inflammation, dryness use 100 per cent minerals and vitamins.

AVOCADO PEAR OIL: From the fruit. Dry skin, eczema Add ten per cent to base oil vitamins, protein, lecithin, and fatty acids.

BASIL: HERB: Whole Plant. Bronchitis, Fatigue, Colds, Loss of concentration, Migraine, Gout, Aches & Pains Depression, Fainting, Mental Fatigue, Migraine, Nausea, Nervous Tension Stimulating.

BAY: Tree Leaves. Sprains, Colds Flu, Insomnia, Rheumatism, Antiseptic, Decongestant, Tonic.

BENZOIN: Tree Trunk. Coughs, Itching, Arthritis, Colds, Sedative.

Bergamot: Peel of fruit. Fevers, Acne, Tension, Wounds, Coughs, Stress, and Antidepressant Uplifting.

BIRCH: Tree Bark. Gout, Rheumatism, Eczema, Ulcers.

BLACK PEPPER: Vine Berries. Colds, Aches, Influence, Flatulence, Rheumatism.

BOIS DE ROSE: Tree Wood. Tonic, Coughs, Headaches, and Anti-depressant.

BORAGE: Seed Oil. PMT, MS Menopause, Heart disease, Psoriasis, Eczema, premature aging, regenerates skin ten per cent dilution. gamma acid, vitamins, minerals.

CAJUPUT: Tree Antiseptic. Pain Reliever, Lung Congestion, Neuralgia, Acne.

CARROT: Root. Seeds Gout, Ulcers, Flatulence, Eczema, Psoriasis, Diuretic.

CARROT OIL: Carrots. Premature aging, itching, dryness, psoriasis ten per cent in base oil vitamins, minerals, beta-carotene.

CEDAR WOOD: Tree Wood. Bronchitis, Catarrh, Acne, Arthritis, Diuretic Lung Congestion, Eczema, Encourages Sexual Response.

CHAMOMILE: Nervous conditions, Insomnia, antibacterial, disinfectant, anti-inflammatory teething, sunburn, psoriasis, eczema, asthma, hay fever, diarrhoea, sprains, nausea, fever, depression Contain azulene (Uplifting), Toning.

CHAMOMILE MATARICARIA: Chamomile Herb. Flowers, Leaves Nerves, Migraine, Acne, Inflammation, Insomnia, Menstrual Problems, Dermatitis Eczema, Psoriasis, Inflammatory Diseases, Burns, Nervous Tension, Neuralgia, Insomnia, Contains Azulene.

CHAMOMILE ROMAN: Athemis Nobilis, Herb, Flowers, Leaves. Nerves, Migraine, Acne, Inflammation, Insomnia, Menstrual Problems, Dermatitis.

CAMPHOR: Tree Wood. Coughs, Colds, Fevers, Rheumatism, Arthritis, Stimulating.

CINNAMON: Anti-viral Antiseptic. Circulatory, Heart, Digestive, Respiratory Stimulant, Antispasmodic, Aphrodisiac, anti-venom eugenol, antiseptic.

CINNAMON: Tree Twigs Leaves. Flu, Rheumatism, Warts, Coughs, Colds, and Viral infections.

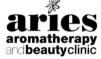

CITRONELLA: Grass. Insecticide, Deodorant, Tonic, Stimulant.

CLARY-SAGE: Herb Flowering Tops. Depression, Nerves, Sore Throat, Aches and Pains, Debility, Sedative Uplifting.

CLOVE: Antibacterial, Antiseptic, Analgesic, Toothache, Digestive problems, Muscular disorders, Asthma, Nausea, Sinusitis, Sedative, Nerve tension, General weakness, Antispasmodic, Do not use undiluted on skin.

CLOVE: Tree, Flower Buds. Nausea, Flatulence, Bronchitis, Arthritis, Rheumatism, Toothache, Diarrhoea, Infections, Analgesic, Antiseptic.

CORIANDER: Herb, Seeds of ripe fruit, Leaves. Indigestion, influenza, Fatigue, Rheumatism, Flatulence, Nervousness, Analgesic.

CORN OIL: Corn. Soothing on all skins, 100 per cent protein, Vitamins, Minerals C.

CUMIN: Herb, Seeds, Fruit. Indigestion, Headache, Liver Problems, Stimulant.

AROMATHERAPY

DINAH SWABY S.P. DIP A. I.T.E.C. Aromatherapy for both men and women helps many conditions from backache to stress. Quality oils, relaxing massage and peaceful surroundings, create a restful experience. Also REIKI , a clothed hands on therapy which utilizes universal healing energy. Telephone: 01420 83919.

HARMONY AND WELL-BEING through essential oils – help restore the balance in your life with professional consultation and application. For more information or to make an appointment contact Rosemary Shackleton on Barnsley 01226 280164 MISPA/IFA member of the caring professions for over 25 years.

THE SANDRA DAY SCHOOL Of Health Studies teaches Aromatherapy to International Society Of Professional Aromatherapists (ISPA) level. Also a variety of massage courses, reflexology, manual lymphatic drainage and one day courses in complementary therapies. TEL: 01706-750302.www.sandraday.com

MRS J EDDY, 5 Tregefeal Terrace, St Just, Cornwall, TR19 7PL. 01736 788934

MRS I WALKER, Foxhill, 103 Clea Lough, Derry Boye, Crossgar, BT30 9LU. 02844 828744

MRS V MULLER, 70 Henderland Road, Bearsden, Glasgow, Lanarkshire, G61 1JG. 0141 563 7086

AROMATHERAPY

MRS M MORRIS, Asteyam@Cswebmail.Com London. 020 8679 8857 / 0958 917537

THE HEALTH & BEAUTY CENTRE, 155 Southband Road, Southport, Merseyside, PR8 6LZ. 01704 233038

NATURES TOUCH, 3 Buccleuch Street, Melrose, Roxburghshire, TO6 9LB. 01896 823782

MS H BARR, 3 Tamfield, Wood Lane, Stoke-On-Trent, Staffordshire, ST7 8PJ. 01782 722095

MS B WILLISCROFT, 3 Church Close, Drayton Bassett, Tamworth, Staffordshire, B78 3UJ. 01827 289714 / 01827 68374

MRS L SEYMOUR, 37 Bunbury Way, Epsom Down, Epsom, Surrey, KT17 4JP. 01372 729661

MS, C PENRICE, Stanley Road, Worcester, Worcestershire, WR5 1BE. 01905 350096

MS K PARRY, 3 Rossefield Rd, Heaton, Bradford, Yorkshire, BD9 4DD. 01274 499554

MS A HODKIN, 65 Dunkeld Road, Ecclesall, Sheffield, Yorkshire. S11 9HN. 01142 364072

P A AROMATHERAPY, 7 Crossway Street, Whetherby, Yorkshire, LS22 6RT. 01937 589188

CYPRESS: Leaves and Shoots. Anti-viral, Astringent, Antispasmodic, Coughs, Rheumatism, Flu, Wounds, Muscle, Nerve, Veins.

CYPRESS: Tree, Leaves, Twig .Menopausal problems, Circulatory conditions, Rheumatism, Colds, Whooping Cough, Nervous Tension, Haemorrhoids, Wounds, Astringent.

DILL: Herb, Seeds, Fruit. Flatulence, Indigestion, Constipation, Nervousness, Gastric Upsets, Headaches.

EUCALYPTUS: Distilled. Cooling, Protecting, Anti-inflammatory, Antiseptic, Antibiotic, Diuretic, analgesic, Deodorising, Coughs, Cystitis, Candida, Diabetes, Sunburn.

EUCALYPTUS: Tree, Leaves, Twigs. Sore Throats, Coughs, Bronchitis, Sinusitis, Skin Infections, Ulcers, Sores, Rheumatism, Aches and Pains, Antiseptic, Anti-inflammatory.

EUCALYPTUS LEMON: Tree, Leaves, Twigs. Dandruff, Scabs, Sores, Candida, Asthma, Fever, Fungal infections, Skin Infections, Sore Throats.

EUCALYPTUS PEPPERMINT: Tree, Leaves, Twigs. Ulcers, Sores, Coughs, Colds, Fever, Respiratory Problems, Viral Infections, Headaches, Flu, Rheumatism, Arthritis.

EUCALYPTUS RADIATA: Tree. Leaves, Twigs. Viral Infections, Colds, Coughs, Bronchitis, Whooping Cough, Rheumatism, Muscular Strains, Antiseptic.

EVENING PRIMROSE OIL: PMT, MS, Menopausal problems, Heart disease, Psoriasis, Eczema, Prevents premature aging, ten per cent gamma lineolenic acid, vitamins and minerals.

FENNEL: Herb, Seeds. Digestive Problems, Menopausal Problems, Obesity, Constipation, Kidney Stones, Nausea Diuretic.

FRANKINCENSE: Tree, Bark. Sores, Wounds, Fevers, Coughs, Colds, Stress, Bronchitis, Laryngitis, Nervous Conditions, Tension. Plant Bark. Bronchitis, Respiratory Problems, Swelling Inflammations, Tension, Nervous Conditions.

GERANIUM: Chilblains, Cosmetic, Endometriosis, Menopause, Diabetes, Throat infections, Nerve tonic, Sedative, Uterine and breast cancer, Frostbite, Infertility, Antiseptic, Astringent, Skin toner,

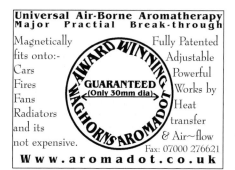

Adrenal Hormones, Relaxing, Uplifting, Moisturising, Toning.

GINGER: Root. Stimulating, Rheumatism, Muscular Aches, Pains, Sprains, Broken Bones, Colds, Nausea, Diarrhoea, Alcoholism, Digestive Disorders.

GRAPEFRUIT: Tree, Rind. Lethargy, Tonic, Obesity, Kidney and Liver Problems, Migraine, Antidepressant, Aid in Drug Withdrawal Treatment.

GRAPE SEED OIL: All skins, 100 per cent base oil vitamins, minerals and protein.

HAZELNUT OIL: From the kernel. Slight astringent base oil 100 per cent vitamins, minerals, protein.

HOPS: Plant, Buds and Flowers. Neuralgia, Bruising, Menstrual and Menopausal Problems, Rheumatism, Nerves, Diuretic, Sedative Analgesic.

HYSSOP: Herb, leaves and flowering tops. Bruises, Rheumatism, Arthritis, Coughs, Colds, Sore Throats, Viruses, Blood Pressure, Circulation, Nervous Tension, Asthma, Tonic.

IMMORTELLE: Flower, Flowering Tops. Bacterial Infections, Rheumatism, Muscle Aches, Weakness, Lethargy, Depression, Respiration, Colds, Flu, Fever, Fungicide.

INULA ODORATA: Anti-viral.

JASMINE: Bush, Flowers. Nervous Tension, Depression, Menstrual Problems, Laryngitis, Anxiety, Lethargy, Relaxant.

JOJOBA OIL: From the bean. Inflammation, Psoriases, Eczema, Acne, Hair care, Penetrates, Ten per cent protein, Minerals, Waxy, collagen-like substance.

JUNIPER: Tree, Bush, Berries. Tonic for nervous system, Digestive stimulant, Diuretic, Acne, Coughs, Ulcers, Fatigue, Rheumatism, Sores, Urinary Infections.

LAVENDER: Burns, Prevents scarring, Antibiotic, Antidepressant, Sedative, Immunoactive, Wounds, Relaxing, Moisturising, Antiseptic, Toning, Eczema, Tension, Insomnia, Asthma, Rheumatism, Arthritis, Bacterial Conditions, Headaches, Dermatitis, Fainting.

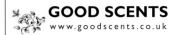

LEMON GRASS: Grass, Whole Plant. Antiseptic, Infections, Headaches, Sore Throats, Respiration, Fevers, Tonic, Insect Repellent.

LEMON OIL: Tree, Rind of fruit. Water purifier, Antiseptic, Antibacterial oil, Verrucas, Insect bites, Tension headaches, Lymphatic tonic, Digestive stimulant, Disperse cellulite, Slimming, Anti-wrinkle Diuretic, Stimulating, Anxiety, Astringent, Antiseptic, BP Vitamin C, Carotene (A) Bioflavonoids.

LIME: Tree, Rind. Fevers, Rheumatism, Sore Throats, Headaches, Anorexia, Alcoholism, Depression, Anxiety Astringent, Tonic.

MACE: Tree, Peel of Fruit. Indigestion, Weakness, Bacterial Infections, Gout, Rheumatism, Arthritis, Circulation.

MANDARIN: Tree, Rind. Insomnia, Nervousness, Liver Problems, Digestion, Anxiety, Tonic, Tranquilliser.

MARJORAM: Herb, Flowering Tops. Relaxing, Sprains, Bruises, Colds, Rheumatism, Intestinal, Cramps, Menstrual Problems, Anxiety, Asthma, Bronchitis, Insomnia, Circulation, Muscular Disorders.

MELISSA: Herb, Leaves. Relaxing, Nervousness, Bacterial and Fungal Infections, Diarrhoea, Eczema, Sedative, Cardiac Tonic.

MYRRH: Tree, Bark/Resin. Antiseptic, Astringent, Tonic, Healing Agent, Dermatitis Coughs, Mouth and skin ulcers, Bacterial and Fungal Infections.

NEROLI: Blossoms, Bitter Orange Tree. Antidepressant, Aphrodisiac, Antiseptic, Digestive Aid, Sedative, Bacterial Infections, Bronchitis, Diarrhoea, Fungicide, Insomnia, Relaxing, Moisturizing.

NIAOULI: Leaves and stems. Melaeleuca Tree Antiseptic, Soothing Agents, Pain Reliever, Decongestant Gomenol. Bush, Leaves, Twigs. Anti-viral, Wounds, Infections, Bacterial Disease, Sore Throats, Burns, Respiration, Acne.

NUTMEG: Tree, Seed. Nausea, Vomiting, Muscle Aches, Rheumatism, Arthritis, Nervousness, Insomnia, Cardio Stimulant.

OLIVE OIL: Rheumatic conditions, Hair care, Soothes, Ten per cent protein, Minerals, Vitamins.

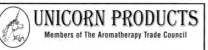
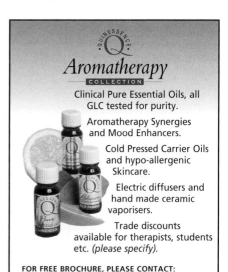

ORANGE: Tree, Rind of Fruit. Depression, Anxiety, Constipation, Nervous Conditions, Muscular Spasm, Tonic, Sedative Antiseptic.

OREGANO: Herb, Leaves and Flowering Tops. Anti-viral, Bronchitis, Rheumatism, Respiration, Muscle Pain, Digestion.

PALMA ROSA: Grass. Skin infections, Anorexia, Tonic.

PARSLEY: Herb, Seeds. Nervous Conditions, Kidney problems, Menstrual and Menopausal Problems, Sedative, Diuretic.

PATCHOULI: Plant. Anti-depressant, Sedative, Aphrodisiac Anxiety, Acne, Eczema, Herpes, Ulcers (Skin), Tired Skin.

PATCHOULI: Plant, Leaves. Skin Inflammations, Fungal infections, Acne, Eczema, Dandruff, Antiseptic, Diuretic Insecticide.

PEANUT OIL: 100 per cent base oil. Protein, Vitamins and Minerals.

PEPPERMINT: Herb, Whole Plant. Inflammation, Nausea, Indigestion, Fevers, Flatulence, Headaches, Migraine, Liver Problems, Arthritis, Stimulant.

PEPPERMINT: Digestive, Respiration, Circulation, Anti-inflammatory, Antiseptic, Gas, Flu, Migraine, Fatigue, Asthma, Bronchitis, Stimulating.

PETIT GRAIN: Tree, Leaves, Twigs. Anxiety, Insomnia, Depression, Antiseptic, Tonic, Aids Convalescence.

PIMENTO: Tree, Berries, Twigs. Flatulence, Indigestion, Cramps, Intestinal Problems, Colds, Rheumatism, Muscular Strains, Depression, Tonic, Tranquilliser.

PINE: Needles, Bark, Berries. Antiseptic, Diuretic, Stimulant adrenal glands, Bladder, Kidney, Chest infections, Infections, Fatigue, Rheumatism, Gout, Flu, Bronchitis, Muscle Pain, Diuretic, Respiration Sore Throats, Colds, Circulation, Muscle pain.

TURPENTINE RAVEN SARA: Bush, Leaves. Viral Infections, Liver Infections, Lung Infections, Respiratory Problems, Antiseptic

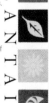 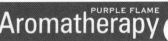

RED THYME: Anti-viral.

ROSE: Flower. Depression, Aphrodisiac, Female organ regulator, Astringent, Sedative, Heart tonic, Stomach Liver, Uterus, Nausea, Headache, Insomnia, Skin Care, Relaxing, Toning, Moisturising, Antiseptic.

ROSE BULGER (BULGARIAN): Bush, Flowers, Petals. Anxiety, Depression, Circulatory Problems, Menopausal Problems, Antiseptic, Tonic.

ROSE MAROC (MOROCCO): Bush, Flowers, Petals, Menstrual Disorders, Depression, Stress, Tension, Circulatory Conditions, Tonic, Sedative.

ROSEMARY: Herb. Physical and mental stimulant, Muscular conditions, Antiseptic, Sprains, Arthritis Rheumatism, Depression, Fatigue, Memory loss, Migraine, Flu, Diabetes, Hair care, Antiseptic Stimulating, Toning.

SAGE: Herb, Plant Tonic. Antiseptic, Diuretic, Blood Pressure, Female Reproductive System, Sores Fatigue, Nervousness, Asthma, Bronchitis, Low Blood Pressure, Bacterial Infections, Rheumatism, Arthritis, Sprains, Fibrosis, Astringent.

SANDALWOOD: Tree. Antiseptic, Tonic, Aphrodisiac, Fatigue, Impotence, Relaxing, Uplifting, Acne, Cystitis, Moisturising, Menstrual Problems, Skin Infections, Fungal and Bacterial Infections, Sedative.

SESAME OIL: Psoriasis, Eczema, Rheumatism, Arthritis ten per cent dilution, Vitamins, Minerals, Proteins, Lecithin, Amino acids.

SOYA BEAN OIL: 100 per cent base oil. Protein, Minerals and Vitamins.

SPEARMINT: Herb, Leaves, Flowering Tops. Flatulence, Indigestion, Intestinal Cramps, Fevers, Nausea, Colic, Haemorrhoids.

SUNFLOWER OIL: 100 per cent base oil. Vitamins, Minerals.

SWEET ALMOND OIL: From the kernel. Itching, Soreness, Dryness, Inflammation, use 100 per cent, Glycosides, Minerals, Vitamins, Protein.

TAGETES: Plant, Flowers. Fungal Infections, Skin Infections, Cuts, Sprains, Strains, Wounds, Circulation, Antiseptic.

TANGERINE: Uplifting.

TEA TREE: Tree, Leaves, Twigs. Anti-viral, Anti-fungal, Anti-bacterial, Antiseptic, Colds, Influenza, Cold Sores, Warts, Verrucas, Inflammation, Acne, Burns, Candida, Shock, Hysteria.

THYME RED (VULGARIS): Herb, Leaves, Flowering Tops. Bacterial Infections, Urinary Infections, Rheumatism, Lethargy, Sores, Wounds, Stimulant, Tonic, Raises Immunity.

THYME RED (VULGARIS): Thyme linalol. Anti-viral, Eliminates toxic wastes, Whooping cough, Warts, Neuralgia, Fatigue, Acne, Hair and skin care, Cooking, Antiseptic powders, Fatigue, Skin Inflammation, Antiseptic Only diluted, Overuse causes thyroid problems.

VALERIAN: Plant, Roots. Sedative, Calming, Nervous Conditions, Trembling, Neuralgia, Insomnia, Palpitations, Sedative, Tranquilliser.

VETIVER: Roots of Grass. Calming, Anxiety, Nervous Tension, Insomnia, Rheumatism, Muscle Relaxant, Antiseptic, Tonic.

VIOLET: Leaves, Plant. Inflammations, Kidney Problems, Obesity, Skin Infections, Fibrosis, Rheumatism Analgesic and Liver Decongestant.

WHEAT GERM OIL: Eczema, Psoriasis, Premature aging, ten per cent dilution. Protein, Minerals, Vitamins.

WINTERGREEN: Herb. Stimulating.

YARROW: Herb, Leaves, Flowering Tops. Inflammations, Cramps, Constipation, Circulation, Rheumatoid Arthritis, Menstrual Problems, Astringent.

YLANG-YLANG: Tree, Flowers. Sedative, Antiseptic, Aphrodisiac, High Blood Pressure, Intestinal Infections, Impotence Uplifting, Moisturising, Anxiety, Depression, Sedative, Tonic.

Carrier oils

Pure essential oils are mostly too strong and concentrated to be used directly on our skin. So they should be diluted with carrier or base oils so that they can be rubbed or massaged onto the skin. Essential oils can be very expensive and will not go very far when full strength, but will cover a large area when diluted and will be just as effective. Oils which are termed 'Extra Virgin, Cold Pressed Oils' are the best carrier oils to use. These are the first pressed oils from a crop. The oils come from the nut or seed of the plants. Although there are hundreds of oil-bearing plants only a few are produced commercially.

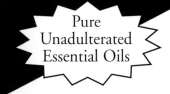

Pure Unadulterated Essential Oils

Scentimental

- **STRICTLY TRADE ONLY**
- **All Oils Batch Coded**
- **Bulk Oil Prices**
- **Stringent Quality Control**
- **24hr Delivery**
- **No Minimum Order**
- **All major credit / debit cards accepted**

Members of N.O.R.A. – The National Oils Research

Orderline: 0800 328 9265

Manufacturers of a Comprehensive range of Quality Home Fragrance Products

Pot-Pourri – Fragrance Oils – Simmering Granules – Incense – Room Sprays – Etc. Etc.

Scentimental

Aromatic House, 46/48, Garden Street, Thurmaston, Leicester LE4 8DS
Tel: 0116 2696 100 Fax: 0116 2696 800
Email: sales@scentimental.com
Website: www.scentimental.com

Oils which themselves have no, or a minimum of, aroma of their own are more suitable for Aromatherapy, to allow the essential oils themselves to work properly. Later extractions can come from heat or solvent processes which can destroy vital trace minerals and vitamins found in the oils.

SWEET ALMOND: The first choice of many Aromatherapists as it is good for all skin types. The best quality oils are cold pressed and filtered. Almond oil diluted with ten per cent of Avocado or Wheatgerm (unless the user is allergic to wheat) is good for people with dry skin, and can help relieve itching, soreness and dryness. Never mix up this oil with the steam distilled essential oil from Bitter almond, (Prunis amygdalis var amara, P. dulcis var amara) as this oil is never used in aromatherapy due to the risk of hydrocyanic acid (prussic acid) forming when the crushed kernels are macerated in water before being distilled.

APRICOT KERNEL: Another good for all skin types, but especially sensitive or prematurely mature skin.

AVOCADO: Used as an addition to other base oils, 10 per cent to 25 per cent. It is good for eczema and dry, dehydrated skin. Should not be kept in the fridge. May be slightly cloudy when cold. This is good as it will then show that it hasn't gone through excessive filtering/refining. It should be a deep green colour. This is not a nut oil.

BORAGE: High in gamma linilenic acid (GLA) Must be stored in a cool dark place to maintain the efficacy of the GLA

GRAPESEED: A good second choice carrier especially for those whose skin seems not to absorb other oils very quickly. It does not leave a greasy feeling to the skin after application. Grape seeds are washed, dried, ground, and pressed with the aid of heat and sometimes refined. Heat is used because the seed has just a 13 per cent oil content.

PEACH KERNEL: Another good for all skin types, along with Sweet Almond and Apricot Kernel oils it is a rich and nourishing oil and similiar in chemical makeup.

OLIVE: Used in a ten per cent dilution for rheumatic conditions, hair care and cosmetics.

SOYA: Can be used 100 per cent on all skin types. Rich in lecithin and one of the few foods to have all 22 health giving amino acids and Vit A and B complex. The downside is that soya is liable to oxidation and can cause acne, allergic reactions and hair damage. Double downside is that much soya is now genetically modified.

SUNFLOWER SEED: Can be used 100 per

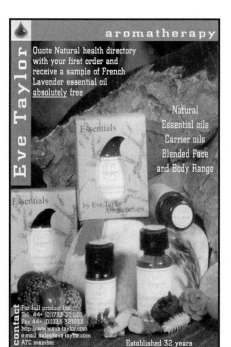

cent. Organic oil is cold pressed. 'Kitchen' oil is probably solvent extracted and is not recommended for aromatherapy/massage.

SEASAME SEED: Used as a ten per cent addition to main oils. Can assist with psoriasis, eczema, rheumatism, and arthritis.

COCONUT: Usually deodorised for use in aromatherapy coconut oil can aid tanning and is reputed to filter the sun's rays. Can cause a rash on some people.

CALENDULA: An infused oil. This oil has an anti-inflammatory, anti-spasmodic, vulnerary (aiding healing of wounds) effect and so is very useful in its own right. The addition of essential oils enhance the effects of the oils together, (a synergistic effect). It also blends well with Hypericum.

CLAUSIACEAE: Macerated oil from St Johns Wort. An anti-inflammatory oil. It is soothing and effective on wounds and is helpful in cases of neuralgia, sciatica and fibrositus. Blends well with Calendula.

WHEATGERM: Used ten per cent in a mixture. Helps eczema, psoriasis, prematurely aged skin, and slows down mixed blends of oils from deterioration.

JOJOBA: A liquid wax rather than an oil, used as a ten per cent addition to other oils.

Consult your Aromatherapist or oils supplier for information on the following:
Camelina, Carrot, Castor, Cherry Kernel, Cocoa butter, Corn, Cottonseed, Evening Primrose, Flaxseed (see Linseed), Hazelnut, Hemp seed, Hydrocotyle (macerated), Kukui nut, Lime blossom (macerated), Linseed, Macademia nut, Meadowfoam, Palm kernel, Passion flower (macerated), Peanut, Pisachio, Pumpkin seed, Rapeseed, Rice bran, Rose hip, Safflower, Sisymbrium, Tamanu, Walnut.

Remember that these oils if used incorrectly or on skin that could be allergic, can cause serious damage. Please consult an expert or professional Aromatherapist before attempting home applications.

Make your own candles
By M. Willcocks PhD

Choose your wax, mould, wick and preferred aromatherapy essence. Melt the wax in a tin or something similar and place in a saucepan of water; heat until it reaches pouring temperature and then mix in a small amount of the essence.

Tilt the tin and pour the wax smoothly down the sides of the mould, fill it to within a couple of inches of the top. Gently tap the mould to release air bubbles in the wax.

Poke a piece of thick wire or thin stick down along the wick occasionally to release air bubbles forming there. Watch for the candle to shrink as it cools. Top off the wax to the original level, put the cooled candle and mould in the fridge for ten minutes or so. Turn the mould upside down over a clean towel and the candle should slide out.

Hold it by the wick only and polish the candle with a nylon stocking, or spray it with candle spray or a clear shoe polish spray.

Untie the wick and trim it to an inch above the top of the candle. Even out the bottom of the candle by heating it on a hot surface and let it melt until the base is level. Be sure that small children are kept out of the kitchen as the hot wax will burn the skin.

Art Therapy

By Margo Sunderland

Why arts therapy? **"Many a person is unhappy, tortured within, because he has at his command no art of expressive action"** – **Dewey, 1934, p65. In arts therapy, clients, both adults and children, are asked to make an image of their feelings, problems or issues, rather than just talking about them in words.**

Using the arts in therapy recognises the limitations of talking about feelings solely in everyday language. Which all too often means going round and round in circles, or using very oblique or minimising references for intense emotional experiences.

People tend to get stuck in the cul-de-sacs of convenient labels such as 'depressed' or 'angry', which often do little more than report feelings, and sometimes, highly inaccurately! Common feeling labels can all too easily 'flatten' what the client is experiencing into something. Which it is not.

Think of trying to describe a beautiful daffodil in literal words, for example. This makes it far less of a daffodil. It is stripped of its essence, its sensuality, and its complexities. and the directness with which it affects us.

Furthermore, everyday words are often sensorially too dry. They can be too flat, too reductionist, too cognitive, missing whatever is of central importance in a client's painful experience, or only making passing reference to it, they are often also just not

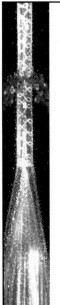

strong enough for the sheer force of some feelings. And when everyday language fails to fully capture what the client is experiencing, she is left frustrated about not really managing to say what she wanted to say. Similarly the therapist can feel that he has failed to really 'empathise in'.

In contrast, art images can speak about feelings with amazing richness. In fact, the mind naturally speaks about emotional Issues through images and metaphors as we see in dreams. In dreams, image and metaphor is the mind's chosen way of processing powerful feelings in our past or present, as well as our fears or hopes for the future. An art image is simply like having a dream while being awake.

Case history

Tessa, aged five, regularly had major temper tantrums on the floor in the supermarket. Afterwards, Tessa was in a very frightened state because of the intensity of feeling inside her. She often had nightmares about monsters that same night. Her mother's response of "you seem very cross" said far too little about what and how Tessa was actually feeling. It failed to convey the full qualitative and energetic aspects of her tantrum experience. The word cross is too vague, too generalised. It is an impoverished word for the actual experience. But in an art therapy session, Tessa drew a picture of floods and avalanches, and a fire that ripped through everything. She then pointed to her picture and said: "Sometimes that's all me."

Tessa had spoken vividly about her vitally lived experience and so the therapist could give her the empathy and the help with emotional processing that she so badly needed.

In the context of therapy, an art image can capture the fuller picture, the deeper realities of a client's emotional experience. It can capture the multi-sensory and essential energetic qualities of a feeling or emotional event, its atmosphere, tensions, tones, intensities, ebb and flows, crescendos and diminuendos, urgencies and dynamic shifts.

In the words of the poet Seamus Heaney, an art image can therefore 'amplify the music of what happens'. When a client makes an art image it is often a profound form of description and evocation of their inner world of image and feeling. In the context of therapy, an art image can enable a client to see, hear, know and feel more clearly, by providing a deeper truth and empathy than is possible through literal words.

In so doing, it can bring hope to a client that can be understood. 'Yes! This is really what I wanted to say', or 'I have told you exactly what it is like to be me at the moment.' The right language of expression frees the client. The wrong language imprisons him or her. In particular, it can be an immense relief for a client to find images and metaphors to express thoughts or feelings, which have previously been nameless and yet craved understanding. In the context of therapy, an art image can enable a client to dare to stay with the disturbing, the too intense or the extremely painful feelings long enough to really think about what is happening, when her first inclination may be to deflect and talk about something easier. This is because an art image provides the means for a client to look at her powerful feelings from a 'safe distance'.

The painting, clay model or sand play picture is out there, so to speak, safely contained on the paper. In the context of therapy, the art image can enable a client to express the many different meanings and feelings about an experience he has had, all at the same time. In so doing, a client can convey a great deal of information, in contrast to reductionist literal statements such as, I'm depressed' or I'm bored.' Feeling words can hide, whereas art images can reveal.

What is Integrative Arts Therapy?

In other words, why offer the client more than one art form? In Integrative Arts Therapy, the client is offered fill access to many different modes of sensory expression. This is because of the following underlying premises:

1 That it is unnecessarily depriving and frustrating to clients to offer them only one mode of sensory expression (for example, just art, or just movement, or just music) when we perceive and imagine through all our senses. We don't experience life through just one sense. Neither do we imagine in just one sense.

2 That it is unnecessarily depriving and frustrating to clients to offer them only one mode of sensory expression, when we remember in a whole array of different images. Some memories are importantly and centrally auditory, others kinesthetic, others visual. Furthermore neurobiologists have found that while adults store important life experiences as event memories and sense memories, infants store their experiences as sense memories only. Their brain is not yet wired up for event memories.

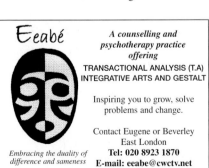

Eeabé

A counselling and psychotherapy practice offering

TRANSACTIONAL ANALYSIS (T.A)
INTEGRATIVE ARTS AND GESTALT

Inspiring you to grow, solve problems and change.

Contact Eugene or Beverley
East London

Embracing the duality of difference and sameness

Tel: 020 8923 1870
E-mail: eeabe@cwctv.net

This has major implications for therapy. If a client is to communicate and explore a pre-verbal memory, only a range of sensory media can fully support them in this. Similarly traumatic memory means an impactive registering of the sensory images of the traumatic event.

When traumatic stress has caused dissociation, again there may be no event memory, no narrative, simply different 'splinters' of the sense impressions of the trauma. Post-traumatic stress is due in part to the meaning given to these vivid sense impressions. Thus if a client is to properly process and work through a traumatic memory, they need a therapist who is open and supportive to working within all modes of sensory expression. One can never assume which sensory mode or modes of experiencing have been dominant during any particular trauma. To be specific, how can a client fully convey, express or explore an auditory memory without using sound, a kinesthetic memory without moving, and a visual memory without visual images or metaphors?

What happens if a client brings a powerful dream of falling and the therapist only offers him/her painting or drawing to capture the dream's vital movement content? What happens if the client brings an image of a frightening mother face, and the therapist offers only movement or music?

What happens if the client brings a haunting impression of someone's piercing tone of voice, and the therapist just offers 'talking about' it? In answer to these questions, with the wrong language of expression for the client's material, too much can get left out, too much can be misrepresented. The client can then end up feeling frustrated, stuck or hopeless in ever being able to say what he wants to say. And while some clients may have only a dim sense of what is wrong, others may be quite clear that they are speaking of something vitally important, in the wrong language.

Moreover, when the client is speaking in the wrong language, the connection with the therapist at that time is inevitably weakened. Having a somewhat blurred or inexact sense of what the client is trying to convey, the therapist may misattune or misinterpret. In so doing, he or she will fail to provide the deep level of empathy, which the client so badly needs in order to fully, process and assimilate painful sensory and emotional experiences.

Finally, as well as the central sensory qualities of the material in any session, the client's feelings about a particular mode of expression must also be taken into account. On one occasion or more consistently over time, a certain art form may offer a particular client more protection than another. One art form may feel too powerful, or too embarrassing, or too exposing to a client, while another art form may feel liberating, bringing the satisfaction of having conveyed an experience with both depth and exactitude.

"All the world's a stage, and all the men and women merely players. They have their exits and their entrances; And one man in his time plays many parts, his acts being seven ages. At first the infant, mewling and puking in the nurse's arms. And then the whining school-boy, with his satchel and shining morning face, and then the lover, sighing like furnace, with a woful ballad made to his mistress' eyebrow. Then a soldier, full of strange oaths and bearded like the pard; jealous in honour, sudden and quick in quarrel, and then the justice. The world's a theatre, the earth a stage, Which God and Nature do with actors fill."

William Shakespeare – *As You Like It, Act ii (abridged)*

Transformational Drama & Dance Therapy
By Christina Artemis

What is Drama, Dance and Voice Therapy? It is the use of drama and related techniques through workshops and courses to heal and transform body, mind, emotions and spirit.

The techniques for training an actor, singer or dancer are used in a therapeutic way; not as in the case of actors who must develop tools for performance, but rather in the 'way of the actor' as a path to profound self-development and personal power. Here, actor is used in the broadest context to include singer and dancer, and both sexes.

Actor training lasts from one to three years, is rigorous, intense, involving not only the physical, mental and emotional sides but also the inner, psychic and spiritual resources.

Even if an artist is lucky enough to make a living, this 'work on the self' never stops. It involves physical work, realigning the body through various forms of training in movement, dance, sometimes fencing to develop control, strength, co-ordination and flexibility.

Secondly, actors and singers must learn techniques for developing a rich vibrant voice, using knowledge of sound, clarity and diction – and at the basis of life itself – breathing.

Thirdly; they must become skilled in using the imagination. At the centre of everything is the actor's need to delve deep into personal emotions – no holds barred, pulling up from deep within that which is needed to put life into a character.

They are expected to 'use' their most private, often upsetting experiences to develop challenging roles. In preparing for a role, they may recall and release bad experiences, but unlike standard therapy, which often talks about them, focusing on the negative, actors are given the space to express their experiences in the work of creating a character.

Certain exercises can be used to bring to the surface, upsetting events from the past, thus resolving emotional trauma; one of the most effective being conscious connected breathing (Rebirthing) used in a very active way. This is one of the most important aspects that makes Drama Therapy so different, exciting, fun and less introspective than other psychology based therapies.

Recently there has been a big focus on physical fitness, with many more people going to the gym. Working with dance as therapy can develop strength, co-ordination and flexibility, and have the advantage of being a wonderful form of self-expression.

Also, human beings often have strong feelings locked in the body (for example, hatred and anger) and dance therapy offers the opportunity to express those feelings in a much safer way. Using Sound in Voice work has a similar effect of healing fears of expressing ourselves, and developing communication skills. Different aspects of Drama, Dance and Voice Therapy affect people in many ways. The benefits however, are fantastic for releasing untold stress and tension which, if not dealt with, will eventually cause pain and disease. This exciting work following the 'way of the actor' helps to bring personal darkness into the light!

However, the difference between actor training and Drama, Dance and Voice Therapy is that we are not requiring people to become actors, singers or dancers, necessarily. So how does this work benefit the 'normal average adult' – if there is such a thing?

Since ancient times drama, or the dramatising of events important to the raising of consciousness of mankind, has been used in one form or other.

Of particular note, the Greek and Roman theatre had great cultural significance, not only in that time but on the development and influence on the arts today. There were big themes; the great Tragedies of life, often seen in a mythological way, were played out in front of huge audiences in vast amphitheatres.

Today, actors are more often than not seen as 'entertainers' even the greats such as Sir Laurence Olivier and Sir John Gielgud.

However, back in our distance past, there were 'medicine men and women' of the old tribes, often called shamans and sorcerers.

These early 'actors' were highly respected and often feared for their powers. Their sacred knowledge was kept passed down from generation to generation. They would have to go through rigorous training, and were particularly skilled in bringing spirit, and other dimensions of reality into a form of performance specifically designed to bring help and consciousness to the tribe.

The community would go to them for advice and healing, and in some cases 'spells' They were often skilled in the use of herbs and, in some cases, they would ingest hallucinogenic plants to take them into an altered state of consciousness.

Their strong affinity with the earth, and her creatures led them to give important attributes and power to the animal and bird kingdoms, and this featured in their ceremonial performances and rituals. Today, the shamans of our indigenous societies, such as Aboriginal and native American Indian could teach us a lot.

I believe we are all magnificent and powerful with a unique purpose to fulfill, but mostly we live quite limited lives within a narrow perspective, based on family and societal conditioning, holding back our full creativity.

We become set in the traditional roles of father, wife, teacher, banker, librarian and so on, and there are parts of our self that we have denied expression, sometimes called sub-personalities.

Drama techniques allow us to play out our unexpressed selves in a safe environment just once removed from actual reality, and this is less threatening. It can be great fun.

In fact, children do this all the time; playing out 'characters' and imaginary situations. I believe they do this to make sense of and understand their world and the people in it.

The child within

Another benefit of drama therapy is the re-connection to the child within us. We have had to 'grow up' and it appears there is not enough time for ourselves, what with work and family commitments.

Often, our imagination has been stifled, a big block to our creativity. In drama therapy we can regain our sense of fun, play, spontaneity, a 'belief in magic' and develop self-expression.

"Ah, every day dear Herbert becomes de plus en plus Oscarié. It is a wonderful case of nature imitating art" – **Oscar Wilde** *(1854 –1900)*

ART, DRAMA & DANCE THERAPY

INTEGRATED ARTS PSYCHOTHERAPY: Explore thoughts and feelings using imagination, imagery, sound or movement; with Therapist acting as guide and mentor, supporting and challenging with respect and compassion. For details phone Janet Branscombe, Bognor 01243 840187

ARTS PSYCHOTHERAPIST: Sensitive work with imagery, personal mythology, dreams, and bodywork. Support in solving your problems, and enriching your life. UKCP reg, holistic healing massage also available. N. London some concessions. Call Fran 0208 8893281.

CREATIVE ARTS PSYCHOTHERAPIST. Bilingual English – Spanish, Experienced working with adults and children. Art forms include; music, drama, paint, clay, puppets. UKCP registered. Hilda Mendoza Tel; 02076030845 Fax 02076032853

POMEGRANATE – ARTS Psychotherapy for people wanting to explore their lives and make choices with greater awareness. We also offer a place to look at relationships to food and body / self image. Pomegranate is based at The South London Natural Health Centre in Clapham. Phone Jo / Allie – 020 7720 8817

ART, DRAMA & DANCE THERAPY

DOMINIQUE PAHUD & David Thorogood, 15 Holmsdale Road, Victoria Park, Bristol BS3 4QL. 0117 904 9726

MS C HOLLIDAY, 55 Sturton Street, Cambridge, Cambridgeshire, CB1 2QG. 01223 511183

MS V WILSON Dip I.A.T.E. Reg. U.K.C.P., 1 Huntshill Cottage, Moons Green, Wittersham, Kent, TN30 7PR. 01797 270621

INSTITUTE FOR ARTS In Therapy & Education, The Windsor Centre, Windsor Street, Islington, London, N1. 020 7704 2534

MS H ROSE, 6 Ridgeway Mansions, Drapers Road, Enfield, Middlesex, EN2 8LS. 020 8366 1721

MS I KEMP, Bunkers, Ashstead Lane, Godalming, Surrey, GU7 1SY. 01483 427754

MS H CRUTHERS, 24 Buckingham Street, Brighton, Sussex, BN1 3LT. 01273 779176

Astrology

By Sue Martin

Astrology is a vast, complex and fascinating subject covering many different areas – the true study of astrology reveals a wealth of information and knowledge – for the birth chart reveals our physical, emotional, mental and spiritual makeup.

Astrology deals in moments in time – each moment in time is unlike any other – just as the planets are all moving at different speeds around the sun, we too, on planet earth are moving in this gravitational force field in a constantly changing pattern of energy. An astrologer calculates a chart based on the individual's date of birth, time of birth and place of birth and from this information the planetary patterns of that moment in time are revealed.

These planetary patterns indicate to a trained astrologer the emotional mental makeup of the individual – the chart also reveals areas of potential natural ability and is a unique individual and just as we each have our own unique finger print patterning – so too, do we each carry our own individual energetic make up – astrology gives access into this hidden world – allowing the individual to utilise their own unique makeup in constructive and positive ways -encouraging the individual to take responsibility for their own personal growth and development. The study of astrology goes back thousands of years – around 400 BC Hippocrates a Greek physician/astrologer/healer recognised, through astrological awareness, that different emotional temperaments could lead to different physical problems.

As we enter the 21st Century – it is to be hoped that astrological insight will once again work along side other complementary/vibrational therapies – bringing the gifts of knowledge and guidance to enable the healing process and to promote true well being.

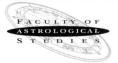
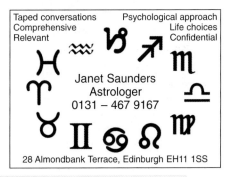

Aura-Soma®
By Aura-Soma® Ltd

Aura-Soma is a non-intrusive colour system of great beauty, which offers you the opportunity for awareness and transformation. It invites you to work from the deeper level of your being empowering you to help yourself through colour.

Aura-Soma brings consciousness and insight from the soul level of your being into your everyday life. Aura-Soma is especially suited for those who wish to come to a new focus in their life and or who wish to develop themselves.

It is a fundamental premise of Aura-Soma that you yourself know what is best for you. Aura-Soma is described as non-intrusive because it is your choice of colours that determines what is explored during the session.

Colour is a universal language understood by all people in all cultures. It is in fact the language of the soul. Your colour preferences, such as your favourite colours or those you like to see next to each other and the pleasure you get from certain colours, are expressions of the inner-self equilibrium. Colour combinations present a medium for the soul to express itself and touch the underlying themes of your life in a way that goes beyond language.

The Consultation – You are the colours you choose

Your choice of Equilibrium bottles is the key to the Aura-Soma Consultation. To

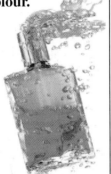

begin you will be invited to choose the four colour combinations to which you are most drawn. During the hour-long consultation that follows you will gain insight into your current situation and the larger pattern of your life story by exploring with a trained Aura-Soma practitioner who will who reveal your gifts, challenges and opportunities. Your colour choice will shed light on your potential for growth and transformation.

Towards the end of the consultation you will identify the Aura-Soma colour products that will be most beneficial for you to apply in the following weeks; this is an important part of helping yourself through Aura-Soma. The consultation provides the insight into your situation, but it is in applying the Aura-Soma colour onto and around yourself that the information discussed in the session may be absorbed and integrated into your everyday experience. The products have an energetic vibration that goes beyond words.

You will also receive a consultation information sheet on which you may make a note of the main details of your consultation, what was discussed and what was recommended. This will provide a valuable record of your ongoing work with AuraSoma.

The products and effect

There are four main products in the Aura-Soma system.

Equilibrium bottles are dual coloured combinations composed of two fractions, oil over water. Each bottle is filled with the living energies of colour, plant crystals and combines the vibrations of the plant and mineral kingdoms in a balanced form that maybe applied directly onto the body. In addition to equilibrium there are the Pomanders and Quintessences. These fragrant tools, composed of 49 herbs, provide protection and support for the aura while you open yourself up to the transformation process triggered by the equilibrium bottles. They are to be passed through the aura around the body.

The background

Aura-Soma was born in 1983, created as the result of an inspiration received by its remarkable founder Vicky Wall. Though blind and in retirement she was inspired by a nightly recurring vision of jewel-like colours sighing their way towards her. This vision led to the creation of the colour combination of bottles that lie at the heart of the Aura-Soma system. These bottles are known as equilibrium. Since those early days the range of equilibrium has grown to over a hundred colour combinations, each combination offering its own gifts and potential.

Although the founder passed on in 1991, the practice continues to grow in popularity worldwide. The current motivation is provided by Mike Booth and a global band of dedicated supporters consisting of 300 accredited teaches and 15,000 students.

The established programme and training of Aura-Soma now has a presence in more than 55 countries worldwide. It is living colour – bringing man the understanding of man.

Professionalism

There is an Aura-Soma code of practice regulated by the A. S. International Academy of Colour Therapeutics. The academy registers and issues practising certificates to those who work according to this code. A current Aura-Soma practising certificate issued by the academy confirms that a practitioner is continuing to be updated in the Aura-Soma system and works according to the practices set out by the academy.

AURA SOMA

CHOOSE FROM 100 BEAUTIFUL dual-coloured bottles. See your own individual rainbow – your diagnosis, your prescription, reveal your special gifts – the purpose of you life's journey; what underlies your challenges – the present & the potential future. Anne is in Enfield 0181 805 0281 email: anne mcg-opendoor@hotmail.com

AURA-SOMA COLOUR THERAPY consultations, workshop, talks and certified courses. Sarah uses Aura-Soma products in Kinesiology massage IHBC sessions. She has trained in Humanistic counselling OCNSEM and is a registered Reiki Master with the School of the Living LightTM . For details of Aura-Soma and Reiki courses, consultations or further information, please contact Sarah Hurst on 01480 382882 St. Ives, Cambs or e-mail: rahhurst@ntlworld.com

AURA SOMA

DISCOVER YOUR TRUE COLOURS with Aura Soma, Colour Healing, Chakra Work and Meditation. Talks, workshops and courses on all aspects of holistic wellbeing. North East area. Ros Taylor: Tel 01388 537534 e-mail: froghall@compuserve.com

MS R IRVING, 33 Linksway, Gatley, Cheadle, Cheshire, SK8 4LA. 0161 428 9675

MR A TILSTON, 17c Church Street, Frodsham, Cheshire, WA6 6PN. 01928 731596

MS I BULL, 23 Greens Close, Bishops Waltham, Hampshire, SO32 1JT. 01489 892382

MR J LENNARD, 12 Riverside, Temple Ewell, Dover, Kent, CT16 3HW. 01304 829557

MS L GRAHAM, 57 Huntingdon Road, Roehampton, London, SW15 5EA. 020 8876 7544

Ayurveda

By Dr. N Sathiyamoorthy

It now seems certain that the stresses of modern life-style (work-related stress and environmental stresses are well known to us all!) has led to an increase in lifestyle-related diseases such as cancer, heart disease and allergies.

And with increasing burdens on the health services, many of us are turning to alternative therapies in the quest for improved health and quality of life and to improve our 'cope-ability'. The ancient Indian system of Ayurveda has been in existence for some 5,000 years and the Sanskrit word 'Ayurveda' means 'Science of Life'. It is the oldest surviving systematic approach to health and health care.

Ayurveda is founded on the principles that every living being is composed of five elements: earth, water, fire, air and ether and these combine to give three basic types (or 'doshas') – Vata (air), Pitta (heat) and Kapha (water). The dominant characteristic determines the physical and psychological make-up of the individual and an imbalance due to an increase or depletion in any of these elements can lead to ill health. Ayurveda treats ailments by correcting imbalances through the holistic approach, i.e. through diet, exercise and general life-style, supplemented when necessary with naturally occurring substances such as herbs and minerals.

The Ayurvedic medicinal system is 100% completely natural and uses complex herbomineral formulations to restore the balance of every body function, preferably before minor imbalances worsen and result in disease. It also helps restore the power of the body to heal itself if a condition has deteriorated, thus ensuring that the treatment is effective and permanent.

The Ayurvedic principles for the various preparations have been carefully laid down over thousands of years. They include formulations consisting of a great variety of plants and minerals in fixed, precise proportions, according to a vast pharmacopoeia and a truly amazing understanding of pharmacology.

In the complex alchemy of Ayurvedic medicine, herbs are combined to achieve truly safe and synergistic effects. Others may buffer one active ingredient whilst certain ingredients play the role of adjuvant, such as to strengthen the digestive system or to help remove wastes. Single herbs, single extracts or isolated active principles are never used in Ayurvedic medicine as it violates the basic tenets of Ayurveda.

An isolated active principle that is not natural to the body will react in undesired ways. No single active constituent has the broad activity of the entire plant and no single plant has the activity and safety of carefully formulated blends.

Bach Flower Remedies

By Stefan Ball- Consultant at the Dr. Edward Bach Centre

The 38 Bach Flower Remedies are medicines for the emotions: simple, natural preparations that are used to treat everyday emotional states such as worry anxiety and lack of concentration. Dr. Edward Bach, a bacteriologist, pathologist and homoeopath whose career took him from University College Hospital to the London Homeopathic Hospital and a successful Harley Street practice, discovered them in the 1930s.

Bach was convinced that the only path to true health was to treat the individual personality, rather than concentrating on the physical symptoms of disease.

He found that specially prepared plants could resolve emotional imbalances, and that well balanced people then got better physically because their bodies were free to heal themselves. By the time he died in 1936 Dr. Bach had discovered 38 remedies, a complete system that could be combined to treat every possible emotional state. The remedies included:

Mimulus to give the courage needed to face everyday fears and anxieties

Gentian to encourage people to overcome setbacks

Larch to give confidence

Olive to give renewed energy to people who had been drained by exertion or illness

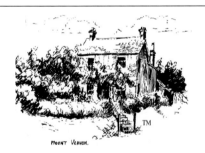
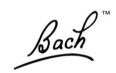

White Chestnut to calm persistent, worrying thoughts

When using Bach flower remedies it is essential to ignore any physical symptoms or disease. Instead the remedies are selected according to the personality of the person being treated.

For example, a kind, gentle person who found it hard to say 'no' to other people would be given Centaury, while someone who always tries to hide his/her worries by making a joke of them would need Agrimony.

Both might be suffering from the same physical symptoms, such as insomnia and frequent colds, but the remedies would be different for each person. The effect of the remedies is to transform negative thoughts and behaviour into positive ones. They do not alter people's personalities or promise instant spiritual fulfillment, instead they bring us gently back to ourselves so that we can go on learning from our lives.

There are two main ways to take Bach flower remedies. One is to put two drops of each selected remedy into a glass of water and sip from this at least four times a day or until the problem has passed.

Alternatively the two drops can be put into a clean, empty 30ml dropper bottle, which is then topped up with mineral water. From this bottle known as a treatment bottle four drops are taken four times a day. Kept in the fridge and used regularly a treatment bottle will last up to three weeks.

The treatment bottle dose is the minimum needed for the remedies to work effectively. You can take them more frequently for moments of crisis, because they are completely safe: it is impossible to overdose on them or become addicted or to build up tolerance.

Bach flower remedies do not affect the actions of other medicines or therapies, nor are they affected by them. This, and the fact that they are free of side effects, makes them an ideal complement to other courses of treatment.

The most famous remedy is a mix of remedies that is best known under the trade name 'Rescue Remedy'. Rescue Remedy contains five remedies; Rock Rose for terror, Clematis for light-headedness, Impatiens for agitation, Cherry Plum for loss of self-control and Star of Bethlehem for shock.

Dr. Bach selected these five remedies because he felt there would be at least something in the mix that would help anyone going through a crisis.

To take Rescue Remedy put four drops in a glass of water and sip as required. In an emergency, if there is no water available, you put the drops straight on the tongue or rub them on the pulse points. Common uses for Rescue Remedy include calming down the victims of accidents and combating pre-operation nerves. Many midwives use them to help mothers through labour.

One range of Dr. Bach's remedies – the ones with his signature on the bottle -are still made at the Bach Centre, Mount Vernon, the Oxfordshire cottage where he spent the last years of his life and completed his research.

Body Electronics

By Peter Aziz

Body Electronics is a deep form of bodywork, which accesses genetic memories from the body to produce fundamental and permanent change, in consciousness as well as in the body.

Suppressed memories, emotions and thought patterns tend to be stored as crystals on the DNA. Many of these crystals are passed down from parents, grandparents and ancestors. Our emotional and mental blocks are associated with these crystals, which will also affect the functioning of the body.

Body Electronics uses a revolutionary method of prolonged point holding, after nutritional preparation, to access and dissolve these crystals. As the crystals dissolve, suppressed memories surface to be re-experienced, not only from your own lifetime, but also memories from your parents and other predecessors. This allows the healing of hereditary problems. As all the emotional and mental blocks are released, the body also heals rapidly. We work with a unity of mind and body: each physical illness will have some stored trauma, emotion or thought pattern associated with it, and we heal the body and mind together.

Body Electronics has been effective in healing impotence and other sexual problems, digestive disturbances, anaemia, cysts, tumours and cancers, immune deficiency diseases, rheumatic and arthritic disorders, and has restored nerve pathways to paralysed areas of the body, following injuries or strokes. It has also freed many people from all kinds of emotional problems and 'stuck' states. A new development is that it is able to mend broken bones in a matter of hours.

There are two ways of practising Body Electronics.

Private sessions usually take two hours, but can be longer, and are suited to those who wish to concentrate on healing a particular illness. For those who wish to go through maximum personal growth and empowerment, including dramatic enhancement or awakening of psychic abilities, the intensive workshops are more suitable.

On the workshops, you will work in a group, which will encourage rapid release of stored memories, working through layer after layer of suppression until total freedom and power are attained. This is facilitated by pressing reflex points all over the body, while teaching psychological release skills.

Books, Magazines & Publishers
By M. Willcocks PhD

Everyone has a book in them, it is said. While this may be true, getting a manuscript ready to be published is a different matter. Any true writer knows that, like painting or music, it takes both talent and a grasp of technique to do it properly.

Talent can't be learned; technique can. It's a sad but indisputable fact that the author is often the last person to see that his work needs revising. Before you start, establish the ethos and format of your book. Research your subject; there are many avenues available for research… libraries, the Internet and book shops. Many societies and associations are invariably willing to help. Next seek expert advice on things like design, reproduction, printing, proof reading and so on. Talk to the professionals; such expertise rarely comes free – and nor should it. You wouldn't expect a car mechanic to replace your clutch in return for a big smile, or a solicitor to draw up your will because it did his soul good. Remember what tends to happen if you pay peanuts.

When you have completed your first section, objective appraisal from someone with no axe to grind is required. This is the most reliable way of establishing whether your work is actually readable. If it isn't, you rob yourself of the most powerful marketing tool of all – word-of-mouth recommendation. Remember, you will need to sell more than a handful of copies to recoup your outlay. If it is readable, not only do you have a good chance of making some money; your determination and self-belief may encourage you to go on to a second and even better project.

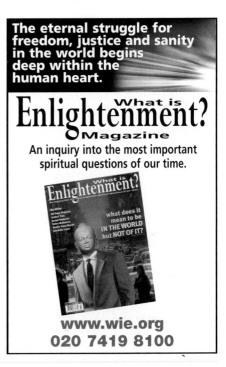

The Bowen Technique
By The Bowen Association

The Bowen Technique is highly effective in relieving many common conditions, such as back pain, sciatica, neck restrictions, sports injuries, knee problems, frozen shoulders, bronchial and asthmatic problems, tennis elbow, menstrual irregularities, headaches and migraines plus stress and tension.

It can also be effective for many chronic conditions such as ME and arthritic symptoms and even for life threatening illness.

Registered nurse and Bowen therapist Joanne Figov of Dorset says: 'Because Bowen can stimulate the body's immune and lymphatic drainage systems, patients with chronic and more serious illnesses can greatly benefit. I've treated patients with ME who regain much energy after a couple of treatments and I'm currently treating a lady recovering after chemotherapy who has found relief from her aches and pains and depression.'

Racked with five years of pain, his face grey with suffering, the car accident victim's last resort before surgery was the Bowen Technique. After a few gentle finger movements across his muscles by Bowen therapist Suzanne Payne of Dorset, the patient felt an energy surge through his body. The chronic neck disorder which had blocked all his movement was suddenly freed.

Emotional with the joy of his release, he said: "It was absolutely wonderful. I fell

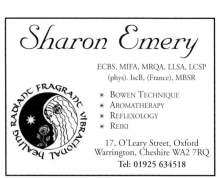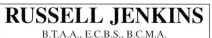
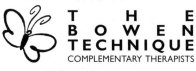
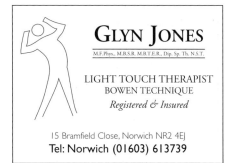

asleep on the couch and then stood up and was able to see the ceiling for the first time in five years!" His recovery is no surprise to therapists world-wide practising this dynamic system of muscle and connective tissue therapy developed in the 1950s by the late Tom Bowen of Australia.

Oswald (Ossie) Rentsch, director and founder of the Bowen Therapy Academy of Australia, once said: "The Bowen Technique is possibly the greatest discovery ever in health care. Bowen training is attracting medical doctors as well as chiropractors, osteopaths, physiotherapists and acupuncturists, all who praise the technique for its power."

How Australian Tom Bowen came by his remarkable technique and put it into action is the stuff of legend. Tom claimed his discovery that tiny movements across muscles effecting remarkable recoveries, was a 'gift from God'. In the small town where he worked in an industrial plant he treated his work colleagues at home in the evenings. He became so busy he had to give up his day job and opened a clinic which was soon attracting patients from all over Australia. Eventually he was seeing over 13,000 a year more than 80 per cent recovering after only two treatments.

Many regard Tom Bowen as a genius, 'the Mozart of healing'. Researchers are still studying exactly how the technique works but it is postulated that every molecule of tissue and cell in the human body is wired directly to the brain. Researcher Dan Amato from New York calls it the 'feedback loop'. And like many others, New Zealand therapist Lou Hassik believes: "The body-mind is one. It's a complex lawful system of interactive processes from head to toe." In other words the Bowen Technique empowers the body to heal itself – the gentle precise moves on specific areas could be said to reset the body's computer.

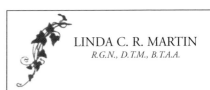
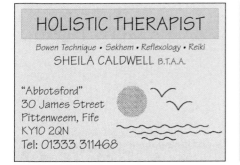

An example of Bowen's ability to help difficult and obscure conditions is Joanne's pilot study on a small section of patients diagnosed with a form of Dystonia called Blepharospasm. This neurological condition is characterised by involuntary muscular eyelid spasms causing forceful contraction of the eyes. The condition can be mild to severe, ranging from twitching to excessive blinking of the eyelids to severe cases where the patient is functionally blind as the spasm forces the eyes shut. Consequently the sufferers are in great emotional distress.

The standard hospital treatment is Botulinum toxin injections that temporarily lessen the spasm by weakening the muscles around the eye. With the permission and encouragement of a hospital consultant, Joanne began treating his patients.

She explained: "Through my work as an ophthalmic nurse and working with these patients I realised that as blepharospasm is primarily a neurological disorder surely Bowen, which works along those principles, could help reset the signal to the brain."

Joanne has a waiting list for patients in the small pilot study which is still in its early stages. The results so far she describes as "very encouraging".

"Because I have to fit the study group around my private practice and my nursing, I've so far been able to work with only eight patients" explained Joanne. "One has recovered completely in four treatments – all the rest have had relief for a couple of days following each treatment session. The lady who recovered completely had suffered the condition for three months – the shortest time, whereas the others were long term sufferers of up to 50 years and they may need many treatments to unlock the deep rooted patterning. What's exciting is that such gentle Bowen moves are obviously addressing a condition which mainstream medical science is finding difficult to resolve."

Because Bowen is holistic in nature, practitioners often find that conditions other than that being treated, are resolved. For example, one 80-year-old woman with a left eye spasm for 11 years also had a chronic back problem. After one treatment the facial spasm lessened for two days but the back pain also disappeared. "She told me she was able to swim for the first time in two years," said Joanne

A 75-year-old woman in the study

wanted to continue Bowen treatments after her sessions ended. Asked why, she replied: "The sense of relaxation and wellbeing are adding so much to my quality of life." Another woman was able, with her doctor's permission, to come off anti-depressants. Bowen's power is not limited to physical conditions and many therapists report vast improvement to patients' emotional wellbeing.

You are never too young for Bowen, therapists report. Even babies in the womb can benefit. Registered midwife and Bowen practitioner Rick Minnery runs workshops to teach Bowen therapists how to help mums-to-be cope with pregnancy and baby care. Rick, from Lancashire, is working towards getting Bowen recognised in hospitals as a gentle technique for pre-natal and post-natal health care.

Sports professionals the world over are being treated successfully with Bowen – its instant results often rival physiotherapy. Tests have shown that competitors having regular Bowen treatments consistently perform better and with an accelerated rate of recovery from injury. Remedial sports therapist Craig Mattimoe from California says: "After five years of treating and preventing athletic injuries I can confidently report that no broad based modality in all of North America comes close to Bowen. I work mostly with athletes, particularly football players who are big business, and Bowen outshines all of the current accepted sports medicine techniques, both traditional and alternative!"

The Bowen Technique is taught in a number of countries around the world by several different training organisations. Courses may be found in: New Zealand, the US, Canada, Israel, Italy, Holland, France, Austria, Norway and the UK. It will soon be taught in South America and South Africa. Because two hands are the only practical tools needed for Bowen it is envisaged the technique will be taught in the Third World to relieve suffering without major expense or technology.

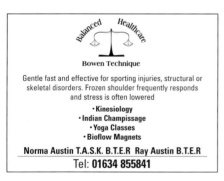
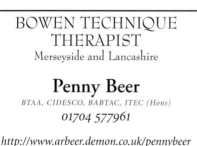
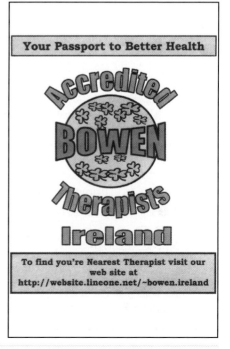

The Bowen Technique

The European College of Bowen Studies
Case histories

Light fingers make many things work, that was the title of an article on The Bowen Technique which appeared recently in the Daily Telegraph. This phrase neatly captures the essence of this remarkable complementary therapy: a gentle and non-invasive therapy for patients and an effective remedial treatment for a very wide range of complaints.

The majority of Bowen patients are those for whom conventional medicine and often other forms of complementary medicine have failed. The Bowen Technique seems to provide the body with the missing key to healing.

To illustrate the diversity of The Bowen Technique, the following are a selection of case histories from Bowen Practitioners who have been trained by the European College of Bowen Studies.

Case histories as published by The European College of Bowen Studies.

Sleeping problems

Little girl, aged 10 days. 1 treatment. M. was a fine, healthy baby weighing 7 lbs. After 10 days, her mother rang the Bowen therapist to say that all was well but that the baby was sleeping all day and awake all night and she wondered if the therapist could do anything that might help to reorganise the baby's body clock. The therapist treated her with a Bowen treatment. That night she slept right through, apart from feeding, and was awake more during the day. She has continued to follow this pattern since that one treatment.

Mental focus

Woman, aged 23. 1 treatment. K. received one Bowen treatment from a therapist at a Bowen Technique stand at a large health show. She wrote afterwards to say, "It made me feel really good and totally relaxed and, after being really 'spaced out', I then felt quite balanced and clear headed."

Lower back pain into hips & right knee

Woman, aged 26. 3 treatments. F. is a very tall (6' 2") nursery nurse, so works with tiny people and furniture all day. She had had this problem for 2 – 3 years. MRI scans had not revealed any cause for the pains and physiotherapy treatment had been to no avail. After the second Bowen treatment she said "it is 99% better than it was". After three treatments, the problems were completely gone and the resolution holding. She now chooses to return for a treatment several times a year as a 'general tune-up and de-stressing'. One session leaves her feeling restored.

Pain with deep breathing

Woman, aged 29. 4 treatments. M. had been experiencing pain in the thoracic area when breathing, from the back through to the front for two years. She had a history of severe asthma and that was linked to this. She had had various manipulations over this period of time via her GP and chiropractors which had offered no relief. After 3 treatments the pain was no longer evident and the breathing was easier. She described

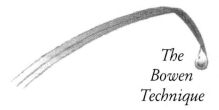

Training Practitioners
in
The Bowen Technique
since 1994

The
Bowen
Technique

European College of Bowen Studies (E.C.B.S.)

"The Bowen Technique is, quite simply, the most down-to-earth bodywork therapy in the book."
- Jane Alexander, in SUPERTHERAPIES

THE BOWEN TECHNIQUE IS REMEDIAL AND HOLISTIC

It is a simple and focused form of 'hands-on' bodywork that can bring remarkable results. The technique prompts the body to reset and heal itself, promoting relief of pain and recovery of energy. The experience of a treatment is gentle, subtle and relaxing. Most of the work can be performed through light clothing. Two to four treatments, at weekly intervals, are often sufficient to achieve lasting relief from even long-standing pain and complaints.

THE BOWEN TECHNIQUE OFFERS GENTLE AND EFFECTIVE TREATMENT

The wide variety of complaints that can be successfully resolved or substantially diminished include:

back and neck pain	sports injuries	frozen shoulder
tennis & golfer's elbows	lymphatic drainage	headache
respiratory conditions	chronic fatigue	stress
fibromyalgia	high blood pressure	AND MANY MORE

The **European College of Bowen Studies** is the professional, experienced organisation which has been preparing UK practitioners in The Bowen Technique since 1994. We strive to offer excellence in every area:

- Structured, modular courses offered throughout the UK, throughout the year
- Experienced, professional and well trained teachers
- Practical, hands-on training with comprehensive Training Manual and Photographic Guide
- Reliable and thorough support service for students and practitioners
- Course fees include emergency cancellation insurance
- preparing confident, knowledgeable therapists, whether using it professionally or for treatment of family and friends

E.C.B.S is a registered college with the **BCMA** and **ALTT** and is linked with professional bodies such as the Federation of Holistic Therapists (**FHT**) and Association of Therapy Lectures (**ATL**) for the purpose of maintaining high training and practice standards in the Bowen Technique.

For further information and Course Prospectus or list of Accredited Practitioners contact:

European College of Bowen Studies (E.C.B.S.)

38 Portway
FROME, Somerset
BA11 1QU

Tel/Fax: 01373 461 873
email: ecbs@cwcom.net
www.TheBowenTechnique.com

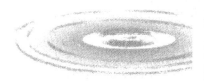

at this stage that she had a lymph drainage problem down one side of her body, mainly in the neck and was prone to lumpy breasts on that side. Her fourth visit was an 'insurance' to make sure that the relief was holding. A month after final treatment, she is free from all discomfort.

Sciatica

Man, aged 40. 1 treatment. P. was unable to put weight on his right foot and the therapist paid a home visit. He was in severe pain and had been all day, from the buttock right down the leg. He was extremely tense and tight. The therapist gave him one treatment of the basic moves and was able to observe his body relaxing during the 40 minutes of the treatment. He was virtually pain free when he got up and was walking normally. Two years later, the therapist reports that the problem has not returned.

Knee and upper back problems

Woman, aged 42. 4 treatments. C. is a practising masseuse who stands for long periods and develops a lot of tension in her back. Her upper back and shoulders were very tight. Also both knees and ankles were giving her trouble. After the first treatment her back loosened. Her knees and ankles were improving after the second treatment. After the first couple of treatments C. told the therapist that she had also been suffering from heavy and painful periods since the birth of her daughter nearly 10 years earlier. The therapist therefore gave her a procedure to address this and C. reported a tremendous change for the better in the next period with reduction of the pain and heaviness.

Neck/shoulder injury

Woman, aged 43. 3 treatments. Y. "I recently had the Bowen treatment for a stubborn and painful neck/shoulder injury, which I have suffered from for over three years. Although I was very sceptical at first – after all, how could so small and gentle a movement make such a difference, when all other treatments I had tried via my GP's recommendations had only eased the symptoms for a short time. I was amazed at the incredible results, even after only the first proper treatment on my neck and shoulders."

Tension back strain

Woman, aged 52. 2 treatments. J. was on holiday visiting family when she heard about The Bowen Technique and consulted a local practitioner. After the first treatment, she reported a lot less tension and stated that something seemed to be working in her body. After the second treatment she returned home saying that she would come back for more treatments when she returned to visit her family again. She sent a postcard to say her back was "brilliant".

Emotional stress

Woman, aged 57. 3 treatments. F. A series of family bereavements and problems over some years had completely drained A of any energy although she is normally an active and energetic person. She was feeling a tight chest, a tight 'band' around her head and her knees and legs hurt. After one Bowen treatment she felt slightly better. All symptoms showed definite signs of improvement after two and after the third treatment she was well on the way to getting back to her original self – including gardening and playing tennis within two months!

Arthritis, whiplash and fall:

Woman, aged 58 series of treatments. J. is overweight and has had arthritis in both knees for 23 years. It had also spread to her neck, right foot and was just starting in the knuckles of her right hand. She had also had a whiplash injury twice and fell at work 11 years ago and pulled the ligaments from the backbone to the hips. Her job requires her to do quite a lot of lifting and carrying. After beginning

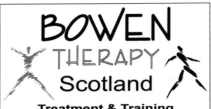

Bowen treatment, she was quite surprised that within a few weeks her knees were feeling much better and after a treatment on her hamstrings the result was amazing. She couldn't remember when she last had that amount of flexibility in her knees. Further treatments brought the same results to other parts of her body. Her neck is much better and she does not suffer headaches from the arthritis as she used to.

Frozen shoulder, head and neck restriction

Man, aged 60+ 2 treatments. N. paid two visits to his doctor for a frozen shoulder and received an injection which seemed to do nothing at all. After the first Bowen treatment there was an improvement and the trouble cleared up after the second visit. A friend of N.'s had suffered from the same trouble for at least one year with little hope of improvement. However, the friend's frozen shoulder was relieved by the Bowen therapist during a treatment given during a visit to the Over-60's Club.

Footballer restored

A letter from Danny Adams to Hella Crawford, Bowen Practitioner Date: May 2000

I was asked to try Bowen therapy by my football physio as I had been having problems with my back, groins and upper leg muscles for most of the season. I'd been to a chiropractor a few times and on my last visit she had advised there was nothing really wrong with my bone structure. I continued to play but still felt restricted in my movements so I decided to give Bowen a try. I didn't really know what to expect but I was determined to keep an open mind and give it a go. I can't explain how it worked but after a couple of treatments the problems I had been having virtually disappeared. I was able to touch my toes with the palms of my hands – something I'd not been able to do for a long while and I seemed to be able to go the duration of a game easily where I had been struggling before. When people ask 'does it work?', I find the best way to tell them about it is my scoring ratio since having Bowen. I'd only scored 5 goals in 27 games before Bowen treatment. From the time I started having treatment until the end of the season, I scored 10 in 12 and from my point of view, that says it all! I also didn't miss a game through injury. Thank you Hella.

BOWEN TECHNIQUE

BOWEN TECHNIQUE and Reflexology Registered practitioner. For an appointment or information please contact Effie Rahs MAR, MBTER, Winchmore Hill, London N21. Telephone: 020 8245 0958

HEALTH VITALICS, Surrey. Cynthia Rigby, S.R.N., an experienced practitioner specialising in a proven range of energetic therapies. I use Bowen, Empulse, Scenar and other technologies to address conditions ranging from frozen shoulder and other muscular skeletal problems to migraine and M.E.. Telephone: 0870 787 3991. e-mail: cynthia@healthvitalics.co.uk

BOWEN TECHNIQUE

ROSEMARY BERRY, DHOM BTAA – Complementary Health Consultant. Holistic treatment using The Bowen Technique, Homoeopathy, Bach Flower Remedies, Allergy Testing and Management. Located in a peaceful rural Devon location with plenty of car parking space. Telephone 01884 855248 or 01884 32320 Email: rosemary@billingsmoor.fsnet.co.uk

MRS A GENTILLI, Greville Mount, Milcote, Stratford-Upon-Avon, Warwickshire, CV37 8AB. 01789 750265

Buqi

By Teresa Leong

Buqi is an ancient almost forgotten Chinese healing practice which focuses on the removal of Binqi – anything that feels wrong in the body. In each generation only a few people knew small fragments of this system, which they passed on secretly to family members.

Dr Shen Hongxun was given some of this knowledge by his Grandfather Shen BaoTai and Professor Yao HuanZhi. It took him a quarter of a century of research in this field to allow the development of a new system – Buqi.

This system uses earth force, vibrational force and mental force to send information into the body to bring binqi out, thus creating the environment and space for restoring one's health.

Treatment is without touch or by just lightly touching the patient. Healing force is sent into the meridians of the patient and in this way the practitioner is able to expel negative emotions.

During treatment, the patient may experience different sensations such as itching, prickliness, heat, cold or blocked pain moving out of the body and afterwards the the body may feel very light.

Taijiwuxigong, the self healing part of the system, consists of exercises to learn to use the earth force, in order to develop spontaneous movements which clear and regulate body and mind.

Comments from clients

"I felt fuzzy electrical pulse's like pin pricks penetrating my skin and something moving out."

"I felt as if water was physically flowing through my body and out of my hands into the ground."

"I went in hardly able to walk due to a bad back. After treatment the pain went and by the next day I was walking normally."

If you enjoy reading and using this book you will enjoy its sister publication The Green Life – available in Waterstones and all good book shops, price £7.95.

You can also find extracts from the natural health series of books at: **www.naturalhealthdirect.com**. *Look us up, there are some interesting links.*

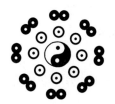

TERESA LEONG

Buqi Healer
Chi Nei Tsang
De-Stress Massage
Cellular Clearing
Medium

London Appointments
Call
020 7381 5709

Business Opportunities

By M. Willcocks PhD

This is a pragmatic guide to setting up in business, be it as a practitioner, shop keeper or any other opportunity you may wish to pursue. You will find that 'product' has been used in a lateral sense.

Each year hundreds of people want to set up in business. There are many reasons:

Loss of paid work; reaction to period of unemployment; identification of opportunity; desire for more money; need for change of lifestyle; no longer wanting to work for someone else.

You may be motivated by one or more of these or have reasons of your own. Take time to think about your own personal reasons for wanting to set up a business.

The first task in setting up a business is deciding why you want to do it. Then you should set yourself clear goals. These should relate to the business and to you personally. For the business you might have goals in terms of the size of the business, the product range, the profitability and the image. For yourself, goals could include financial rewards, free time, lifestyle and status.

Write your goals down – they will help motivate you when the going gets tough.

Businesses falls into three main categories:

• Manufacturing   • Service   • Retail

All three areas offer opportunities. Manufacturing generally is in decline yet probably offers the most opportunities because so many of the goods we buy are imported and because the European Single Market offers great export opportunities. The service sector has grown rapidly.

Finding an idea

You can find a business idea in many ways. Whatever your idea, you need to be sure that people will buy from you or use your services. You also need to be certain that you can make sufficient money from it to run the business successfully and give you the financial return you need to earn a living

Personal budget

Draw up a personal budget for all the things you need money for – mortgage and/or rent, rates, clothing, food, car, holidays etc. When you've totalled that up, add on another ten per cent for contingencies. If your business can't give you that amount of money at least then you should re-consider your decision to start.

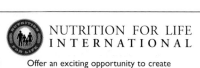

Thinking ahead

Even at this early stage you should also be thinking of how your business idea might change or be improved over the next few years. Will you be able to add new features or benefits, will you need to extend the range of products or services you offer. Running a successful business means always planning ahead.

You as a business owner

Not everyone can be a successful business owner but many people can and do run good, profitable businesses. There is no such thing as a typical business owner. Successful business people are male and female, young and old. They come from a wide variety of backgrounds – educated, illiterate, highly skilled, employed, unemployed, rural, inner-city, disabled and able-bodied.

There are no tests to pass to become a business owner and you don't need particular qualifications but there are some characteristics which are common to many business people. It's useful at this stage to have a look at your own personal strengths and weaknesses, your skills and experience and the resources which you can bring to the business.

Support

Starting and running a business requires a lot of support. So what is involved in setting up a business? Whatever your business idea, there are some steps you will have to take:

- research your market
- check out your sources of materials/ supplies, their availability and cost
- look at your production requirements – premises, machinery and labour
- work out your total costs
- estimate your selling price
- plan how you will achieve sales
- decide the legal framework of your business
- check out any legislation which might affect you
- estimate your total financial requirements and where you might raise the money
- produce a business plan.

One of the key factors in business success is often support from the family. How does your family feel about you starting a business? Will they support you? And how?

Research your market

The aim of market research is to tell you if there are enough people to buy your product to make it into a business which can pay you at least a living wage. There are many ways of researching the market and a fairly straightforward method is suggested below. Start by asking yourself who are your potential customers. They may be: children, old age pensioners, motorists, people with disabilities or perhaps all of those and more. It can help to write down who you think your customers will be.

Where are the customers?

Next, ask yourself where are the customers? Are they in your local housing estate, in your city , in every town and village of the UK? You need to decide on the area you can comfortably service. It may be too expensive, for example, to offer to collect clothes for dry cleaning outside a ten-mile radius from your workplace. The area you can reasonably service is therefore your marketplace.

Write down where you see your marketplace. Now ask yourself how many customers, as described above, are in that marketplace? Then ask how much these customers spend or might be prepared to spend on your product. Ask who is presently supplying these products and, finally, ask yourself why you will be preferred rather than your competitors? When you have answered these questions you should be in a position to estimate the potential success of your enterprise.

Finding the Answers

How do you go about answering these questions? You can do this in two ways:

• using information other people have gathered
• finding out information for yourself

Once you have decided on your marketplace you can find out the number of potential customers for your product by consulting the census return for that area – that will give you numbers of people, numbers of households etc. If your customers are likely to be businesses you could consult yellow pages or a trade directory such as that produced by the local council. To find out how much these customers spend on your particular product/service you can consult:

• Family Expenditure Survey   • Social Trends
• Specialist market research reports   • Business monitors

To find out who is currently supplying similar products you can consult a whole range of trade directories and yellow pages.

Doing your own research

In some cases, if you are researching a new product, published information may not be available. You may also want to add to the information you have gathered. In both these cases you will need to carry out research yourself. This means talking directly to potential customers. You can do this in several ways:

• face to face interviews • telephone interviews • postal surveys.

To do this you will need to draw up a market research questionnaire. This is not difficult but requires careful thought. It's useful to get some help from your Local Enterprise Agency. The questionnaire should help you answer questions such as whether or not people would be interested in your product, how often they might buy it, what they're prepared to pay for it, why they buy it, when and where they buy it.

Properly carried out, the questionnaire will give you very valuable information. You need, of course, to think about the number of people you should contact before you can draw conclusions. For example, if there are 1,000 households with gardens in your town you would need to contact at least 100 to be in any way sure of the market for gardening services.

What the research should tell you

The research should help you identify a very important factor – your unique selling proposition (USP), or why people will actually buy from you. You can identify this by looking very carefully at why people presently buy. What benefits are they looking for? Are there any extra benefits you could offer? You can also look at your competitors – what are they not doing well? Perhaps, it's their service, quality, design, range or after sales service. What could you improve on?

The research should also help you identify your price. You need two very important pieces of information – what price will the market bear and what will it cost you to make your product, including all expenses?

Many people believe they have to set a price which is lower than the competition. You should resist this temptation. If you offer a cheaper price you will reduce your profit and will have to sell more to compensate. It makes much more sense to fix a reasonable price which is good value for money and to offer a unique selling proposition which is attractive to your customers.

If you think this is not possible you must ask yourself if it is worth marketing your product at all. The final outcome of market research should be that you can make a realistic assessment of your level of sales for the first year of your business.

Checking out resources

To get started in business you will normally need:

- Materials   • Equipment   • Premises   • Labour

Materials

You must, of course, shop around for where you can buy materials at the right quality for the best price. You should try to buy direct from the manufacturer, if possible, as that is always cheapest but it may not be practical. As a start-up, your level of orders might be too small or the manufacturer may be outside the country so you can't see samples of his full range. Try at all costs to avoid buying from a retailer as you will then be paying the dearest possible price.

Equipment

Do you buy new or second hand equipment? You will end up buying what you can afford but it can be very worthwhile to shop around today for used equipment. Scan the classified columns of the newspapers and look out for auctions. You can often pick up used tools and equipment which are in good condition for less than half the price of new ones.

Premises

Finding premises is a key priority. Your options could include:

- working from home   • renting premises
- buying premises   • using mobile premises.

The best option depends very much on the type of business you plan to operate.

Working from home suits many people who are making small products or who are providing a service or consultancy. It's obviously the least expensive option but it has drawbacks. Do you really want customers calling to your home at all hours? Do you want to be so close to your business all the time? You must also, of course, consider if you will need planning permission and check if your house insurance policy has any clauses e.g. about storing certain materials, which might be relevant.

Renting premises is the option most people choose. Again, it depends on your business, but an attractive choice is to rent space from your Local Enterprise Agency. It offers a variety of sizes of units at reasonable rents on a licence basis – that means you don't have to sign a long lease and can get in and leave easily without too many legal requirements. The agency will also offer central services such as typing, telephone answering, photocopying and fax. You also have at hand the advice and guidance of the agency staff. Another choice is to rent premises from the private sector. This is what you'll probably do if you plan to open a shop or start a larger business. The private sector landlord will almost certainly want you to sign a lease. If so, take this very seriously. Once you sign, you are committed for the full term of the lease and can be compelled to pay rent even if your business stops trading. Get professional advice from a solicitor before signing any lease.

You may choose to buy premises but as this ties up a lot of capital, few start-up businesses take this route. You may decide that being mobile suits your business best – a van or other vehicle will allow you to go where the business is or you can set up your business at a market stall in a different area each day. There are fairly strict regulations about street trading so check with the local council before you start.

Whichever option you choose you must be sure that your choice of premises suits your business. Is it in the right location? Is it the right size? Does it offer all the services you need? Can you use it all the times you plan to use it?

Labour

In terms of resources, you may need labour, other than your own, to get the business going. Many start-ups solve this problem in the early stages by taking on a family member or close friend. Often this is quite successful but sometimes it is not. It can be difficult to ask family and friends to make a commitment over and above the level of wage you can afford and what do you do if your wife's brother is always late or your husband's best friend is just not cut out for the job? You will have to take a business decision but friendship or good family relationships can lose out.

It is best to draw up a job description for every job you have and then be sure you recruit the best person you can afford to fill that job. Start as you mean to go on and treat all workers alike. You will be very dependent on your workforce so it pays to treat them well. Be sure they are trained to do the job, be sure they have the right tools to do the job. Reward effort and penalise carelessness and laziness. There is a considerable amount of legislation now surrounding the employment of workers. Your local Training and Employment Agency office will help. They are also a very good source of potential workers and can advise you of all kinds of schemes on offer to make it easy for you to recruit and train your workforce – often at little cost to you.

Costs

Once you have decided what resources you need, it is then possible to start estimating your costs. You will need to cost very accurately: Material costs, including any waste; labour costs; overheads or operating costs; start-up costs.

Material costs

You can usually estimate material costs quite accurately by measuring the raw material needed to make a product but don't forget to allow for waste. For example, if you have to buy a full sheet of plywood but the bookcase only needs three quarters of the board and the remaining quarter is not really useful you need to charge the price of the full board to your bookcase. Other less noticeable examples of material costs include charging for packaging or for sundries like thread and buttons, which look like very small costs until you add them all up.

Labour costs

To work out your labour costs you need to know how long it takes to make a product. Then you need to know your wages and all other related costs like National Insurance, employees' insurance, holiday pay and so on. Divide your total wage costs by the number of hours you expect the employee to work (and remember, in a 40 hour week only 30 hours or so might actually be productive) and divide the number of hours into the total costs. This will give your hourly labour rate. Multiply this by the time it takes to make your product and you have your labour costs.

Operating Costs

Adding these two costs together gives you what is called your "direct" costs. If you take these away from your selling price you are left with your gross profit. You then need to calculate your overheads or operating expenses. These vary from business to business but will probably include: Rent, rates, electricity, advertising, insurance, telephone, postage, stationery, transport costs, audit fees, bank charges and interest, repairs and maintenance.

You will also have to make an allowance for depreciation. An easy way to think of this is as an allowance you set aside each year from the business to allow you to replace equipment or vehicles when they need replacing.

Will your business be viable?

When you have calculated all the costs it is possible to estimate if your business will be viable. Start with your sales forecast. Deduct your direct costs. Deduct your indirect costs. The balance is your net profit before any tax. If you included a wage for yourself in the direct costs then the profit is yours to do with as you wish. Be sure you've included all the money you've drawn from the business including your expenses. It's obviously prudent to keep as much of the profit as possible in the business, certainly in the early years.

Achieving sales or selling your services.

Without sales you don't have a business, so the first priority in business is to sell. Sales don't just happen – a number of factors have to come together: You must have the right product at the right price in the right place at the right time and you must promote that product to your customer. Putting this together can take a lot of effort – it is called your marketing plan and, if you don't bring all the ingredients together in a sensible way, you will find it difficult to achieve sales.

Product

Having the right product means making sure that you are offering a product which is of the right quality, the right design and the right colour. It may mean offering a range of shapes/sizes. In other words, it is giving the customer what he/she wants.

Price

The right price is what the market will stand, i.e. what people will actually pay for your product. If they will pay £5, why should you sell it for £4? Obviously you need to watch the price your competitors are charging but remember you don't always have to charge less. It's possible sometimes to charge more for what is essentially the same product and yet sell more. Why? Because people look at your total offering, not just your price, and if they think they're getting overall value for money, price may not be a deterrent. Whatever you charge, make sure it covers your costs and gives you a profit.

Place

The right place is deciding where and how it is easiest for your customer to buy from you. There are a number of options:

- direct – straight from your premises or by you calling at your customer's premises
- retail – in a shop or supermarket
- mail order – through the post or in a catalogue
- through agents or wholesalers

Choose the option or options which suits your business best. If you are making pastries it may be possible to sell them through shops and through hotels who buy them for their customers.

Legal framework for your business.

You have a choice of the legal form for your business.

SOLE TRADER – you are a self-employed person and submit an annual set of accounts to the Inland Revenue. You also pay National Insurance. You will usually pay Class 2 contributions but if your earnings are low you can apply for exemption. If your earnings exceed a certain limit you will also pay a percentage based on your profits. You do not need to register your business name but be careful you don't choose a name which is too close to someone else's name. If you use a trade name your stationery must also have your own name and so must your premises. You are personally liable for all debts incurred by the business.

PARTNERSHIP – very similar to sole trader except there are two or more people involved. The big difference is that all the partners are jointly and severally liable for all the debts. This means that if, for example, one partner disappears, and the other is liable for all, not half, the debts. It is essential to have a proper partnership agreement drawn up by a solicitor. Even if you and your partner(s) are very friendly, things can go wrong. The agreement will set out in writing all the matters of importance such as banking and cheque signing arrangements, roles of each partner, profit/loss sharing and so on. While you're certainly not planning to fail the reality is that failure may happen and so it is wise to draw up the agreement with failure in mind.

LIMITED COMPANY – a company is a separate legal entity, which is distinct from you, even if you are a director. A company must have at least two shareholders, a director and a company secretary. A company can sue and be sued and can borrow money. The money raised by the owners of the company to set it up is divided into shares and each shareholder receives shares in proportion to the amount of money invested. Profits or dividends are usually paid in proportion to the shares held.

Limited companies can offer some protection to the owners in that their liability to meet the company's debts is limited to the amount of their shares. However, it is normal practice now for banks to look for personal guarantees from the company's shareholders or directors if the company needs to borrow. This removes the limited liability protection of the company. Limited companies are strictly controlled by legislation. They must make an annual return to Companies House and submit annual accounts. If you plan to set up a limited company take professional advice.

The law and your business.

Business activities are controlled by a number of laws. If you are in any doubt consult your solicitor. Many of the departments mentioned below have free information guides which you should obtain.

Inland Revenue

You must tell the tax office you have started to trade and you must send in the annual accounts of your business. If you employ people, you will have to deduct tax from their earnings.

VAT

A successful business venture is soon likely to reach the point where its level of sales take it beyond the turnover at which VAT registration is required. Once registered, you must charge VAT on all taxable sales and claim VAT back on any taxable purchases you have made. You must make a quarterly return to the VAT office.

National Insurance

You must pay National Insurance contributions for yourself and any other employees.

Health and Safety

You must ensure the health and safety of your workforce and maintain a safe working environment. You may also need to ensure that your premises have a means of escape in the event of fire.

Employment Law

There is a wide range of legislation here including contracts of employment, equal opportunity, fair employment, union membership and more.

Insurance

You will need employers' liability insurance if you employ people and obviously any vehicles you have must be insured. You should also consider public liability, product liability, fixtures, fittings and stock cover, personal accident, sickness and so on. A reputable insurance broker will advise you. It is wise to get two or three quotes.

Working capital

The money you need to pay bills and wages before you receive payment for goods you have sold. To estimate this figure you will need to produce a cash flow forecast. This means estimating on a monthly basis when you expect to be paid for your goods. You must also estimate wages, materials and overheads. Take this total from your sales income and the balance, if it is in deficit, is the amount of money you need to keep the business going. This is usually financed by a bank overdraft. When you come to estimate your working capital, look at the picture over at least 12 months and identify your peak requirement for working capital. Then ask yourself – what would be the figure if, for example, sales didn't reach the amount we'd hoped for or if costs increased? Your working capital requirement would increase. That's why it can be prudent to ask for a little more money by way of overdraft. Whatever you do, do not ask for less than you will actually need. And of course, remember that more sales means more working capital, not less, so while it is good to grow the business, make sure you have the money in place to finance the growth.

There are basically four ways to raise money for your business: Invest yourself; borrow it; persuade others to invest; obtain grants aid.

Your own investment

This must come first as no-one will provide 100 per cent of the money you need. You must show your own commitment to the business.

Borrowing

Most borrowing is from banks but there are other sources such as credit unions, local enterprise agency loan funds, hire purchase companies and youth enterprise organisations. It's one thing to borrow money but quite another to pay it back. Before you borrow, check your business can afford the repayments. Shop around for the best deal on interest rates. You may be asked for security – what do you have that you are prepared to put up as security? If you won't do that, why should a bank lend to you?

Finally, it's wise to match borrowing to needs. For example, a car should last 3-4 years – finance it over that period. A rule of thumb is: short term finance for short-term assets, long term finance for long-term assets. In other words, finance debtors by way of a bank overdraft – money from debtors should come in quickly and a bank overdraft is usually reviewed annually. You should finance assets like cars or machinery or buildings over a period roughly equivalent to their lifespan. In other words, hire purchase a car over 2-3 years, mortgage a building over 15-25 years.

Investment from others

You may be able to persuade others to invest in your business. These may be family or friends, but could be a venture capital company. This is a company which specialises in investing money in businesses. Usually this will happen only in limited companies and investors will expect to receive shares for their investment. They will also usually want a return on that investment.

Grants

The main source of grant aid in UK for small businesses is through redevelopment and regeneration schemes. There are other grants for people who have been unemployed for more than six months; check with your local Chamber of Commerce and the DSS. The Prince's Youth Business Trust offers grants for the under 29s.

Controlling the finance

Once you've raised your capital, you'll need to set up a book-keeping system. It doesn't have to be complicated – a range of user friendly computer software is available for small businesses. Get advice from your accountant.

The business plan

You should now try to bring together in a business plan all the areas discussed in this advisory text. You will need this plan if you are approaching a bank or other funding agency but quite apart from that, it is a good exercise for you yourself to prepare a plan. It is a very useful tool which can help you control your business.

Buteyko method

Asthma- How to beat it, naturally
by Margaret Brooks

The Buteyko method allows the sufferer an effective drug free management of asthma, emphysema, allergies, migraine, chronic fatigue (ME) and many others. The Russian Ministry of Health officially approved the method after clinical trials in 1985, proving it an effective drug free treatment for bronchial asthma. In Australia, clinical trials in Brisbane claimed more than a 90 per cent success rate, providing positive results for asthmatics.

The method is taught by a qualified practitioner in classes of up to nine people, on a four-five session daily basis or over a weekend giving ten hours of tuition. A set of specific exercises are learned and refined. These are practised when you leave the course on a daily basis.

During the class you are taught how to unblock your nose, if you are a mouth breather, and other aspects are covered such as how to breathe through your nose while you are asleep and factors that increase your breathing, such as emotions, foods, the weather etc.

You are shown how to exercise correctly, how to manage colds and the flu – the most worrying time for anyone with asthma, emphysema or any other breathing related disorder. It is also important to look at the whole body and the support of the immune system is vital if you are to get completely well. After the course there is full follow-up support and a follow-up questionnaire is sent after six months.

The Buteyko method deals with the cause of the problem rather than just treating the symptoms and it takes patience and perseverance to change years of poor breathing. Like anything we learn, to be successful we need to apply ourselves diligently to what we are taught. Only then can we reap the rewards of our endeavours and live a healthy life.

Thousands of people have successfully been taught and are now experiencing control over their asthma without having to resort to harmful medication. In time, it is thought that the Buteyko method will be incorporated into mainstream orthodox medicine. Change sometimes can be painfully slow.

Dr. Buteyko made his discovery 47 years ago and it has taken all this time to get from Russia to the UK.

In Russia the method has been taught to millions of asthmatics and is also used by athletes to gain extra speed and stamina. It may sound too simplistic to say that if we were to breathe properly we would not have asthma, for this is the very thing that asthmatics can't do. Anyone who has asthma knows how difficult it is to keep the breathing under control when you are struggling to get your next breath. The harder we struggle, the tighter our chest seems to become. Could our body be trying to tell us something? Breathe less and our airways seem to relax. Could deep breathing too much, in fact, be harmful?

For all of our lives we have been told that we need to breathe deeply, so that we get plenty of oxygen into our lungs and to expel all of the harmful carbon dioxide. But the truth is there is no scientific evidence at all that deep breathing is beneficial to us. In fact there is lots of evidence to show that it is positively harmful. Carbon dioxide (CO_2) is as beneficial to our body as oxygen. Indeed without 6-6.5 per cent CO_2 in the lung alveoli, the gas exchange cannot function properly and, most importantly, CO_2 dilates the airways naturally.

Professor Konstantin Buteyko and others have understood the importance of CO_2 and its relationship to asthma. He discovered that only one in ten people breathe correctly. He noticed, whilst observing sick patients, that those who were sick breathed more than those who were healthy. He believes that some 200 diseases are linked to breathing. He maintains that the cause of asthma is over-breathing and that asthmatics 'hidden hyperventilate', over-breathing three or more times more than the body needs.

When this happens the body starts to develop defence and compensatory mechanisms such as asthma, a blocked nose and an increase in the production of mucous, histamine and cholesterol. This is in response to a fall in the level of carbon dioxide caused by over-breathing.

The function of our respiratory system is to maintain a correct ratio of oxygen to carbon dioxide as well as moving air in and out. We need to change our perception of asthma and understand how and why it occurs. Thinking of asthma as a disease is stopping us from understanding this message from our body.

Professor Buteyko devised a system to re-train the mechanism that regulates breathing and normalise the levels of carbon dioxide. The Buteyko Method teaches us how to raise CO_2 levels back to normal (6.5 per cent). At normal levels, asthma can't exist.

As the CO_2 starts to return to normal, asthma attacks become fewer and bronchodilators (blue inhalers) are therefore used less. When you return to a normal level of carbon dioxide and are able to maintain it, symptom free, then you can speak to your doctor about reducing and eventually stopping, your steroid prevented (brown inhalers).

The Buteyko method can be taught to anyone over the age of four to adults in their 80s and beyond.

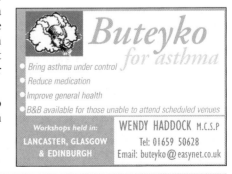

Cancer Care

Complementary Approaches to Cancer
By the team at New Approaches to Cancer

Cancer is probably as old as life itself. It has been found in fossils and in Egyptian mummies. Every human body contains about ten billion cells, controlled by what scientists call DNA (deoxyribonucleic acid). DNA is the raw material of life; it provides the computer programme for each cell in the body.

Sometimes, and no-one knows exactly why, the DNA fails to stop a cell dividing at the right time and it runs amok. About 100,000 of these malignant cells are formed in us each day and are usually destroyed by the natural immune system.

But if the immune system is weakened in any number of ways, cells invade the body tissue and prevent its proper healing function.

This is what we know as 'cancer' and it can occur in its several hundred forms, so there is unlikely ever to be one miracle cure or magic bullet.

It is probably true that most cancers can be avoided by a change of lifestyle; that it is the conditions we ourselves create which provide the soil on which it grows. There is a huge element of chance whether it will get out of hand in any one of us.

Human cancers in particular seem to thrive in a climate where the need to compete, removal of taboos, loss of religious belief, has become too much for us to handle. Stress such as divorce, guilt, fears, bereavement, redundancy etc. probably do not cause but they may help cancer develop later in life.

Of course cancer can be ugly, degrading and painful. Frequently it is none of these. So take heart.

The statistics may look bad, therefore turn the statistics on their head. One in four of us die from cancer – true. That means three out of four survive.

Everywhere, on buses, escalators and in supermarkets we pass people living with cancer. It is not always the relentless killer we dread. Hope is better for the optimist who banishes all negative thoughts and gets on with the business of living well.

The Holistic Approach

There is more understanding, more help, more hope for cancer patients today than ever before. Cancer is talked about, publicised; its conquerors and patients tell their stories on television and in the press. The old taboos have gone.

Public awareness of medical matters has put under the spotlight the rift between traditional methods and the increasingly popular holistic approach.

This sees the person as a multi-

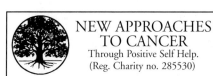

dimensional being, not a machine; the protection of health as a matter, not only for the body, but also the mind and spirit. Each depends upon the other and sickness occurs when that inter-relationship goes wrong. This is not a new idea. It was urged by the father of medicine, Hippocrates, 2,500 years ago!

The holistic practitioner believes that traditional medicine can be greatly enhanced by the knowledge of complementary therapies. Acupuncture, herbalism, homeopathy, reflexology and so on are not necessarily 'alternative'; they can be complementary to surgery, radio and chemotherapy.

There is no need for patients to abandon the family doctor when they decide to utilise complementary and natural medicines. The largest cancer hospitals use diet and meditation as an optional therapy for cancer patients.

Medical experts of all persuasions should pool their knowledge and encourage the patient to join the team and assume responsibility for his/her own well being.

Take control. It's your health. Your body. There is often a sense of confusion and isolation after a cancer diagnoses.

Sharing the burden not only eases the strain on physical and emotional levels, it also gives the family courage and hope to realise that there are so many ways they can learn to help themselves.

Cancer support groups are in the main cheerful and unself-pitying- there is laughter and honesty.

Groups vary in size and purpose. There are those run in private homes, rather like clubs, which offer counselling, practical help and the comfort of being with others coping with similar problems.

There are some with purpose-designed premises and a team of specialists working more like a medical centre. All try to liaise with local GPs and hospital consultants. Most offer classes in relaxation meditation and nutrition and advise on complementary therapies.

Access to complementary therapies is easy, with many hospitals and NHS practices offering aromatherapy, massage and healing to those who are ill, and complementary therapy centres are ever more common in our high streets.

There is help for those who need it all one has to do is ask!

MGN-3 arabinoxylan compound
By Andrew Paterson

I t has been well known for many years that large polysaccharide molecules can stimulate immune responses, in particular, a group of them called arabinoxylan compounds.

These particular polysaccharides have now been manufactured via a unique process in Japan, involving the enzymatic breakdown or 'predigestion' of rice bran, which greatly enhances this immunomodulatory function.

The resulting substance, known as MGN-3 arabinoxylan compound (the first three letters referring to the scientists that developed it) has been available as a food supplement in Japan and the United States for a few years now, and has recently arrived in Europe.

Although nobody knows exactly how it does it, MGN-3 arabinoxylan compound can stimulate a weak immune system more powerfully than any other agent, natural or unnatural. It does this by increasing the activity of white blood cells, especially the NK (Natural Killer) cells.

Comprising 15 per cent of the white blood cells, these Natural Killer cells form the backbone of the immune system with their ability to go through the body engulfing and destroying bacteria, viruses and infected or abnormal body cells (such as cancer cells). When the body is in a diseased state, the immune system becomes overloaded and the activity of these cells is compromised.

This is often compounded by medical treatment — such as chemotherapy in the case of cancer — which further depresses the immune system.

It is extremely important to both disease prevention and disease treatment, therefore, to stimulate the immune system and more specifically NK cell activity, as any boost in this activity can greatly increase the chance and speed of recovery.

This is why MGN-3 arabinoxylan compound has already attracted so much interest amongst doctors in Japan and the United States: it can not only stimulate NK cell activity, often by as much as 300 per cent, but does so without any toxicity or other adverse side effects.

It can also promote up to three times higher replenishment of the white blood cells, further increasing immune resilience.

Unlike most natural supplements, there has been substantial clinical research, including human trials, carried out on MGN-3 arabinoxylan compounds, the results of which have been published in peer-reviewed medical journals.

This research has taken place at UCLA/DREW University in the United States and various universities and medical research institutions in Japan

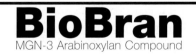

Biobran
MGN-3 Arabinoxylan Compound

THE REALLY HEALTHY COMPANY
www.healthy.co.uk
Tel: 020 8480 1000

including Chiba University, Kobe Women's College, Jichi Medical School, Nipon University, Kyushu University, Nagoya University, Kyoto University, Toyama Medical University and Kawasaki Medical University.

The main researcher on MGN-3 has and continues to be Dr. Mamdooh Ghoneum, a professor at the Department of Immunology at Drew University of Medicine and Science in the United States.

Dr. Ghoneum, now an internationally recognised authority on cancer immune therapy, received his Ph.D. at the University of Tokyo in radio-immunology and did his post-doctoral work at UCLA in immunology.

Over the last 20 years he has been researching various substances that can enhance the immune system, and says that "MGN-3 is the most powerful immune complex I have ever tested!" So impressed was he with the results that he has now devoted his entire research efforts to this compound.

Research papers on MGN-3 arabinoxylan compound have been published in conjunction with a variety of diseases ranging from cancer and diabetes to viral infections such as AIDS and hepatitis B & C.

However, it is clear that there is a need for more trials (especially double blind trials) to scientifically pinpoint exactly how effective MGN-3 arabinoxylan compound is in increasing actual survival statistics for the various disease states mentioned.

In the meantime, this food supplement is a promising addition to the arsenal of 21st century doctors.

Case history

SUBJECT: Male, aged 48

Clinical Record and Treatment: In early March 1996, the patient felt unusual languidness and was diagnosed with chronic hepatitis (non-viral) and slight diabetes.

After rest and an intravenous injection for Major Minofargen C, his liver function came to a temporary lull and he left the clinic after one month. Thereafter, the patient experienced periodic deterioration in his liver functions despite continuing intravenous treatment for Major Minofargen C, and suffered from chronic hepatitis until the beginning of March 1997. The patient then started taking 3g of MGN-3 per day (1g/dose) and his level of liver function increased to nearly the same level as at the beginning of therapy 12 days earlier. The level gradually decreased, reaching the lowest value after one month. The patient's GOT and GPT levels returned to normal one month later. Presently, the patient's liver function has returned to normal, and the patient is experiencing no other health-related problems.

Changes due to MGN-3: The patient's energy level increased after MGN-3 administration, and his unusual fatigue, especially in the afternoon, gradually abated. The patient was able to sleep and wake normally, had a good appetite and looked healthy.

Evaluation: As indicated, GOT and GPT levels temporarily increased after the administration of MGN-3, before steadily decreasing and returning to normal. During MGN-3 administration, no special treatments were performed; therefore, it is possible to conclude that these changes were due to MGN-3. These results suggest that MGN-3 protected the patient's liver and its immunopotentiation function was effective.

Children & Baby

Parenting: a natural start

There are natural alternatives and choices for all parents. From the first decision to attempt conception, through pregnancy, post natal care and childhood, there are many exciting and rewarding therapies, treatments, natural products and practices that can be used.

We can only summarise some of the choices here, and each parent will need to contact an individual practitioner or manufacturer to find out more about those therapies or products that seem most suitable. There are so many ways in which we can give our children a natural start in life.

Pre Conceptual Care

Effectual parenting can start well before conception. A potential mother to be can naturally take care of herself to give her child the best possible start. This care will ideally include diet, stress management and general health care.

In particular it is important to ensure a high intake of Folic Acid for at least three months before conception. The expectant mother needs established stores of Folic Acid in the body because as soon as conception occurs these stores will be drawn upon to assist with the formation of the new child. Folic Acid deficiency has been linked to Neural Tube Defects, such as Spina Bifida. Pharmacists and Health Stores stock Folic Acid supplements, the recommended dosage is generally four hundred micrograms a day, but it is always wise to check with a health practitioner. Effective natural sources of Folic Acid include some breakfast cereals, Brussels sprouts, yeast extract, granary bread, broccoli, spinach, kale, spring greens, green beans, or cooked black eyed beans. There are also moderate amounts of Folate in oranges and orange juice, potatoes, cauliflower, peas, natural yoghurt, bread, eggs, brown rice, wholewheat pasta, cooked Soya beans, chick peas and parsnips. If these

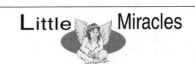

foods are organically produced so much the better, as this will minimise the intake of any toxins. Some complementary therapies can be useful at this time too. Acupuncture is used to promote fertility, by stimulating the flow of chi around the female reproductive organs. Acupuncture should not be undertaken during the first two days of menstruation; your practitioner will advise.

The male parent to be can also supplement his diet to aid conception. Zinc promotes mobility in sperm; it makes them better swimmers! Healthier sperm will mean an increased chance of conception. Other therapies such as Aromatherapy are used in pre-conceptual care, but it is important to take full advice as you may already have become pregnant and some oils can be detrimental in early pregnancy.

Ante-Natal Care

Once pregnancy has begun there are many natural treatments that can help make the time more enjoyable for both mother and child. The main problem in early pregnancy is nausea or sickness. This is down to the massive hormonal changes taking place in the mother's body. Various alternative therapies can help. Acupuncture, Shiatsu and Acupressure are safe to use at this stage of pregnancy, provided your practitioner knows you are pregnant. At the same time the mother can gain relief from backache, tiredness, constipation, varicosities, carpal tunnel syndrome and heartburn. There are natural approaches to reducing nausea, such as eating ginger.

Hypnotherapy has been used for mothers who have had difficulty in feeling the movements of her unborn child. It can help the mother to become in tune with her baby, thus adding to the well-being of both. Hypnotherapy can also be used both before and after the birth, particularly to aid relaxation. Stress management is important during pregnancy, especially as effective management can avoid high blood pressure, which can otherwise lead to complications such as pre-eclampsia.

Of course there are many ways of managing stress, from visiting a practitioner to burning the correct Aromatherapy oils. Yoga and relaxation classes learnt now during pregnancy will also give breathing and other techniques for use during and after childbirth. There are also midwives who specialise in counselling. They will focus on the anxieties, stress and the psychological difficulties associated with pregnancy.

The pregnant woman is undergoing many changes and the healing power within is especially active during pregnancy. This is therefore an ideal time to treat the mother to be, as well as the baby to be, whether homoeopathically, through Reiki, or with other natural healing systems. There are many natural products for use during pregnancy too. For instance, ice cold Aloe Vera gel is good for relaxing tired legs, while

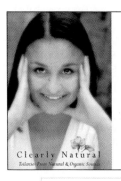

other creams may include cucumber or camomile. These natural soothing products are good at all times, but especially when the body is bearing extra weight. Natural forms of low impact exercise are also ideal during pregnancy. Aquasize and swimming are great for relieving the problems of weight carrying while keeping the body oxygenated, giving your baby a better blood supply and keeping her or him active too. Walking and cycling can also be effective in this way, if care is used.

Nearer the time of birth, Acupuncture can be used to turn a breach baby to cephalic presentation, so that the head is down, ready for a natural delivery. It can also stimulate the body into labour and is used to varying degrees as part of the care offered by the HHS in some areas, as well in private midwifery practice. If induction of labour is necessary, then Acupuncture can be less invasive and traumatic for both mother and baby than other medical intervention.

Childbirth

Before this point the mother will have made her choice of place of birth and the type of birth she prefers. If, after taking appropriate advice, a water birth is wanted then a birthing pool can be hired. For other deliveries birthing chairs, birthing stools and other equipment can all be hired, whether for home or hospital use.

A natural birth is often regarded as one undertaken without the aid of artificial pain relief. Methods of natural pain relief and aids to relaxation applicable include Reflexology, Acupuncture, Shiatsu, and various forms of Massage, as well as yoga. Immersion in water can also alleviate pain, even if full water birth is not the aim.

Transcutaneous Nerve Stimulation (TNS) may also be considered as natural pain relief, as by stimulating the body's endorphins, it can avoid the need for pharmaceutical alternatives. Some of these methods will work better for some people than others, but all are proven to be effective.

Tea Tree Oil is used as a natural antiseptic. During labour many women like to have this in the water they may be using as analgesia (pain relief). Burning tea tree oil can also be beneficial, but is not advised in hospitals because of the proximity of piped oxygen supplies creating a fire hazard. At a home birth the burning of oils may be more practical. Otherwise, drops of Tea Tree oil can be added to a paper tissue and inhaled during labour. Other oils may be recommended by a practitioner. Clary Sage may be used to help stimulate uterine contractions in the latter stages of pregnancy and during childbirth. Lavender and Rose are often used as natural aids to relaxation. Again all of these benefits will be for both mother and baby.

Homoeopathic advice may also be taken prior to labour. Arnica may be recommended as a way of reducing bruising and trauma during the birth. Homoeopathic remedies have no side effects for mother or baby and you cannot become addicted to them. This is because only a minute amount of the active ingredient is used. Reflexology can be used to aid a smooth, uncomplicated delivery. As a pleasant and relaxing therapy it helps the body to rebalance and rejuvenate. Reflexology encourages the body's own healing processes, by improving circulation, energy flow and muscle tone, whilst reducing tension and stress.

Manipulation, such as chiropractic or osteopathy, is useful before and after childbirth, as it is during this time that ligaments become naturally relaxed Manipulation is particularly useful for back and symphysis pubis pain, as well as for re-adjusting pelvic position.

Post-Natal Care

After the child has been born the parents can gain benefits from natural products and therapies for both themselves and the newborn. Perhaps the most exciting and widely used treatment for new babies, particularly if birth has been traumatic, is Cranio-Sacral Therapy. The infant skull allows small amounts of movement, helping the baby's head adapt to the pressures of leaving the mother's body. When birth is either unusually rapid or slow, the baby's head may not have recovered fully from this natural distortion. Problems as diverse as colic, feeding difficulties and disturbed sleeping patterns can all be linked to this.

Gentle manipulation and treatment of babies using Cranio-Sacral Therapy is accepted as an excellent way of realigning the infant's skull so that the bones can take their natural, correct shape. Some hospitals now offer Cranio-Sacral care as part of post natal care, either through visiting therapists or midwives who have chosen to train in the therapy. Cranio-Sacral Therapy can be used from the first week after birth, but is also effective for relieving problems in later childhood, such as hyperactivity.

Acupuncture is used for breastfeeding problems, while Acupressure is often used on babies, with the Acupuncturist applying fingers rather than needles. Kinesiology can be used to treat childhood disorders such as asthma, eczema, recurrent ear nose and throat infections, food intolerances, sleep pattern disorders and behavioural problems in infancy and childhood, as well as dyslexia.

Baby massage is another natural tool for optimum, natural child care. This can be learnt ante-natally by parents so that massage can be given at home whenever appropriate. Baby massage encourages positive touch, this is especially important if the baby was born early, as bonding with the mother is enhanced in this way. Massage can also help with more immediately evident problems, such as colic. Aromatherapy massage is especially good for baby's relaxation, and for treating colds and snuffles. Products such as oil burners that attach to light bulbs give more lasting benefits.

Complementary medicine has much to offer parent and child. Various therapies will be effective in dealing with childhood disorders, as well as creating the best possible, natural surroundings for child development. If you are concerned about chemical sensitivities then decorating and furnishing your home is a responsible task. Chemical free paints, furniture, fabrics, flooring and bedding may be considered particularly important. The added responsibility of parenthood may also provoke you to take a new look at other facilities in your home. Is your water effectively filtered? Is your heating system creating the minimum amount of air disturbance in the home?

Organic and cotton nappies are more than just an old-fashioned alternative no longer applicable in the modern time-starved world of parenthood. A vast proportion of modern waste is created by so-called disposable nappies, which actually take an extremely long time to decompose. This suggests that cotton nappies are a better ecological choice. They may also be better for your child. Cotton nappies reduce the incidence of nappy rash and do not include bleaching and other chemical agents. Cotton nappies are natural, and much kinder to your child's skin.

Natural choices are never ending for the parent: organic food, natural wood toys – from an environmentally sustainable source – even that the placement of savings for the child is ethically sound. The great news is that the opportunities, therapies and products are there to give children the natural start they all deserve.

Chinese Herbal Medicine

By Robert L. White & Professor Yilan Shen

When our bodies are in full balance (yin and yang) we are healthy but when that balance goes out of harmony (either way) we become ill. Every day our bodies generate billions of new cells mainly when we relax and sleep. This regeneration is supplied by what we eat, drink or breathe in.

So when we are ill something in this process is not working properly, either because of something lacking in our diet or a process not working correctly as when cells grow abnormally and become cancerous. In the Traditional Chinese view our bodies consist of five organ systems (Zang-Fu) which are all interconnected and work by stimulating or suppressing each other. When we are healthy these systems are in balance. The two sides of the balance are well known as yin and yang. When the balance is disturbed, either by physical injury or overactivity of a system or underactivity of another, then we become ill. At other times the balance will be naturally altered, such as during pregnancy.

Any treatment must restore that balance to allow the patient to become healthy again. The five elements (Wu Xing) are characterised by gold/metal, wood, water, fire and earth and the comparative organ systems are: GOLD – lung and large intestine; WOOD – liver and gall bladder; WATER – kidney and bladder; FIRE – heart and small intestine; EARTH – spleen and stomach.

These are all interlinked by a series of channels called meridians and collaterals. During diagnosis these links and their activity are tested by taking the 28 pulse readings that can find blockages or overactivity. Further tests are made by examination of the eyes (where colour alteration and pressure is noticeable) and the tongue, which is very reactive to the health state.

All herbal medicines or pharmaceuticals supply the missing elements either directly or by stimulating an organ into action or suppression. Pharmaceuticals are recognised as stronger but with more side effects. A side effect is described as the required curative effect working in another or wrong place. Herbal medicine is more natural and gentle and closer to our normal foods so is more easily ingested and digested. Acupuncture by comparison uses only the stimulus of the bodies own system of communication and no drug or herbal stimulus therefore no side effects. Because it can have such a direct effect on the nervous system it is particularly effective in illness involving pain by suppressing the pain and letting the body relax and therefore repair itself. It is also good for stopping the signals of craving such as hunger or the desire to smoke.

Relaxing and stress removal can be very effective for skin diseases or asthma. Stimulating the circulation can be another way of curing illness. Stimulating the phlegm system is the way the body clears out toxins, viruses and unwanted elements. Most people do not realise that this natural waste disposal system runs right throughout the body from the tips of the toes to the hairs on the skin. It is the knowledge of the links through the body, the meridians and the acupuncture points that tell of the expertise of the doctor. Herbal medicine, acupuncture and moxibustion are the three medical fields of Traditional Chinese Medicine taught by the State Administration of Traditional Chinese Medicine (TCM) in China and are used to treat illness by the most natural method possible. Because acupuncture and moxibustion are drug-free practices they have many uses not available to any other branches of medicine.

Today throughout the world more people rely on herbal medicine than any other medical system. All the member doctors of the Society of Chinese Medical Practitioners in UK have at least ten years experience in Chinese hospitals and are expert in finding the best treatment. The average clinic will use herbal remedies in 74 per cent of cases, acupuncture in 15 per cent of cases, and a mix of acupuncture and herbs in seven per cent. The remainder, some four per cent, will be treated by moxibustion or creams and wash liquids and shampoos.

Herbal medicine has been developed over 3,000 years of clinical experience to find natural organic medical products that provide the necessary elements our bodies need to provide energy (Qi). This vast databank of plant material and their effects form the basis of all herbal remedies. A prescription will include the main agent or principal herb and perhaps three or four associate herbs to activate the cure. There can also be an adjuvant herb that will reinforce the principal herb's effect or moderate its toxicity and messenger herbs that activate the reaction to a particular organ or area of the body.

Research presented to the Royal Pharmaceutical Society conference on Traditional Chinese Medicine showed that all these elements were necessary for the best effect and that trying to limit remedies to just one or two active ingredients only reduces effectiveness. This is why modern pharmaceuticals have to be much stronger and therefore more toxic. Traditional Chinese Medicine was first described in the Yellow Emperor's Canon of Internal Medicine (a book of two parts, 'Simple Questions' and 'Miraculous Pivot') which records discussions between the Yellow Emperor (2696-2598BC) and his minister Qi Bo. Miraculous Pivot is so detailed that it is known as the 'Classic of Acupuncture and Moxibustion'.

Moxibustion is a heat treatment that uses a rolled up Moxa herb stick rather like a cigar. The Moxa herb is Mugwort or Artemesia vulgaris. When lit it burns slowly producing heat treatment. Modern research has now identified 409 acupuncture points, of which 361 are on the 14 Meridians plus an extra 48 points. As modern science knows the signals stimulating or suppressing the various parts of the body are electro-chemical messages. By pressing on these identified points it is possible to either stimulate or suppress those messages. Simple external pressure is called acupressure. Actually touching the point with a very fine needle is called acupuncture. The effect can be further enhanced by vibrating the needle or applying a small electric current. An alternative is to apply heat either externally with the moxibustion stick (similar to acupressure) or internally through the needle, which is why acupuncture and moxibustion are usually taken together.

Finally, there is the patient history, diet and statements of sensation such as pain, nausea, dizziness, grief and depression to be assessed. The doctor's ability to interpret this diagnostic material is based on thousands of years of carefully recorded case histories giving symptoms and remedies which act as a guide to diagnosis.

CHINESE HERBAL MEDICINE

Mr Thierry March BSC. MSC. MNIMH. MRCHM Registered Western And Chinese Medical Herbalist. Brabant House, Portsmouth Rd, Thames Ditton, Surrey. 0208 3987592. Lifestyle Natural Health, Hershorn Centre, Walton, Surrey. 01932254624.
www.herbalist-thierrymarch.co.uk
01372 811605

Chiropractic
By The British Chiropractic Association

Chiropractic is a profession that specialises in the diagnosis and treatment of conditions which are due to mechanical dysfunction of the joints and their effects on the nervous system.

Chiropractors use their hands to adjust the joints of the spine and extremities where signs of restriction in movement are found, improving mobility and relieving pain. The body's own healing processes will then be able to get on with the task of improving health. This treatment is known as 'adjustment' or 'manipulation'.

Poor, inadequate or incorrect function in the spine can cause irritation of the nerves that control our posture and movement. This spinal nerve stress (which may be caused by factors such as accident, poor diet, lack of exercise, poor posture and anxiety) can lead to the symptoms of discomfort, pain and even disease which are a warning that your body is not functioning properly.

By manipulating joints, chiropractors stimulate the joint movement receptors – your body's position sensors, which provide feedback to the brain on where the joint is in space. This stimulation can affect the way your nervous system works. Depending on where the nerve irritation has occurred in your spine, your symptoms may include headache or migraine, neck pain, back pain, chest or abdominal pain, shoulder, arm, wrist and hand problems, leg, knee, ankle and foot problems.

This is because the irritation of the nerve in one area can sometimes lead to pain (known as 'referred' pain) in other parts of the body. Painful symptoms are a warning sign that should not be ignored. Your chiropractor is trained to diagnose the cause and, if indicated, treat using manipulation. Chiropractors do not prescribe drugs or use surgical procedures. A chiropractor will begin a first consultation by taking a full case history. Then standard orthopaedic and neurological tests will be given and the movement of the spine and joints will be checked.

If a chiropractor identifies an underlying condition for which other treatment is appropriate, the client will be referred to a GP or other specialist without delay. Chiropractic can, however, be helpful in providing additional relief, even for conditions such as these. As well as using manipulation, a chiropractor may use ice or heat treatment, as well as other techniques, having first explained exactly how they

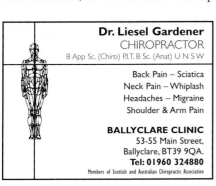
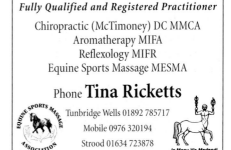

work. Chiropractic treatment is suitable for everyone, including newborn babies, the elderly, pregnant women and sports enthusiasts. A chiropractor will also help to maintain health, and keep the body working as it should, by offering exercise and lifestyle advice to follow after recovery from a specific problem.

Case history

HISTORY: A young lady complains of neck discomfort and stiffness, after being in a recent car accident.

FINDINGS: Painful and restricted movement of head and neck. Neck and upper back muscles very tight and tender to the touch. Pain experienced neck and arm with light pressure applied to the top of head, exacerbated when leaning head to the side and compressed. Reflexes sluggish on the left and none found on the right. Dizziness and nausea experienced on frequent movement of head. Neck X-rays reveal a total loss of normal neck curvature, but there are no signs of fracture, degeneration or other pathology. This is a typical X-ray finding associated with a whiplash injury. It is known as a 'soft tissue injury' because there is no fracture of the spinal bones, only the softer tissues of the spine such as ligaments, discs and muscles are damaged.

ASSESSMENT: These are typical findings for a patient involved in a rear-impact collision. She has suffered a condition known as a 'Cervical Acceleration-Deceleration' or 'CAD' injury. In lay terms,whiplash.

TREATMENT: Early treatment is vital, but it is not enough to just receive any form of care. A successful resolution to a CAD injury requires the right kind of treatment. More than anywhere else, this is the realm where a doctor of chiropractic that specialises in personal injuries is preferable to all other forms of medicine without question. According to a study by the British Medical Journal, whiplash or cervical strain patients were treated with various common forms of medical care. They found that patients treated by chiropractors fared much better than others in the study.

Colloidal Silver

By Vida Butcher

An antibiotic that can give hope in this new Millennium, yet has been known since ancient times, is making a come back. With the rise of the M.R. 'Superbug' in hospitals and the allergic reactions experienced by thousands to the antibiotics prescribed in the doctor's surgeries, we must look to a natural alternative.

Colloidal Silver, used by the early Egyptians, Greeks and Romans, is regaining the attention of the medical profession. In times past, silver utensils and drinking goblets were everyday items for the privileged, who also often put a silver coin in milk to stop it souring. Colloidal silver has many distinct advantages over antibiotics. Illness-causing organisms do not seem to build up a resistance to Colloidal Silver in the way that they do to pharmaceutical antibiotics, which are becoming less effective as resistance grows.

An ordinary antibiotic kills perhaps a half dozen different disease organisms, but Colloidal Silver is known to be successful against more than 650 illness-causing micro-organisms. Biomedical research has shown that no known disease-causing organism; bacterial virus or fungus can live for more than a few minutes in the presence of even minute traces of silver. It is rapidly fatal to parasites without being toxic on its host, and is quite stable. Thus Colloidal Silver is safe for humans, including children, the elderly, animals, reptiles, plants and all multi-celled living matter.

Colloidal Silver is manufactured to the highest quality; the finest is comprised solely of 99.9 per cent pure micro-fine silver suspended in demineralised water.

It can be gargled, dropped into the eyes, used vaginally and anally as well as atomised and inhaled into the nose and lungs. Taken orally, the silver solution is absorbed from the mouth into the bloodstream, then transported quickly to the body cells. Swishing the solution under the tongue briefly before swallowing ensures fast absorption. It is impossible for single-cell germs to mutate into silver-resistant forms, as happens with antibiotics, and Colloidal Silver cannot interact with other medicines being taken. It is a truly safe, natural remedy for many of humanities ills.

Benefits personally experienced include curing of mouth ulcers, cold sores, sore throats, eye problems, ear infections, heat rashes, water infections, thrush, colds and 'flu' symptoms. It is also useful in dealing with cuts, bruises and sores.

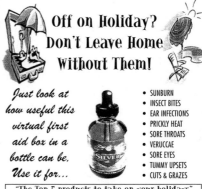

Colonic Hydrotherapy

By Dr. Milo Siewert

The colon, or large intestine, is an important part of the digestive system: some five feet in length and 2.5 inches in diameter, situated at the end of the alimentary canal, it completes the digestive process and handles food waste and much other bodily waste.

It is normally populated by billions of friendly bacteria which assist in detoxifying waste, synthesise certain vitamins and help us guard against infection. These same bacteria make up 70 per cent of the dry weight of our faecal waste.

The colon structure is of smooth muscle and is broadly divided into three segments: the caecum and ascending colon into which food waste enters in a fluid state through the ileo-caecum valve, the transverse colon where water, minerals and vitamins are re-absorbed and the descending colon where mucous is secreted to coat the faeces prior to defecation through the rectum and anus.

In health, bowel transit time from eating to defecation is 24 hours or less and the bowel movement is at least once daily.

In disease, poor digestion, yeast overgrowth, spastic colon, irritable bowel syndrome, chronic constipation and diarrhoea are usually accompanied by auto-intoxication, literally 'self-poisoning' – the re-absorption of soluble wastes into the bloodstream- which places a heavy burden on the other eliminative organs of the body, the kidneys, the skin and the lungs.

Chronic constipation can lead to further direct complications: diverticulitis, haemorrhoids, fissures, atonicity, spasticity, prolapse, colitis, and even bowel cancer as well as chronic toxic conditions in the rest of the body, like the skin (e.g. acne and eczema), the cardio-vascular system, the nervous system and the liver.

Correct function of the colon is a necessity for health, for truly 'disease can begin in the colon'. It has been said that colon malfunction can lead to 80 per cent of all diseased states.

What is Colonic Hydrotherapy?

Colonic Hydrotherapy is an internal bath that helps cleanse the colon of poisons, gas, accumulated faecal matter and mucous deposits. Such techniques were first recorded in 1500BC, and have been used in traditional and naturopathic medicine since that time. Using sterilised equipment, filtered water is gently introduced into the rectum, which progressively softens and expels faecal matter and compacted deposits.

Why Colonic Hydrotherapy?

Conducted by a trained therapist, filtered water at a carefully regulated temperature is introduced under gentle gravitational pressure through the rectum into the colon. With special massage techniques, the water begins to soften and cleanse the colon of faecal matter and old deposits, which are piped away with the wastewater.

The therapist works progressively round the structure of the colon allowing water alternatively to flow in and release. The whole process takes about 30 minutes.

Herbal preparations may be used for certain conditions, and regular colon implants of Lactobacillus acidophilus are given to assure normalisation of bowel fibre. The modesty of the patient is preserved to the utmost during the process.

Is any preparation required?

No special measures are necessary prior to colonic hydrotherapy, although results may be more rapidly achieved by following a colon cleansing programme

Is it safe?

Yes, equipment is disposable or sterilised using hospital approved sterilisation solutions, which kill all prevalent bacteria, viruses and fungi in minutes. Countless thousands of colonics have been given safely, the water pressure is very low, so there is no danger of bowel perforation and the water is pre-filtered. Unlike regular uses of laxatives, colonic hydrotherapy is not habit forming and in fact improves colon muscle tone.

And the results?

The Colonic International Association maintains high standards of qualification for its registered therapists. Most people quickly experience improved mental clarity after colonic irrigation. With their toxic load diminished and elimination improved, a greater feeling of well-being and lightness is felt. Obvious relief from bloating and constipation, toxic headaches, painful haemorrhoids and skin problems. In the longer term, bowel disease risk is also diminished and nutrients are better absorbed leading to improved all round health.

Who can benefit from colonics?

Essentially anyone with a condition aggravated or caused totally or in part by autotoxity, and where the resulting improved elimination aids healing.

Most diets include mucous forming foods like eggs, sugar, flour and tofu and even those people on relatively good diets and who have regular bowel movements have old hardened accumulations of mucoid deposits which hinder proper elimination and need periodic cleansing.

How many treatments?

Depending upon the condition being treated, the individual and the initial results, anything between six and twelve treatments may be recommended spread over one or two months.

Deposits built up over a lifetime cannot be shifted in one or two irrigations only.

Following the course, it is a good idea to have a treatment every six months to maintain inner cleanliness and good elimination.

Colour Puncture

By Angelika Hochadel

The correct application of colour puncture can overcome blockages and treat chronic complaints as well as acute condition. An essential advantage of this gentle method is that it combines well with any other treatment and that it can be used at home or during journeys in a simplified form with therapeutic instructions.

It is particularly suitable for treating children as it is free of side effects or pain. The colour therapy is ideal for supporting well-being and can be used as a preventive treatment to stabilise and stay healthy.

Colour is the primary source of life and health. It is a 'language' which our cells understand and through which they can communicate with each other.

Rudolf Steiner and Dinshah Ghadiali attribute great importance to colours. They claim that every disease originates from either the lack or the surplus of colour in the body. A balancing of this colour discrepancy would equal healing.

The more modern colour therapy is closely linked with the names of Finsen (who received the Nobel Prize for his work on the therapy with light and colour in 1903) and Rollier. Both achieved, by work, the basis for today's medical colour light therapy, which was generally limited to the known red and blue light treatments until 20 years ago.

In 1978, Peter Mandel began to transfer the light therapy onto the Chinese meridian system in order to find out whether acupuncture points are suitable for colour treatment.

Latest discoveries in biophysics lead to the conclusion that the complete cell metabolism and the communication between cells and groups of cells would simply be unthinkable without light. Colours – as pure vibrations – represent nothing but the various frequencies of visible light. These colour vibrations cause directly as well as indirectly the most different reactions in the body. Their effect is indisputable. But it depends on the choice of medium, through which we 'receive' the colours how they affect us.

Within colour puncture, the medium is the skin which, according to latest research, is able to take in light and colour impulses, just like the eyes. On the surface of the skin we find areas and points which have a higher receptivity. Many of these consist of acupuncture points and reflex zones known for their special relationship to colours and their ability to conduct impulses to the inside of the body.

It was Peter Mandel's task to investigate the colour receptivity of all acupuncture points and skin segments. For many years, every single point and zone has been exposed to various, exactly defined colour vibrations in order to test and determine the resonance attitude between colours, zones and the respective organs, body segments and layers of consciousness systematically.

This resulted in superior zones, segments and points, which are called somatologies or reflex fields. These reflex fields are in hierarchical order, i.e. from coarse to the subtle superior emotional/mental sectors. The combination of points and zones and a specific choice of therapy colours have a balancing, regulating effect through the light-conducting systems of the body with ultimate benefits for the area of the complaint.

Did you know?

Colours contain the energy of the Sun made visible on different wavelengths and, together with music and fragrance, are the quickest means nature has of getting into contact with the subconscious. Light and Colours have an effect on the total energetic system of the body. Colours communicate directly with the cells and have an effect on the endocrine system and the energetic structure of the brain.

COLOUR PUNCTURE

COLOURPUNCTURE, COLOUR Therapy, Dr Jacob Liberman's Therapy with Light and Colour and Reiki. Diploma Colour Therapist, Spectral Receptivity Practitioner Margit Wyllie MIAC, Smithy Croft, Clachan, Tarbert, Argyll PA29 6XL. call 01880 740640

JENNY STIFFLE (ITEC DIP., MIFA) – Treating all physical, mental & emotional problems with COLOURPUNCTURE, Aromatherapy, Indian Head Massage, Manual Lymph Drainage, Reiki Healing. Practicing in Surrey. Office 'On-Site' treatments available. Tel 020 8643 2949, (fax/e-mail available).

COLOUR PUNCTURE

COLOUR HEALS. Colour flows along channels in your body, carrying information for repairing the cells. Quartz is the conductor light and is the source. For more information or to make an appointment please call Velvet on 0370 846134. (Wentworth Surrey) Also beautiful Crystal Healing.

MR R WILLIS, T.F.H. Practice at Fareham and Waterlooville, Hampshire. Colour Puncture, Acupuncture (Ac.Cert.China), Allergy Testing, Shiatsu, Kinesiology. For more information please call: 01329 317065.

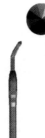

"Better to hunt in fields, for health unbought,
Than fee the doctor for a nauseous draught.
The wise, for cure, on exercise depend;
God never made his work for man to mend"
JOHN DRYDEN

Colour Therapy

By Michael Grevis

How can colour benefit health? The psychological effects of colours in our built environments are quite marked. Colour needs to be understood to be applied in a way which supports activity or rest, agitation or calm.

The colour language is universal and rooted in our biology. Red stimulates the sympathetic nervous system which raises our readiness for action. Blue simulates the complementary system, the parasympathetic, which lowers blood pressure and induces calm. Other colours invoke various degrees of these extremes of action. Colour is understood by the unconscious mind whether the stimulus is applied directly to the skin or through the eyes. In this way, bodily response patterns can be shifted and harmony can be restored by the judicious use of coloured light in therapy.

What colour therapy systems are there?

Treatment lamps are the standard traditional method. In the influential method of Theo Gimbel (England) colour is always accompanied by a lesser amount of its complementary, and appropriate shapes are built into the masks of the stained glass filters (broad bandwidth).

Colour may also be applied by the use of gels, coloured silks, solarised water and crystals, or applied mentally through healing hands and visualisations. There is now a

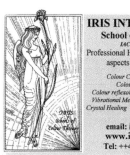
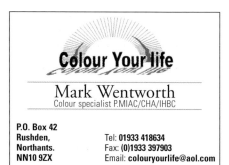
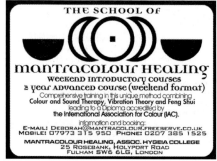

treatment lamp which uses monochromatic, dichroic filters and can be programmed to radiate any parts of the body which the therapist deems necessary.

Since the earliest known civilisations, colour has been used to communicate aesthetic ideas. The use of colour in the monumental works of Egypt and then Greece was extended into the Christian iconography of early oil painting where colour was used as a rich symbolism in its own right. Medieval stained glass made a huge impact on worshippers of that time because vivid colour speaks to our intuitive and feeling capacities.

Nature has evolved some extraordinary feats of colour communication. Colour perception is widespread in animals and insects, and human perception uses cortical processes based on complementary colours. Nature seems to have understood a great deal more about light and colour than human beings did before the modern scientific age. Butterflies and birds arrayed themselves in spectral colours made by interference from microscopic diffraction gratings in their cells. Insects and flowers evolved to share the same colour and form language. Deep marine creatures often make their own light.

What can light do for our health?

In northern climes, winter often brings the blues. A simple and proven remedy is the use of powerful light. Seasonal Affective Disorder is readily cured by sitting in front of bright light for about half an hour twice a day. The effect is brought about by activation of the pineal gland in the brain which modulates the production of melatonin and serotonin – the molecules responsible for sleeping and waking.

Until the 1960s, babies born prematurely suffered a life-threatening condition of jaundice, which may have necessitated a blood transfusion. Now, all that is required is exposure to light. This cure results from the chemical breakdown of bilirubin by light. Dyslexia sufferers are now enabled to read comfortably with tinted glasses or overlays; black and white is often too harsh for them to see clearly.

Another recent use of light therapy involves shining light onto a non-visual part of the retina to prevent sleepiness over a period of 48 hours. The use of strobed light in a sleeper's eyes has been found to stop snoring.

Is ultraviolet dangerous?

It is important to note that there are three divisions of UV light: A,B and C. It is UVC which is the most dangerous radiation. It is almost entirely filtered out by the ozone layer of the atmosphere, when that is intact. UVB is useful for vitamin D production but it is not good to get too much exposure. UVA results in skin tanning but fair-skinned people need to protect their skin from over-exposure. The healthful benefits of sunlight are usually thought, in temperate regions, to outweigh the danger of skin cancer.

Aura Soma is a very popular method of gaining self-insight and using colour in a gentle way: through looking at bottles containing twin-coloured liquids, or by applying the shaken mixture to the skin, or around the body via an atomizer. Vicky Wall was the originator of the widespread Aura Soma approach, of which others have subsequently developed variants. An increasing number of therapies are incorporating colour. The classic example is colour and acupuncture (acucolour or colourpuncture). This work has been developed over several years and many companies make low-level lasers for the purpose.

There is also Chi Lite a non-coherent light emitting diode (LED) resonating at 660 nanometres which can be used by acupuncturists – and for home use – to stimulate the DNA within the cell to accelerate the process of healing. Another company makes a lamp for localised application of halogen-derived broad bandwidth light or glass filtered colours which also has researched evidence of its effectiveness. Some of these systems use newly created patterns for colour application, some are for topical application, and others use the very ancient Chinese acupuncture meridians which have been plotted on the body for 10,000 years.

In the west, it is common practice to apply the rainbow colours to the eastern concept of energy centres or chakras. This is then applied in healing with colour, and colour can be applied to yoga postures which work on specific centres. Red is considered to be the foundation colour concerned with the physical status of the person and related to the first or base chakra. The colour of harmony and balance on all levels is green, and the related chakra, the heart, at the crown is violet, shading off into the colour of free spirit magenta.

Reflexologists use the Native American healing tradition which maps all parts of the body onto the hands and feet. Treatment is applied with finger pressure as a rule, but a colour torch on the parts of the foot relating to the spinal chakras has been found to work equally as well. A full understanding of the workings and potential of colour has still to be discovered. At present, colour is being applied in so many ways that no overall philosophy can be discerned. However, psychological and physical healing certainly takes place as a result of colour treatment, and colour certainly assists wellness when it is used wisely in our surroundings.

Complementary Health Care

By John Fuller, The British Complementary Medical Association

Most complementary therapies in use today have been in practice for thousands of years in other parts of the globe. So why has the proliferation in the western world been so great? A prime reason is that complementary medicine is fulfilling the health expectations which orthodox medicine has not met.

People feel frustrated and are turning in ever-larger numbers to complementary medicine to ease their distress and to benefit from its holistic approach.

Now complementary medicine is accessible to everyone. At least one in five people in the UK are using complementary medicine and the numbers are growing day by day. It is one of the most rapidly expanding fields of private medicine, with practitioners now outnumbering orthodox GPs.

Let us get it clear from the beginning that 'complementary' medicine is quite different to 'alternative' medicine. These are terms used for therapies not previously taught in western medical establishments, and which are derived from a wide range of beliefs and attitudes about health and well being.

Alternative medicine is conducted by practitioners who are trained to the same standards as registered medical practitioners. This qualifies them to diagnose and to take clinical charge of the patient and includes specialists such as osteopaths, chiropractors and acupuncturists. Alternative treatments favoured by the public include such therapies as; osteopathy for treatment of back pain; acupuncture for treatment of smoking, acute back pain and osteo-arthritis; homeopathy for anxiety, insomnia, hay fever and rheumatoid arthritis.

Complementary therapists on the other hand, will work with registered medical or alternative medical practitioners wherever possible. They do not, however, make medical diagnosis, they do not assume responsibility for the patient and they accept that the doctor remains in full clinical charge of the patient at all times.

Complementary, or natural holistic medicine is just what it says. It is complementary to orthodox medicine. It is not used 'instead of' and it does not conflict with it.

There is now a vast range of

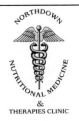

NORTHDOWN

NUTRITIONAL MEDICINE

&
THERAPIES CLINIC

Specialising in combining normal allopathic medicine and complementary therapies

Specialities include:-

Nutritional medicine, Stress management, Pain management, Sports injuries & nutrition, Male health, Natural HRT, advice on Holistic care for Cancer and Medico-legal problems.

Associate Therapies include:-
Consultant Nutritionist
Osteopath & Cranial
Osteopath (Adult & Paediatric)
Reflexologist
Massage Aromatherapist
Allergy Testing
Nurse & Aloe Vera
Information Centre

Call 01795 842588 or Freefone 0800 652 1123
www.virtual-nutrition.co.uk
www.nutrimedline.com

complementary therapies to choose from in the UK. Some have been scientifically tested and some have not. For anxiety or insomnia problems, for example, people may seek help from aromatherapy, reflexology or Chinese medicine.

Those who have a problem with smoking, sleeplessness or obesity might turn to hypnotherapy and those who suffer from asthma or eczema may find that homoeopathy or Chinese medicine will help their condition. In conventional medicine an increasing number of doctors and nurses are recognising the value of complementary therapies and the advantages they offer.

A few GPs are both using and practising alternative and complementary medicine. Around 40 per cent will provide access to some form of complementary therapy for their NHS patients, if requested.

The integration of complementary and orthodox medicine

The increasing demand for complementary medicine is very much patient driven and the call for it to become available on the NHS is growing. The Patients Charter acknowledges its benefits and supports patients who wish to be referred to a therapist by their own doctor.

Often a patient turns to complementary medicine after having found a deficiency in the NHS. In common law the patient has the right to make this choice. Integration of complementary medicine within the NHS would seem to be the next logical step.

The British Complementary Medicine Association is looking at ways to ensure the delivery of safe and efficacious complementary medicine to the public. It is working to secure the agreement of minimum common standards across all therapies as a basis for self-regulation.

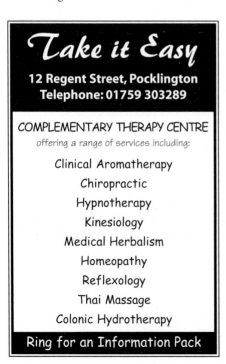
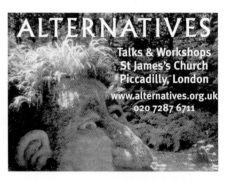
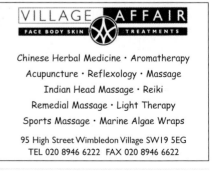

To protect the public the BCMA has a strict code of conduct and disciplinary procedure in place, which is mandatory for all its members. It is vital, however, that complementary and orthodox medicine develop a mutual respect and understanding so that complementary medicine can work in partnership with the established healthcare system of this country and is not submerged by it.

True integration requires that we appreciate the perspective of other professionals. While it must be admitted that there are misunderstandings in the medical profession about the significance of complementary medicine, their existence has generated a great deal of goodwill for co-operation and innovation. A number of doctors either incorporate complementary therapists in their practice team or are happy to refer patients to therapists they can trust.

Huge amounts of money are being spent to shore up the NHS. The Government's ten year NHS Plan, launched in July, is far reaching but it does not allow for complementary medicine.

It does admit that the NHS has failed to keep pace with our society. One of the most significant changes is the steady growth of complementary medicine with a quarter of the population using it, many of the on a regular basis. An estimated 75 per cent want it to be available through the NHS. Hence, it is absolutely essential that it becomes freely accessible in hospitals and doctors surgeries throughout the country – to all who need it, not just those who can afford it.

The Department of Health says its aim is to secure the provision of high quality care for all regardless of their ability to pay, or where they live. The BCMA considers that the integration of complementary medicine within the NHS will enable this provision to be more widely extended into areas where at present orthodoxy fails.

The cost advantage offered by complementary medicine is that it treats the patient holistically. It will usually reduce or eliminate the necessity for expensive clinical drugs or other specialised treatment.

One of the hallmarks of complementary medicine is that it encourages patients to accept responsibility for their own health and to develop a lifestyle, which would considerably reduce the demand on NHS resources.

The embodiment of complementary medicine within the NHS would contribute substantially by reducing costs (especially drugs) and improving the cost efficiency of the NHS for the future. There are over 49,000 complementary therapists in this country providing a variety of solutions to many of our current health problems.

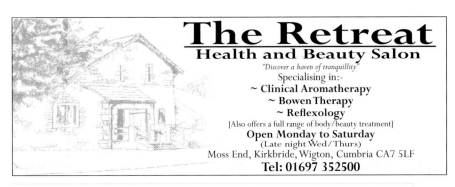

People want to feel confident that the treatment they get is reliable. Complementary therapies are safe and a qualified therapist will recommend and encourage their patients to maintain their relationship with their doctor. The result of such teamwork means that there is less likelihood of a recurring need for medical intervention.

With the confusing proliferation of medical self-help data on the Internet there is a desperate need for accurate and trustworthy details on complementary medicine. This is another area of opportunity for complementary and conventional medicine to work together to improve the standards in information technology. In this situation the BCMA has now taken positive steps to ensure that its website information is accurate (visit www.bcma.co.uk) and it is also linked with the Internet Health Library (www.internethealthlibrary.com)

As the major multi-discipline umbrella body for complementary medicine in Britain, the BCMA believes in self-regulation and knows it can work. It strongly urges greater collaboration and co-operation between all forms of healthcare with complementary therapists, doctors, nurses and patients working together to achieve optimum health for the nation.

The majority of complementary therapies originate from Asia and the Far East. There are between 100 and 130 different types currently on offer in the UK. As a general rule Chinese medicine is mostly herbal in nature, while Japanese therapies are mostly of the bodywork/massage type. There are also a number of therapies emanating from other countries such as Australia, America and Europe, which have been developed more recently.

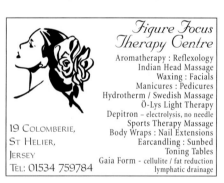
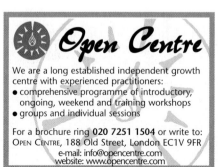

Holistic healing therapy is an inner process through which a person is made whole. It works on the physical, emotional, mental and spiritual levels. Practitioners of complementary medicine will use their skills to guide their patients along the road to self-healing. This holistic approach treats the whole person, not just the disease and deals with the cause not the symptoms. It is specific to each individual and aims to assist the patient's own inner healing process, helping him or her to find their personal path back to health.

There is now a plethora of health information available in books, magazines, and the Internet, plus self-help phone lines, all of which can be quite bewildering to any one seeking advice that has no medical knowledge.

Among the vast range of complementary therapies on offer, some have been scientifically tested and some have not.

Many have regulatory bodies who ensure high standards of practice among their practitioners and who regulate standards, education training and ethics within their particular profession.

Drugs or surgery are not used in these treatments and most are not invasive but completely safe.

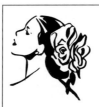

A unique concept in complementary care

The Bristol Health Co-operative has been formed to pursue standards, education and service in the development of complementary medicines.

The purpose of the Co-operative is to make complementary medicines available to all.

The growing membership of the Co-operative is made up of complementary practitioners who recognise the benefits and support that working together can bring.

○ Directory of Practitioners and Services
○ Telephone advice and referral service
○ Treatment services in the community
○ Corporate occupational health care
○ Professional development and training

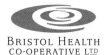

BRISTOL HEALTH
CO-OPERATIVE LTD

FOR FURTHER INFORMATION CALL NOW ON

0117 958 5058

COMPLEMENTARY HEALTH CARE

SUPPORTIVE CARING THERAPEUTIC Breaks with Holistic Therapies, in Magical Cornwall, for people with health problems and life difficulties. Penwethers Holistic Care Centre, 57 Killerton Rd, Bude, Cornwall EX23 8EW. Tel 01288 354 256. www.holisticcare.org.uk

SOUTH LONDON NATURAL HEALTH CENTRE. A centre for the promotion of natural health in all its aspects, including Floatation, Acupuncture, Massage and Homeopathy. We also run a concession clinic and popular lifestyle treatment programmes. Tel: 020 74986526

COMPLEMENTARY THERAPIES Information Service, South Manchester/Cheshire. Do you know what therapy you need? For free information and a register of qualified and insured therapists ring Chris or Kate on Tel 01625 522613/525329

RUSSELL MAY BELMORE CENTRE, Lower Road, Stoke Mandeville, Bucks HP21 9DR. For the best in complementary treatments and beauty therapy. Also available; courses & classes, floatation therapy & sunbed. Easy access, open 7 days a week. Call our friendly staff on 01296 612361

GOLDINGS HILL CLINIC

Goldings Hill Clinic of Natural Medicine, 1 Lower Road, Loughton, Essex.

Tel: 0181 508 7514

FOR A PROMPT AND PROFESSIONAL SERVICE

• ACUPUNCTURE •
• AROMATHERAPY •
• BOWEN TECHNIQUE •
• CHINESE HERBAL MEDICINE •
• COUNSELLING •
• HYPNOTHERAPY •
• INDIAN HEAD MASSAGE •
• NATUROPATHY •
• OSTEOPATHY •
• REFLEXOLOGY •
• REIKI •
• SHIATSU •
•SPIRITUAL HEALING •
•THAI MASSAGE •

NEW DAWN
Soul Therapy Centre
Eva J Day

27 Matlock Crescent, North Cheam, Sutton, Surrey SM3 9SS

Tel/Fax: +44 (0)20 8715 3006;
e-mail: translingua@btinternet.com

ASTLEY CLINIC OF COMPLEMENTARY MEDICINE

Our intention is to help you find the best choices that Complementary Medicine and Natural Health can offer, either at our own clinic or by referring you.

We have registered practitioners in many therapies and have strong links with the medical profession.

You may prefer an initial health check which will give advice on foods which may be advantageous or detrimental to you and which supplements and remedies are beneficial to you.

This advice can also be given by post on receipt of a hair sample on our special form.

Home visits are also available.

For forms and more information, contact:

The Astley Clinic (at food For Thought)
26/28 Astley Road, Seaton Delaval, Northumberland. NE25 0DG
Tel: 0191 237 5935 Fax: 0191 2375621 E.mail: sandra@smichelson.freeserve.co.uk

KAILASH

Centre of Oriental Medicine

Indian Ayurvedic Medicine, **Tibetan** Herbal Medicine,
Chinese Herbal Medicine, **Japanese** Herbal Medicine.

Acupuncture, **Healing** (Bio-energy, BuQi),
Osteopathy (Craniosacral Therapy),
Massage (Indian Panchakarma, Mongolian Chua-ka,
Japanese Shiatsu, Thai Yoga, Chinese Tui-Na, Reflexology)

Meditation, Yoga, Tai-Qi, Qi-Gong

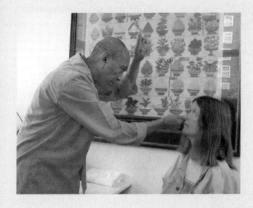 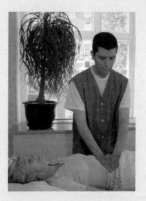

Free 15 Minutes Consultation

7 Newcourt Street, London NW8 7AA
(just off St. John's Wood High Street)

Tel 020-7722-3939 Fax 020-7586-1642
info@orientalhealing.co.uk

www.orientalhealing.co.uk

Therapy Centres and Practice Clinics

A multiplicity of practitioner clinics and complementary centres have sprung up around the country in recent years to meet the increasing demand from the public for complementary medicine.

Apart from a small number that have charitable status, the majority of these are privately run and funded without financial support from Government or grant aid. The type of facility will depend on how therapists set up their practices, either as a group or as independent practitioners.

In addition to the therapies and treatments on offer, complementary therapy centres will generally include other activities such as workshops, short courses and lectures. A healing sanctuary will sometimes form part of the complex. These facilities tend to be linked with various forms of self-development to encourage clients to achieve an optimum holistic lifestyle. The size of such centres will depend on their location and the facilities available. They can vary from a custom-built centre to a converted church hall.

Clinics are usually purpose designed with each therapy room or bay being furnished with separate facilities according to the therapy being practised. A large clinic may consist of a suite of rooms, converted premises or even a complete building housing a number of practices.

The state of the art in therapy clinics has to be Westminster University's new Polyclinic. Opened last year by HRH The Prince of Wales, it is the first centre in

Europe to provide a wide range of low price complementary therapies alongside facilities for teaching and research.

Strict hygiene standards will be observed whatever therapies are being provided. There will usually be a central reception area where clients can wait or make appointments with the therapist of their choice. Some practitioners work independently and may rent a room in a clinic or work from home with a room set aside for use as a clinic. Alternatively, they may undertake home visits for clients who are unable to visit the clinic.

Valuation of a therapist

Orthodox medicine has not met your expectations, so you decide to try something else, but you are worried about quacks and unqualified therapists exploiting you for your money. How can you be sure that the therapist you go to is genuine?

Don't accept what any one individual says to you. Check that the therapist is registered with a recognised professional association, which holds a public register, code of conduct, effective disciplinary procedure and complaints mechanism. Get the address of the organisation and contact them for information on their training criteria and practice standards. Be discriminating. The object of self-regulation in complementary medicine is to ensure that patients are not harmed.

What happens when you first consult a therapist? They will be prepared to spend more time with you than a GP. They will take your medical history and ask questions about your lifestyle, diet, work and leisure pursuits, as well as the condition for which you are seeking treatment. The cost of treatment per session will vary depending on the therapist you chose and the type of treatment you are offered.

What type of health problems lead people to seek help from complementary medicine? Muscular-skeletal problems, allergies, digestive, respiratory as well as stress, depression and psychological disorders.

If you are considering using a complementary therapy find out what is involved before embarking on a course of treatment. You need to be aware of unqualified practitioners. If in doubt consult the British Complementary Medicine Association or the British Holistic Medical Association for further guidance and obtain from them a list of their member organisations.

All the principal complementary therapies have training programmes requiring high standards of achievement. The basic student-training period lasts from one to three years depending on the therapy being studied. To qualify each therapist must meet the criteria and standards demanded by that therapy and will be assessed at the completion of the course by a recognised and accredited examining body.

Once qualified they will normally apply for membership of the organisation representing their therapy. That association may itself be a member of a multi-discipline umbrella body such as the BCMA. The therapist must also be properly insured to practice privately or in a registered clinic.

The benefits of natural health care

Good health is a precious commodity at any time of life and the treatments to which our body is subjected can have a damaging as well as a beneficial effect. Conventional medicine gives scant thought to what is the driving force that keeps us alive or how the different parts of our body integrate.

Doctors view their patients simply as a collection of organs, limbs and cells, with little attempt to understand the person as a whole. The present medical establishment is still based on science, but a human being exists on many levels.

We have feelings. We get stressed and depressed. We get aches and pains. We suffer health problems with un-diagnosable symptoms. Yet all we really need is a better understanding of the illness and a willingness to develop our own natural healing ability. To take responsibility for our own health.

What are the benefits offered by complementary medicine?

Overall it can change the energy balance in our body, improve mental and physical well being and general health. It may not lead to throwing away the crutches and dancing in the street, but it can help us to use our body more efficiently, assist relaxation and reduce stress.

Complementary medicine is holistic and most therapists take the whole body approach to treatment. Good health means integration and wholeness between all the different levels of our being. It helps us to keep stabilised and in harmony with ourselves and flexible enough to grow and develop the in-built self-healing systems, which already exist within us.

Complementary medicine in the 21st century and beyond

Steeped in the wisdom and practice of the ancients as complementary medicine surely is, there seems little doubt that technology of the future will validate the practices handed down through the ages and continue to enhance the work of therapists through the 21st century.

Complementary medicine is certainly here to stay. Patients are voting with their

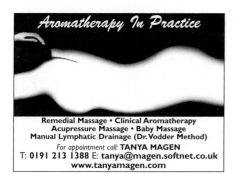

feet as practitioners and agencies look to the future. Many divisions between professional groups are already beginning to fall away. In the medical world nurses and pharmacists are taking on responsibilities once only associated with doctors, while health care assistants are doing much of the work that nurses used to do.

There is a growing recognition that healthcare is about teamwork, rather than individuals working in isolation. Many therapists are now multi-disciplined and the majority of complementary health centres offer a variety of different treatments which complement each other.

The future of healthcare points to more openness between patients and practitioners as well as the regular interchange of useful data between different professional bodies, with common standards of practice shared across the professions.

One possibility is a single umbrella body that covers all health care professions and has authority to undertake investigations of multi-disciplinary teams, linked with an ombudsman.

This would mean better protection for the public from unsafe practitioners with healthcare professionals working to the same standards of conduct and having a shared code of ethics.

Ongoing research is currently being undertaken by a number of Universities in Britain. Although a substantial amount of research already exists, it needs to be greatly extended, to determine the genuine therapeutic benefits and dispel the orthodox view that these therapies merely produce a 'placebo' effect.

The evidence exists to show that complementary medicine can produce positive results. In the final analysis it is the 'outcome' that counts and this is different with each patient, depending on the cause of their condition, and not the symptoms on which conventional medicine is based.

The future is bright for complementary medicine. All the signs are there.

No one has all the answers but there is much common ground on which complementary and orthodox medicine can and must work together given the will.

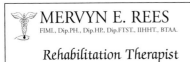

COMPLEMENTARY HEALTH CARE PRACTITIONERS

ELAINE ARTHEY: Multi-dimensional healer. Transformative work through the mind-body-spirit connection. Healing, Shiatsu and Massage on land, in water and under water. Expessive Arts, Aromatherapy, Aura-Soma, Bachflowers plus lesser known modalities. Call 01473 827636.

BLUE JASPER: Reflexology, Healing, Crystal Therapy, for health, well-being and balance. Individualised courses for acute and long term health problems, fatigue, stress, tension etc. Also crystal and healing workshops. Caroline Lawrie, North London, 0181 881 9785. E-mail blue.jasper@virgin.net

MARIETTE LOBO M.A.: Tui Na (Chinese Massage), Reflexology, Reiki (Master), Lymph Massage, Aromatherapy. Tel: 0141 339 5591 {answer service} for clinic details. Proven experience in the fields of sports injuries, cancer, paediatrics, geriatrics, using complimentary therapies.

MICHAEL VILLEMIN ITEC, MGCP, MMLD UK from Santé au Naturel. Trained at the respected Rawworth College for sports Therapy and Natural Medicine. Practices in Swedish Massage, Thai Traditional Massage, On –Site Massage (Seated Acupressure), Manual Lymphatic Drainage (Vodder), Reiki Healing and is also a certified infant massage instructor teaching parents how to promote the development of their babies/ toddlers. Evening and Weekend Consultations, Home visits and personalised gift vouchers available for all occasions. For a relaxing & energising treatment to leave you feeling refreshed and alert contact Michael Villemin at Santé au Naturel on 01962 890420/ 0468 061959 fax 01962 890322 email: santeaunaturel@yahoo.com

COMPLEMENTARY HEALTH CARE PRACTITIONERS

DR. S. TREFZER MSC MBBCH DMS med MF Hom. Physician in General Practice and Hospital Medicine. High Tree Hopuse, Eastbourne Road, Uckfield, East Sussex TN22 5QL, practicing General Medicine, Chiro-therapies, Acupuncture, Colour- Acupuncture, Homoeopathy and Herbal Medicine in Central London and Richmond-Surrey. (Tel:0973- 702461)

AROMATHERAPY & REFLEXOLGY – SOUTH LEEDS. Sue Chapman, BSc (Hons), DipSysPrac, GNSR. Aromatherapy Massage - £25 (first session - £30). Reflexology - £20 (first session - £25) For an appointment call 0113 2775002 or 07721 067711 (Mobile)

ANGELA CHAN, N.D.D.O. (1982), (Qualified & Experienced Practitioner). Gentle effective treatment for Backaches, Neck Tension, Sports Injuries and Stress. Tel: 0208 2989064 (Kent) Tel: 0208 244 8138 (London).

MEDICAL HERBALISM – Your personal formulas. Iridology – What do your eyes reveal about your health? Skenar Therapy – Russian statistics claim healing results between 60 per cent & 90 per cent. Free Introductory consultation Jutta Blumenthal, MH., Ir. 0117 9428948

MRS D CHILD, 9 Gravel Hill, Emmergreen, Reading, Berkshire, RG4 8QN. 01189 47 5772

MRS B J HARDING, 26 Red Lion Street, Boston, Lincolnshire, PE21 6PZ. 01205 354066

MRS C CARTER, Essential Training Solutions, PO Box 5116, Badby, Daventry, Northamptonshire. 01327 312444

MS E REID, Rosewood Aromatherapy Room, 41 Rosewood Avenue, Paisley, Renfrewshire, PA2 9NJ. 0141 884 1811

Words of **Wisdom**

"*Poisons and medicine are oftentimes the same substance given with different intents*"

PETER MERE LATHAM

Counselling and Psychotherapy

By Bridgitte Scott

"My belief is in the blood and flesh as being wiser than the intellect. The body unconscious is where life bubbles up in us. It is how we know that we are alive, alive to the depth of our souls and in touch somewhere with the vivid reaches of the cosmos" – **D.H.Lawrence**

A lot of people are stuck in the freeze position, feeling powerless, trapped and depressed. Others are caught in the chronic state of fight or flight. When we are trapped in the freeze, our body functions are lowered and we cannot see a way out. The healing work would include finding a way Emotional Therapy

Depression? Unhappiness? Relationship Problems? Tired, Can't Cope? Any of these symptoms and more can be caused by suppressed emotions where a fight or flight reaction is imaginable and to feel the power in the body again (feeling literally able, in the legs, to run away, fight with the fists, dare to stand up in a conflict).

With chronic fight or flight reactions the body is in a chronic overcharge, there is a permanent feeling of being under stress. The immune system becomes over stimulated and states such as chronic high blood pressure, heart problems, allergies, or chronic tension in the muscles can occur. A physical and emotional reaction has to be stimulated and a safe solution for the mind has to be found in order to get back to the natural cycle of charge, discharge and recuperation. The autonomic nervous system can then become balanced in its 'alert' and 'relaxing, digesting' response.

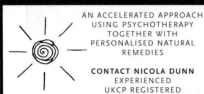

When we freeze in a conflict, or through an overwhelming experience, we normally don't allow ourselves to release the charge fully. Usually we just get on with life, pull ourselves together and pretend that nothing has happened. We have learnt not to trust or to ignore our body's language.

We learn socially to inhibit our emotional responses (e.g. 'big boys, big girls don't cry'), which means a break down of the physiological repair mechanism too. When we re-educate ourselves that it is okay to listen to the body, honour its natural functions and its expression of feelings, we can become free.

We control our free expression of our life, as we are in conflict between the instinctual self, the social self, and the concept of what we 'should' be.

I want to show you a way in which it is possible to free the frozen conflict and how to deal with it on a physical, emotional and mental level.

As we look at animals in the wilderness, we see that they live an instinctual life. Only mammals have a brain that allows feelings and choice of social groupings. We, as humans, have a further choice with our intellectual brain. We can read and write. We can choose where we want to live, have the conscious use of tools and fire and can choose to be hunters or gatherers.

Still, we have the instinctual animal nature, which interferes with the decisions of the mind. When threatened, the body reacts according to the instincts. Then the body reacts towards flight or fight. If there is no escape and the experience is too overwhelming, we freeze. An animal in the wilderness will drop as if dead when it cannot run away from the predator. If it is not killed, it will recover from the shock by shaking and trembling until the body returns to its healthy physiological function.

I work with people who come to me for help, initially with Cranio-Sacral Therapy and Biodynamic Massage. We work towards strengthening the body, to encourage the body's own healing capacity. Eventually the emotional and instinctual content of the trauma will come into the open and can be integrated.

Body Unconscious, the place where the hidden stories of life are showing in the body, where the truth lies, where conflicts, unresolved traumata, are trapped and where the truth and healing can be retrieved.

It can take time, sometimes years, to free a healthy response and regain vitality. It is not enough to work towards relaxation, as the instinctual responses have to be allowed freedom, which can become quite a lively process. Safe and stable support from the therapist is essential if a profound change is to happen.

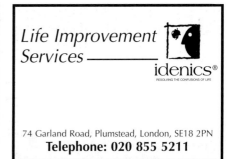

Biodynamic Psychotherapy

By Margaret Barnes.

Biodynamic Psychotherapy is a branch of body psychotherapy developed by Gerda Boyesen, a Norwegian psychologist, Reichian psychotherapist and physiotherapist. Based on a biological theory of psychology, it is concerned with the organic link between the body and the psyche.

While a significant part of the therapy may be verbal exchange between therapist and client it differs from most other branches of psychotherapy in its interest in bodily phenomena and non-verbal sources of information and communication. Orthodox verbal psychotherapy is combined with a range of specially devised massage techniques, breathwork, body awareness exercises, regression and emotional expression work to help to resolve physical as well as psychological problems.

The term 'biodynamic' refers to the concept of life energy flowing naturally and spontaneously. Life energy (known as chi in Chinese medicine and bioplasma energy in contemporary research) is the force that moves us and brings us to life on all levels: physical, mental, emotional and spiritual. 'Mind' and 'body' are not seen in hierarchical relationship but as inter-functioning aspects of the whole person.

The theories, philosophy and methods of Biodynamic Psychotherapy were developed and refined over many years, Originally trained as a clinical psychologist, Gerda Boyesen worked in several psychiatric hospitals in Norway. She trained and worked in private practice as a Reichian psychotherapist then took the highly unorthodox step of also training as a physiotherapist, working in Norway's leading physiotherapy clinic, where advanced neuro-muscular massage techniques were achieving remarkable results with patients from psychiatric hospitals. With this unusual background Gerda Boyesen combined her clinical knowledge and analytic training, observing in detail the relationship between psychological and bodily processes in her psychotherapy patients.

In particular she became aware of the intestinal sounds during psychotherapy sessions, particularly at moments of insight or emotional release. Intrigued by this connection she began to listen to her own intestinal sounds and those of her patients.

Finding that she could initiate these sounds by massaging different parts of the body she discovered that the quality of her touch influenced the strength and quality of the sounds. This visceral feedback told her where the patient's nervous tensions were located, giving her the means to reduce fear, depression and psychosomatic symptoms. After sessions patients typically felt light and at peace with themselves.

Gerda Boyesen had discovered something unique and revolutionary – that the intestines have two functions: the digestion of food and the digestion of nervous tension. This latter function she called 'psycho-peristalsis'. Despite achieving remarkable results with her patients Gerda Boyesen had difficulty getting her radical theories and methods accepted. In 1968 she left Norway and moved to London where she found greater acceptance. Here she set up the Gerda Boyesen Centre for Biodynamic Psychology and Psychotherapy where, for 25 years, she has trained hundreds of therapists in her theories and methods.

In 1999, in her late 70s, Gerda Boyesen decided to focus on writing, teaching and research work. She asked colleagues to set up a new school to carry on her work. The London School of Biodynamic Psychotherapy (Gerda Boyesen Method), whose directors and trainers have an international training background, will ensure the continuation of established training standards as members of the United Kingdom Council for Psychotherapy (UKCP). Gerda Boyesen acts as adviser and participates in training.

In our individual families, groups and society generally, the spontaneous expression of certain feelings is not welcomed. There may be prohibition, disapproval or punishment, so the individual learns from an early age to repress or restrict instinctual responses. Conflict and confusion are accompanied by muscle tension which hold back the expression, remnants of which remain long after the original urge has been forgotten. These physical and psychological responses are movements of the life energy. When we deny or repress them we deny or repress our life energy, who we are, on a physical and psychological level and the result can often be seen as distortions in posture, muscle tone and psychosomatic symptoms as well as in psychological disturbances.

Biodynamic Psychotherapists work with the whole person using language, imagery, non-verbal expression and touch, to work with sensitivity and at the client's pace, to create a safe environment in which client feels able to deal with their deepest concerns.

There is no pre-determined agenda and therapists select from a wide repertoire of methods appropriate to the client's need at a particular moment. Whatever that need emotionally, physically or verbally the therapist works with what is uppermost for the client at that particular moment.

Psychotherapeutic massage plays an important role – for instance, massage of the muscles which have held back an urge to strike someone may release old feelings of anger to be reassessed.

Massage may also be used to cleanse the tissues of the remnants of stress hormones, or to relax and harmonise the client after a period of emotional expression.

The aim of the therapy is to help clients come to terms with past traumas and upsets – while history cannot be changed, the client's feelings about themselves, the situation and its bodily effects can.

Clients are encouraged to develop awareness of what is happening in the body so that they are aware of the effect a situation is having on them.

They can choose whether to express what they are feeling or to suppress it and perhaps give it expression at a more appropriate time.

The aim is also to help the client move towards a position of health in both body and psyche so they are better able to deal with their everyday lives, to achieve greater autonomy, self assurance, empowerment, freedom and self realisation.

Biodynamic Psychotherapy ultimately enables clients to achieve greater balance, joy and contentment in their lives.

COUNSELLING & PSYCHOTHERAPY

MR D TANGUAY, Flat 1 Langley Mansions, Langley Lane, London, SW8 1TJ. 020 7582 4287

MR G GAD, 25c Vauxhall Grove, London, SW8 1SY. 020 7735 4513

MS D WEBB, Bath, 01225 461361

COUNSELLING & PSYCHOTHERAPY

PAULINE DALBY M.A.S.C. Qualified therapist working in York, using holistic healing therapy, stress management and counselling. Bringing balance to emotional and physical aspects of peoples lives, 'Helping you to help yourself'. Palmistry analysis also available. Tel 01904 670553 appointments only.

HUMANISTIC/ TRANSPERSONAL COUNSELLING AND WORKSHOPS. Warm, supportive environment provided for exploration of issues blocking well-being and Self development. Creative ways of working on offer including shamanic work. Scilla Alvarado BAC Accredited Counsellor MA, Bed (Hons) North London 020 7359 6783. scilla_alvarado@telinco.co.uk

BIODYNAMIC PSYCHOTHERAPY (humanistic approach) Specific emotional issues or for self-exploration. Short and long term. Also Biodynamic Body Therapy. Clinics in Central London and North London. Hartmut Wuebbeler, Dipl.-Biol., M.Sc., D.I.C., M.T.I. For information and appointments 020 7326 5324

MRS KATHLEEN HUNT BSc, Sidmouth, Devon EX10. Tel 01395 516091. Well qualified and very experienced therapist. Flexible hours and negotiable fees. Help for all emotional problems to individuals, couples and families.

CHRISTINE LOMAS, M.S.E.C.(Prac) BFRP, B.R.C.P., B.Ed(Hons). Counsellor/Teacher. Mind, Body, Spirit approach to healing the past, awareness in the present and future growth. Individual sessions, evening/daytime talks, courses and meditation. Ring 020 8852 7748.

LONDON SW11 (BATTERSEA) : Experienced Biodynamic Psychotherapist / Counsellor. For an appointment or an exploratory chat call Rus Gandy on 020 7223 4269 or Email: rus@sadhippo.com (Rail: Clapham Junction, Tube: Clapham Common)

RICHARD CLEMINSON MSc, UKCP registered biodynamic psychotherapist working with individuals, groups and organisations. He offers stress counselling, verbal psychotherapy, biodynamic massage and group therapy. Research interests: creative blocks, frustration. Sussex 01273 500797

DR ELYA STEINBERG (MD, UKCP) synthesises knowledge and experience in conventional and alternative medicine to allow the person energy to develop. Bioenergy, Healing, Holistic Reflexology and Biodynamic Psychology and Psychotherapy. North London. 020 8455 7572. Hebrew and English.

Craniosacral Therapy

By Michael Kern DO, RCST, MIGA, ND

Craniosacral Therapy takes a whole-person approach to the healing process, recognising the interconnections of mind, body and spirit, and how the body can reflect our experiences and retain memories of any trauma.

It is an effective form of treatment for a wide range of illnesses, helping to create conditions for optimal health, encouraging vitality and a general sense of wellbeing. It is suitable for people of all ages, including babies, children and the elderly, and can be effective in acute or chronic cases.

Intrinsic health

Craniosacral Therapy is a hands-on approach, which involves 'listening through the fingers' to the body's subtle rhythmic motions and any patterns of congestion and resistance. The practitioner becomes skilled at listening to these rhythms and learns to therapeutically relate to patterns of inertia. The emphasis of treatment is to encourage and enhance the body's own self-healing and self-regulating mechanisms, facilitating the expression of intrinsic health, even in the most acute resistances and pathologies.

Life as motion

Life expresses itself as motion, and there is a clear relationship between motion and health. All healthy, living tissues of the body fully 'breathe' with the motion of life

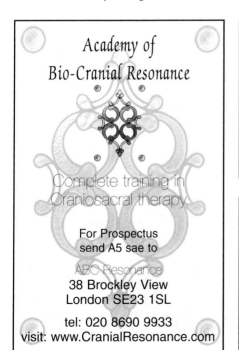

producing subtle rhythmic impulses, which can be palpated by sensitive hands. These rhythmic movements were discovered by Dr. William Garner Sutherland, after he had an insight whilst examining the sutures of cranial bones. Dr. Sutherland realised that these sutures were, in fact, designed for motion. During many years of research, he demonstrated the existence of this motion and concluded that it is essentially produced by the body's inherent life force, which he called the 'Breath of Life'. From an early stage he understood that he was exploring a subtle and involuntary system of rhythmic movement, which is important for the maintenance of health.

A gentle facilitation

The work is gentle and non-invasive. With a skillful touch, the practitioner can assist the body to resolve its patterns of inertia, thereby encouraging a revitalisation of the body's tissues with the healing resources of the breath of life. Subtle suggestions can be introduced through the practitioner's fingers to help restore a balance in tissues that have been holding some restriction or disorder. In this regard, the quality of therapeutic presence of the practitioner can become a reflective mirror for the patient and their potential for change.

An expression of health

The subtle motions produced by the breath of life initially arise at the core of the body and involve the central nervous system, the cerebrospinal fluid and the surrounding tissues and bones, including the bones of the skull. These motions are expressed as tide-like rhythms, which help to maintain balance and integration throughout all the body systems, distributing the healing and ordering properties of the breath of life. They can be felt throughout the body and may yield a wealth of information to an experienced

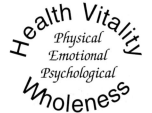

touch. Dr Sutherland referred to the rhythmic expressions of the breath of life as primary respiratory motion. He saw that the healthy expression of primary respiratory motion was fundamental to all other physiological functions of the body. The body, with its patterns of health and disease, is organised in relationship to how these essential ordering forces of the breath of life are able to manifest

Inertial patterning

If primary respiratory motion becomes congested or inertial, then the manifestation of the body's basic ordering principle is affected and the expression of our intrinsic health becomes compromised. Sites of inertia may result from any experiences, which overwhelm the body. Stresses, strains, tensions and traumas can accumulate over the years creating inertial patterns, which become retained in the tissues, and affecting the rhythmic motions of primary respiration.

Some common causes of inertia and any consequent disturbance are physical injuries, emotional and psychological factors, birth trauma and toxicity. The way in which our bodies become patterned is thus a unique expression of our health history and experience. Craniosacral Therapy seeks to free any areas of inertia so that the ordering principle of the breath of life is expressed through the tissues. When this happens, it is marked by the restoration of balance and symmetry in the rhythms of primary respiratory motion.

Alternative medicine should be available on the NHS

IT has always been a subject close to his heart. Now Prince Charles, anxious to share his views on alternative medicine with as wide an audience as possible, has written:

"For years, the NHS has found complementary medicine an uncomfortable bedfellow – at best regarded as 'fringe' and in some quarters as 'quack'; never viewed as a substitute for conventional medicine and rarely as a genuine partner in providing therapy.

"The response to the recent Guild of Health Writers' Award for Good Practice in Integrated Healthcare, held in association with the Foundation for Integrated Medicine, of which I am proud to be president, suggests that integrated medicine is more widespread than expected.

"At last there are signs of a genuine partnership developing as more and more NHS professionals and complementary therapists find themselves working alongside one another."

CRANIOSACRAL THERAPY
JOHN CASSELL RCST

34 Northover Road
Portsmouth
01705 664720

The Grove Natural Therapy Centre
Southampton
01703 582245

MONICA ANTHONY
UKCP RCST MBSH LRAM

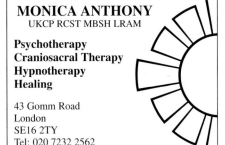

Psychotherapy
Craniosacral Therapy
Hypnotherapy
Healing

43 Gomm Road
London
SE16 2TY
Tel: 020 7232 2562

Michael Lloyd-Wright
Ph.D., DC., RCST.

**Registered McTimoney Chiropractor
& Craniosacral Therapist**

Natural Remedies,
35 Brecknock Road,
London N7 0BT   Tel: 020 7267 3884

Helen E. Francis
M.A.R., I.T.E.C.

*Massage, Metamorphic Technique,
Reflexology, Cranio Sacral Therapy*

The Bryn,
Bryn Lane,
Newtown,
Powys SY16 3LZ   Telephone: 01686 626948

Crystal Healing

By Sue Richter

There are many ways in which the healing properties of crystals can be implemented therapeutically. One of them is the ancient art of 'Laying-on-of-stones'.

While the client reclines in deep relaxation, the therapist gently lays the selected crystals on and around the body, often creating intricate patterns or mandalas on the energy points, or chakras. By activating the chakras in this way, the crystal energy can reach every level – physical, emotional, mental and spiritual – to harmonise and heal where appropriate.

Crystals are power tools; they are friends. Indeed, whichever way you view crystals, Crystal Healing remains a beautiful, gentle experience, using some of the most exquisite examples of the earth's natural resources.

Crystals are limited only by the restraints of our own imaginations. They are all things to all people at all times. To some they can be subatomic particle transducers, to others a subtle energy that can help relieve pain on any level. They can help us to connect with the Angelic realms, or they can help relieve some of the tensions and stresses of everyday 21st century life.

Treatment can, additionally, take the form of crystal colour lamps, thus emphasising and amplifying the qualities of colour through the energy of crystal. For some conditions crystal massage or crystal reflexology may be used as an alternative

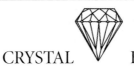

form of treatment. Gem elixirs or oils may also be prescribed. All beings have an energy field, or aura, and this includes minerals. So by introducing the very specific vibration of a crystal's energy field into our own aura, profound changes in our energy field are implemented. Just by holding or wearing a crystal, healing can take place.

The therapeutic properties of minerals are governed by several factors, the most obvious of which is probably colour. An excellent illustration of colour's important role is seen in comparing the similarly structured stones amethyst and citrine.

Amethyst is violet, the colour of the crown chakra. Cool and calming, amethyst is often used in cases of stress and tension, especially when this manifests in the physical as headaches or insomnia. It is also used to aid meditation, helping to create a calm meditative state quickly and easily.

Healing, using crystals, is among the most ancient of all known therapies, and references to their use can be found in the Old Testament, as well as among the ancient Egyptian hieroglyphs. Millions of years old, crystals' extraordinary beauty has been a source of wonder and mystery throughout the centuries.

Crystals have been used in numerous civilisations for a myriad of purposes, from amulets, symbols of authority and, notably, for their healing powers.

Due to their perfect molecular structure, crystals vibrate at a constant rate. It is this property that makes them ideal components for many modern technological developments, from quartz watches to the fastest of computers. And it is this unique quality that makes crystals the ideal tools for balancing and harmonising the body, so allowing the body's natural healing abilities to work more effectively.

Additionally, all crystals and gemstones vibrate at different frequencies, so by carefully selecting the crystals with the correct vibration for their client's needs, the crystal healer can guide the therapeutic properties to go to the deepest level of their being, to energise and re-balance the body to create a state of harmony and well-being.

However, when amethyst is subjected to a heat source (whether naturally deep within the earth, or artificially- even the heat from a candle flame) it changes colour, from purple to yellow or orange, and thus 'becomes' citrine. With this change of colour, (and name!) its energy changes also. It is no longer a gentle, passive – albeit powerful – crystal. It is now vibrant and dynamic, bringing in the quality of sunshine and joy.

Tradition can also teach us a lot. Turquoise, for example, has long been used by many of the old civilisations to ward off evil spirits. The Aztecs, Egyptians and Native Americans all used it for protection, whether from malevolent gods or mortal enemies. Turquoise, as a colour, is today associated with the thymus chakra, governing the immune system. Thus one of the healing qualities of the gem turquoise is to boost the immune system, the 'protector' of our physical bodies.

Of course, this is a simplistic example, and needs to be seen in the light of the many other factors involved. Crystalline structure and formation, mineral and elemental content, all play an essential role when considering the healing qualities of gemstones.

Many people have the ability to tune in to the Devas within the crystal, thus enabling them to utilise the spiritual aspects of the stones. It is only when one understands the synthesis of all these energies that the true and full healing properties of a particular crystal can be fully appreciated.

One of the beauties of working with crystals is their ability to adapt themselves to enhance many of the healing arts and therapies practiced today. They can bring power to the fingertips of the reflexologist, or astounding subtlety to the wonderful art of the aromatherapist. For those who work with Feng Shui, crystals can direct, enhance or disperse qi, as required.

Many people now 'channel' information, and find crystals can bring clarity and focus to their work. A quartz cluster can be programmed, for example, to keep a room or area clear of any disharmonious energies. Think of the advantages of having such a cluster in a therapy room, whatever one's discipline, or in a counselling practice. The possibilities are endless.

YOUR OWN CRYSTALS

The coming together of two minds, two spirits and two physical bodies, both 'vibrating' on the same beautiful frequency, is like falling in love for the first time.

Crystals and gemstones should be chosen with the same emotions. It is so important that the stones we choose and use should 'vibrate' on a frequency as close as possible to our own. So, when choosing your own stones, here are some practical tips:

Close your eyes, then open your eyes quickly and select the first stone that catches your eye. Run a hand over the stones available for selection; the one that sticks to your skin is your stone.

Intuitively, you will instinctively 'know' which stone to choose and which is 'right' for you! You might feel as if the stone is jumping up at you. Or you might sense or even 'see' a strong crystalline white light radiating from the stone and attracting you like a magnet.

'Into Every Life a Little Crystal Shall Fall'
from the Book of Aesclepius

CRYSTAL HEALING

MS J ROBERTSON, 8 Jubilee Cottages, Station Rd, Marston Mortain, Bedfordshire, MK43 0PN. 01234 765604

MS R PAYTON, 2 Tregarrick Cottage, St Tudy, Bodmin, Cornwall, PL30 3PJ. 01208 850542

MR I MARTELL, Wood House, Shotley Bridge, Conset, Durham, DH8 9TL. 01207 255220

MISS J WARD, 97 Lumley Rd, Chuckery, Walsall, West Midlands, WS1 2LH. 01922 646069

MS J NICHOLSON, 185 Warminster Road, Sheffield, Yorkshire, S8 8PP. 01142 580322

Dowsing

The art of dowsing and the healing arts
By Michael Rust – The British Society of Dowsers

To the man in the street who has actually heard of dowsing it is usually known as something to do with finding water with a twig. True; but what is rarely realised is the relevance of this strange practice to searches for many other things – underground caverns, tunnels, pipes and services, missing objects, energy patterns from standing stones and its use as a diagnostic aid in the search for good health.

Dowsing is a controversial subject, which simultaneously arouses awe and disdain, depending upon the disposition of the enquirer. Material science, developed with the impetus of our current Western civilisation from the Greek natural philosophers onwards has brought innumerable benefits to life and we, in the rich countries of the world, are the inheritors of these many blessings. From time to time scientists investigate the dowsing phenomenon and it is only in rare circumstances, such as the researches of Betel, that, from a scientific standpoint, justification for the claims of dowsers is found.

Ideas and theories about the nature of dowsing abound but those scientists who claim that dowsing success is no better than chance or is a chimera have to face the fact that the track record of the best dowsers is impressive and, it can be justly argued that people generally do not continually pay good money for a service if it is not delivering sound results.

It is quite possible that the methodology of material science is not an appropriate tool with which to investigate dowsing. Many deep thinking scientists are now ready to admit the limitations of their craft and realise that it may not be able to reveal the truth about everything.

This is not to suggest that scientific enquiry should not be brought to bear upon dowsing and dowsers. Future developments may increase our understanding.

As an adjunct to the healing arts, dowsing has now a considerable history. From the early twentieth century French dowsers such as Turenne were pioneers in this field and the word radiesthesie or radiesthesia was coined, meaning medical dowsing. This frequently involved the use of simple instruments? such as a pendulum allied to samples of disease states, bodily organs and remedies in conjunction with charts.

Various methods are employed in the presence of the patient to determine the causes of ill health or imbalance and to seek the remedies best suited to lead to a cure. Frequently, a sample from the patient, such as hair or a blood spot is taken to act as a focus so that the diagnosis can be carried out in the absence of the patient. This fact is sometimes difficult for patients to accept but the technique is well established and proved as a practical and efficient approach.

The American doctor Abrams carried out his researches in California early in the 20th century using techniques very similar to dowsing and his findings were endorsed by the Horder Report in this country in 1925. Dr Guyon Richards followed up this approach in his medical practice. A lay practitioner, Vernon Wethered, wrote of his own researches and developments as did Tansley.

Eventually Dr George Laurence, Dr Aubrey Westlake and Carl Upton were instrumental in developing further medical techniques incorporating the use of dowsing. Today the use of dowsing, which has been compared with the use of the stethoscope insofar as both require the subjective interpretation of indications by the practitioner, is embraced by a number of qualified medical practitioners as well as many alternative or complementary therapists.

In adopting this approach to the healing arts, just as in any other field of dowsing, it is axiomatic that the best and most reliable results will be obtained when the practitioner has proper and detailed knowledge of the subject to which his dowsing is being applied. Dowsing results should be tempered with professional knowledge and common sense. The British Society of Dowsers, a registered charity, exists to further knowledge about all forms of dowsing and organises each year an active programme of meetings and courses as well as publishing its respected quarterly journal.

You can try Dowsing

You will need two metal rods, each about 50cm (20in) in length. You can use an old shirt hanger as a source of wire. You need to bend the wire to obtain two identical rods with 'handles', so that there is a straight angle (90 degrees) between the handle and the main part of the rod.

The handles should be approx. 10cm (4in) long. You may find it helpful to place several wooden beads on the handle. These beads should rotate easily. You can add a tightly fitting bead at the bottom of the handle to prevent other beads from sliding off the handle. This way balancing and holding the rods is much easier.

Now is the time to test your new rods. Start walking slowly along a straight line holding the rods as described below.

It is crucial to hold the rods properly. You should place the handle of the dowsing rod in the middle of your palm, then close your hand. Do not squeeze the rods too tight, they will not move. Hold them in such a way that the main part of the rod is parallel to the ground and attempt to keep them in that position at all times.

You may notice that your rods move 'by themselves' and cross over certain points. Remember the location of these points and walk over them again; if you get same results repeatedly you probably have talent for dowsing.

Earth Healing & Earth Acupuncture

By Ali Northcott

Earth Acupuncture works much in the same way as acupuncturist's work on the human body. The practitioner will locate areas that are blocked, stagnant or depleted (usually by dowsing) and then, by becoming sensitive to the flow and quality of the energy, work with needles to restore the balance of the energy.

The needles are formed by working with the five elements of fire, earth, metal, water and wood. Intention and ritual is a key part of the process, as is being responsive to the land. Clearing the energy may also include tools for shielding and protection.

Our health and vitality is strongly influenced by the quality of the Earth's energy. When we live in areas of balance, our energy system is supported and we benefit from the nourishing and healing energy of the Earth. However, in areas where the energy field is out of balance our overall wellbeing is adversely affected and over a period of time our health can deteriorate. These fields of disruption are known as geopathic stress. Earth Acupuncture or Earth Healing detects, clears and heals areas of geopathic stress, much in the same way as an acupuncturist restores balance to the human body, detecting areas that are blocked or stagnant and then introducing techniques to restore a healthy flow.

Beneficial energy

Earth energy, when in balance, has a generative quality which exerts a positive influence on our energy and supports our immune systems, encouraging us to function better on all levels – physically, emotionally, mentally and spiritually. Places with clear Earth energy have different qualities, depending on the source, and are experienced in many ways, calming, grounding, even sacred and holy, uplifting spirits, inspiring creativity.

Disrupted energy

In areas where the Earth's energy has become disrupted, the Earth literally becomes sick and geopathic stress occurs. People and places do not tend to prosper when situated on areas of geopathic stress as it inhibits health, stability and growth. Buildings situated on areas of geopathic stress tend to have a history of inhabitants who suffer from misfortune, ill health and problematic relationships. In some areas, where the energy is particularly disturbed, it may feel unpleasant. It promotes negativity and affects our ability to relax and focus properly. Over a period of time it can break down the immune system and make us vulnerable to disease. Illnesses associated with geopathic stress vary but include headaches, tiredness, ME, candida, eczema, infertility and even diseases such as cancer. It can also delay recovery from illness and aggravate old conditions.

History of Earth Healing and Earth Acupuncture

Earth Acupuncture is born out of the ancient tradition of Earth healing, found in the history of cultures throughout the world. For many years, ancient cultures recognised the fundamental link between the health of the environment and the wellbeing of the people living there. Earth healing is part of a body of knowledge known as Geomancy, the basic principle being to promote a harmonious relationship between humans and the environment, the internal and external landscape. It is a rich part of our heritage, currently undergoing a revival, and includes dowsing, sacred geometry and the creation of sacred space. Places such as Stonehenge and Avebury, follow these principles and are associated with power points in the Earth, places for healing and spiritual growth.

Surveys

Geopathic stress can be detected in a variety of ways; the traditional method is by dowsing to survey land and building. This will locate the various sources of Earth energy including streams, ley lines, geomagnetic grid crossings, and indicate areas that are disrupted. A survey should include recommendations for correcting and balancing the energy wherever necessary; you should also be advised on maintenance.

Consultations

If you feel that you may be experiencing geopathic stress, then this can be diagnosed during a visit or by map dowsing. Some natural health practitioners are aware of geopathic stress and will indicate when there is evidence that is affecting the health or recovery of their patient. An Earth Acupuncturist will work on site to clear the area. Working with the land is important and honours the physical and spiritual relationship between humans and the Earth. Some practitioners specialise in certain aspects of geopathic stress and there is a tendency to work mainly with streams. It is helpful to find out if the practitioner is experienced with all the various sources. Recommendations may be given on the layout of your home and the long-term maintenance of the energy. You should also be advised if further treatment may be needed. You may be invited to become involved in the process, which is a positive way of working with the energy. People find this process connects them to the Earth, which in itself is therapeutic.

The benefits

Earth Acupuncture is a deep healing process which works in harmony with the land, transforming the energy of the earth into clear, harmonic resonances so that the land and those living there benefit from the generative energy, which nourishes us, supports our immune system and promotes good health and a sense of wellbeing.

EARTH ACUPUNCTURE

EARTH ACUPUNCTURE: Ali Northcott for consultations Tel. 0115 9856058. For more information about energy transformation and training in Geomancy try our website; www.earth-healing.co.uk. Also see features written by Ali Northcott on Earth Acupuncture, Geopathic Stress and Space Clearing. Main advert in the Feng Shui section.

Ali Northcott practises Feng Shui, Space Clearing and Earth Acupuncture. She has worked with Earth healing and energy transformation for over 11 year. Ali is currently running The Earth Healing School, providing training in Earth Wisdom and Geomancy. Tel 0115 985 6058.

The 64 hexagrams of the wisdom of the I-ching

The entire wisdom of the I-ching is expressed with eight basic trigrams; heaven, earth, water, fire, mountains, wind, lake and thunder, by pairing them to make hexagrams, or six line signs. This produces these 64 signs of wisdom.

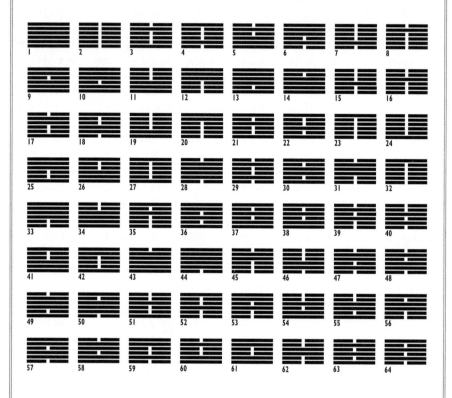

1 CREATION	17 FOLLOWING	33 RETREAT	50 CAULDRON
2 RECEPTION	18 REFINEMENT	34 POWER	51 SHOCK
3 DIFFICULTY	19 APPROACH	35 PROGRESS	52 KEEPING STILL
4 YOUTH	20 CONTEMPLATION	36 DARKENING	53 DEVELOPMENT
5 WAITING	21 BITING THROUGH	37 FAMILY	54 BRIDE
6 CONFLICT	22 GRACE	38 OPPOSITION	55 WANDERER
7 ARMY	23 DEPARTURE	39 OBSTRUCTION	57 WIND
8 UNION	24 RETURN	40 DELIVERANCE	58 THE JOYOUS
9 RESTRAINT	25 INNOCENCE	41 DECREASE	59 DISSOLUTION
10 TREADING	26 TAMING	43 BREAKTHROUGH	60 LIMITATION
11 PEACE	27 NOURISHMENT	44 MEETING	61 TRUTH
12 STANDSTILL	28 DOMINATION	45 GATHERING	62 DEFERENCE
13 FELLOWSHIP	29 UNFATHOMABLE	46 GROWING	63 COMPLETION
14 POSSESSION	30 OPPOSITION	47 OPPRESSION	64 NOTHINGNESS
15 MODESTY	31 INFLUENCE	48 THE WELL	
16 ENTHUSIASM	32 DURATION	49 REVOLUTION	

Education

Aspiring therapists seeking a career in Complementary Medicine (CM) may well ask 'Am I entering a minefield?' Sourcing a positive study and training programme may not be as easy as it appears for the would-be CM practitioner. The British Complementary Medicine Association has expressed alarm that the qualifications of teachers often fall short of what is required to ensure the health and safety of the public.

Complementary therapy courses are now being included in the curriculum of further education colleges but in some cases do not employ properly qualified practitioners in the subject being taught. Such studies are not official Government courses, but are vocational in origin. Often qualifications achieved are well below existing standards of individual BCMA member associations and less than 'A' level achievement, which puts their credibility in doubt. Tutors need a minimum of three years practical experience in the therapy they teach, yet some have no experience at all.

Courses offered by these colleges are usually short, between ten and 20 weeks, providing no more than 20 to 40 hours tuition. This compares with the recognised minimum of nine months and around 250 hours tuition for a single therapy.

For many Complementary and Alternative Therapies the minimum period of practical training is two years or more. This goes further than a theoretical study course in that it deals with patients' health problems, management, administration and supervision of clinics and therapy centres, records, report systems, assessments

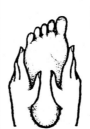

and customer care. It would seem that for some Further Education colleges filling classrooms to achieve a commercially viable curriculum takes precedence over safeguarding the health and safety of the public. This is inadmissible in such a sensitive area of the public domain. The result is that poorly trained and unqualified therapists are unleashed to practice on an unsuspecting public.

So, how does the aspiring therapist plot a course through this malaise? While there are National Occupational Standards (NOS) in Complementary Medicine which have been established by the Care Sector consortium, these apply to Aromatherapy, Reflexology, Homeopathy and Hypnotherapy only.

Training in these therapies at Level 3 and Level 4 are equivalent to 'A' Level or above. They meet the criteria laid down by the Government for practitioners in the UK and provide a common basis for standards of good practice. There are many other therapies for which no recognised NOS standards exist. Beauty therapy, for example, has an NVQ in basic Aromatherapy, but this is a beauty treatment only and does not qualify the beautician to treat patients' health problems.

National Occupational Standards differ from professional and educational standards. Professional standards, codes of conduct and guidelines usually focus on individual practitioners. Education and training standards are designed to provide direction and guidance to those who offer education and training. By contrast, NOS are concerned with the outcomes which individuals have to achieve when they are delivering services to users. The range of therapies available in the UK is extensive. Let us look more closely at some of them:

ACUPUNCTURE is a traditional Chinese medicine based on the idea that the body has

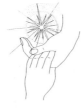
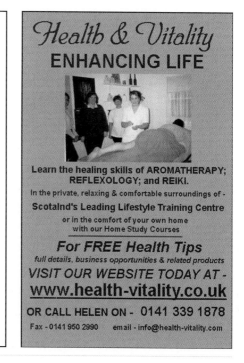

a network of energy pathways called 'meridians'. Illness is seen as a blockage or imbalance of energy along the meridians. Fine, sterile needles and / or moxibustion (burning herbs) are used to gently stimulate certain energy points in order to regulate energy flow and restore health.

AIKIDO means 'way of spiritual harmony'. Its founder, martial arts expert Morihei Uyeshiba, consolidated martial arts techniques and perfected the fundamental religious philosophy into 'Aikido', making it a true spiritual discipline.

ALEXANDER TECHNIQUE is an educational approach to a sensible use of the body, which can help many problems, such as back, neck and shoulder pain, stress related conditions and fatigue. By showing the client how to release unwanted tension, the Technique enhances their overall sense of balance and well-being.

ALLERGY THERAPY is used to diagnose a patient's allergies. There are various methods of diagnosing an allergy. Once the cause has been found, the foods or substances, which cause the allergy, can be eliminated from the diet or environment alternatively, treatments to neutralise the allergy may be used.

AROMATHERAPY employs aromatic essences ('essential oils') extracted from wild or cultivated plants for beauty treatments and therapies to improve health and prevent disease. They are administered by massage, inhalation, compressions and in baths.

ASTROLOGY is the study of planetary influence on human affairs. Astrologers use this knowledge to guide people in an understanding of their talents, challenges, and to highlight favourable or less favourable times to come.

AYURVEDIC MEDICINE is the traditional medicine of India. It incorporates medicinal, psychological, cultural, religious and philosophical concepts. The system aims to balance

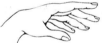

the elements and energies of the body. The wide range of treatments may include herbal medicine, exercises, diet, breathing techniques, massage and yogic cleansing.

BACH FLOWER REMEDIES offer a simple, safe and effective system of medicine to promote emotional wellbeing. It is a system of 38 flower remedies, formulated from the flowers of wild plants and trees. Each remedy treats a different emotional state.

THE BOWEN TECHNIQUE is a simple and gentle form of 'hands on' therapy that is safe and effective for people of all ages. It is a series of gentle movements on the muscles and connective tissues along the whole body, using the thumb and fingers. There is no manipulation or adjustment of hard tissue and treatment is gentle, subtle and relaxing.

BUQI uses natural human forces, which one develops through exercise. Buqi healers consider self healing a precondition to heal others. Treatment is without touch or by lightly touching the patient. Healing force is sent to the meridians of the patient enabling the practitioner to expel negative factors.

CHINESE HERBAL MEDICINE treats the person as a whole in order to maintain general health as well as treating the particular condition. It is frequently used in conjunction with acupuncture. Herbs based on prescriptions used and tested over thousands of years are specially adapted to suit the individual.

CHIROPRACTIC healthcare is concerned with the diagnosis, treatment and prevention of biomechanical disorders of the muscular skeletal system. Treatment consists of a range of manipulative techniques designed to improve the function of the joints, relieving pain and muscle spasm.

COLONIC HYDROTHERAPY is a method of cleansing the large intestine using purified water to flush away toxic waste, gas, accumulated faecal matter and mucus deposits.

COLOUR THERAPY is a subtle art using the healing energy of the colour spectrum or coloured light for therapeutic purposes. There are various ways in which a therapist may determine which colour a person needs and ways in which the colour may be administered, e.g. being bathed in coloured light.

COMPLEMENTARY MEDICINE complements allopathic methods of medicine; not to be confused with an alternative treatment, and encompasses a wide array of therapies.

COUNSELLING & THERAPY involves the Counsellor listening to, caring and supporting the client. Generally, Counsellors will not give advice, but rather help the client to understand how they can help themselves.

CRANIO-SACRAL THERAPY is based on the discovery that every cell in a healthy body expresses a rhythmic movement, which is fundamental to life known as Cranio-Sacral motion. Therapists are trained to feel this subtle motion in the body. They use their hands to reflect back to the body the pattern it is holding.

EASTERN HERBAL MEDICINE is a body of knowledge and practices that maintains health and endevours to restore it whenever it is lost.

FENG SHUI can be simply translated as meaning 'environment' but more usually, it refers to the 'feel' of a place. The art of Feng Shui takes its omens from the earth and, through a structured approach gives ways of balancing and harmonising the features and elements of a home, workplace, public building or of a wider environment.

FLOATATION CENTRES provide a pool or tank filled with ten inches of warm water saturated with Epsom salts. The pool is enclosed in a sound and lightproof cubicle. The saline solution supports the body so it floats without any effort. This combined with the warmth, peace and darkness enables deep relaxation.

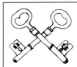

FLOWER & TREE ESSENCE THERAPY 'Vibrational' or 'Energy Medicine' is a combination of flower remedies / essences and gem elixirs which contain the vibrational frequency, or 'life force' of the flower, crystal or mineral being used. Essences are taken orally to rebalance the system and restore harmony.

HEALING is given through hands or thought, without manipulation or the use of instruments, drugs or remedies. Healing is the balancing of energies within the body, mind and spirit. In well-trained hands, this profound system of medicine is both powerful and gentle.

HERBAL MEDICINE is the practice of using plants to treat and prevent disease. Herbal formulas have three basic functions; elimination and detoxification, health management and maintenance, and health building. Treatment may be given in the form of fluid extracts, tinctures, tablets or teas.

HOMOEOPATHY is based on the principle of using like to treat like. A substance, which in large quantities causes the symptoms of an illness, can be used in an extremely diluted form to relieve the same symptoms. Derived mainly from plants and minerals, homoeopathic remedies are safe, effective and non-addictive. The practitioner administers remedies tailored to the individual.

HYPNOTHERAPY is a combination of two words hypnosis, in which a trance state is induced, and therapy, which is where problems and conflicts are resolved. Trance is a state of deep relaxation where learning and openness to change are most likely to occur. A person in a trance is fully conscious during a session and is always fully in control of their actions and thoughts.

INDIAN HEAD MASSAGE is a safe and highly beneficial therapy, which uses Ayurvedic

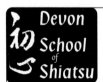

Healing system techniques to reduce stress, rebalance energy flows and leave the receiver soothed, comforted and revitalised.

IRIDOLOGY pronounced eye-ridology is a study of how the health of the body and its organs are reflected in the eye.

KINESIOLOGY is a manipulative therapy which uses 'muscle testing' to discover and correct energy blockages and imbalances within the body. The practitioner uses light touch, deep massage and gives dietary advice. Kinesiology is a system of treatment based on the principle that certain muscle groups are related to specific parts of the body.

LIGHT TOUCH THERAPIES could be described as those therapies that are non intrusive and that are able to restore equilibrium structurally, energetically and emotionally.

MANUAL LYMPHATIC DRAINAGE uses a range of specialist and gentle rhythmic pumping techniques to move the skin in the direction of the lymph flow. It can be used as a preventative or as a remedial therapy.

MASSAGE aims to improve and maintain body systems. Stress causes muscle tensions and chemical reactions: The therapeutic touch of trained hands can release tension, improve circulation, assist the drainage of toxic waste and leave one feeling relaxed.

McTIMONEY CHIROPRACTIC differs from other types of manipulation. McTimoney Chiropractic comprisies a variety of techniques using only the hands of the practitioner. It is renowned for its gentle approach. At every consultation the whole body is assessed and treated as needed. McTimoney Chiropractic is also used to help animals.

MEDITATION is one of the oldest relaxation techniques. Quietening the mind can quiet the body. A relaxed meditative mental state has a corresponding effect on the body.

METAMORPHIC TECHNIQUE is a simple massage technique of the feet, hands and head that helps to promote self-healing and personal growth. The practitioner acts as a catalyst. The power of life within guides the person's innate intelligence to discover which direction they wish to take in their lives.

NATUROPATHY is a compilation of a wide variety of natural measures used to restore the body's own healing potential through nutrition, fasting, vitamins, minerals, manipulation, exercise and relaxation. It is based on a belief in the healing power of nature and views the individual as an integrated whole.

NEURO LINGUISTIC PROGRAMMING (NLP) is the science and art of personal change. It teaches using the mind in powerful and effective ways to bring about results in all areas of life. NLP can create changes in thought patterns, feelings and reactions, leading to a more positive outlook and increased self-confidence.

NUTRITIONAL THERAPY is the science of working out what nutrients are right for you. Concentrating on your symptoms, your lifestyle and your diet a nutritional therapist will design a program for you including dietary and supplement recommendations, as the belief is you are what you eat.

OSTEOPATHY is a manipulative therapy, which focuses on keeping the body in structural balance so it can heal itself. The spine and joints are manipulated to restore the bones, muscles, ligaments and nerves to their true alignment and so restore health.

PAST LIFE REGRESSION By the use of deep relaxation and guided visualization, one is able to recover memories of a life one appears to have lived before. These past life memories can be vivid or simply impressions of a different time, place and personality. Phobias, unexplained fears and physical pain can be released, and patterns of behavior explained.

PILATES is a unique and versatile form of body conditioning that works the body through variable resistance on a series of mat and stretching exercises. Pilates Method unifies the eastern emphasis on mental concentration and the western emphasis on physical activity.

POLARITY THERAPY uses gentle touch and pressure applied to the reflex points on the 'meridians', or 'energy lines', of the body. Subtle energy blockages are released, restoring balance and vitality. Exercise, counselling and diet aid the process of healing.

PSYCHOTHERAPY is a process of self-discovery based upon a caring and supportive relationship between therapist and client. By exploring the sources of emotional conflicts and stress, and gaining insight into unique strengths and abilities, one can learn to live a more meaningful life.

QIGONG is the phonetic transcription of two Chinese characters. Qi means air which represents energy flowing through the body, Gong is the great effort put into the Qi practice. The system now referred to as QiGong consists of specific movements and patterns that bring an increased sense of health and well-being.

EDUCATION

'BREATHING SPACE: TRAINING & SUPPORT' provides Tailor Made Programmes for individuals, groups and teams in areas such as Personal And Professional Development, Life Coaching, Stress Management, Relaxation, Reiki (all levels), Self Help Skills. Tel/Fax 015395 36995

BURTON MANOR COLLEGE, Burton, Neston, Cheshire, CH64 5SJ. Residential/Non-Residential/Day Courses. Diploma in Aromatherapy starting October 2000. Also Post Graduate courses for Aromatherapists plus wide range of Complementary Health courses. For brochure contact. Tel: 0151 3365172. e-mail: enquiry@burtonmanor.com

LOOKING FOR A COURSE in complementary medicine with recognised qualifications leading to a career? The Bristol School offers high quality training in Aromatherapy and Reflexology. Contact us on (0117)9874430 Or www.coursesltd.com

RADIONICS is a method of healing at a distance through the medium of ESP. A trained practitioner can discover the cause of disease within living systems, human beings, animals or plants. Suitable therapeutic energies can then be made available to the patient to help restore optimum health.

REBIRTHING or 'Breath-work' is a term covering breath By simply changing one's normal breathing pattern slightly, in an easy to learn and safe way, it is possible to obtain deep relaxation and an opening of the mind. Breath-work is designed to be used as a tool for personal healing and well-being.

REFLEXOLOGY practitioners work on reflex points of the feet to correct imbalances in the body. Reflexology is preventative care, which improves blood circulation, removes toxins / impurities friary the lymph system, balances the whole body, revitalises energy and reduces tension and the symptoms of stress.

REIKI is the Japanese term, which translates as 'Universal Life Energy'. Reiki makes it possible for a person to re-attune to the Universal Life Force enabling them to heal themselves, other people, animals and plants.

ROLFING is the sculpture of human structure. In a Rolfing session the practitioner works with his hands to untangle the web of tissues, while the client is asked to relax and assist by making slow movements.

SHIATSU uses non-invasive manipulation methods to stimulate the circulatory and lymphatic systems, releasing their energy flow to the organs, muscles and joints, thus promoting healthy function and flexibility.

SPINAL TOUCH is a gentle therapy to restore postural balance. Posture is assessed to see where the body has stress or strain. Then, by using light touch on specific points, correction takes place. It is painless and does not involve manipulation of bones but corrects muscle tension and distortion to help a wide range of complaints.

STRESS MANAGEMENT is holistic and a number of techniques such as hypnosis, behaviour therapy, bio-feedback and massage may be combined with advice on diet and exercise. 'Cognitive Restructuring' is also used, which is a method that teaches new ways of interpreting what they themselves and others do and say. Practitioners have a wide variety of approaches and put varying emphasis on treatments.

T'AI CHI CHUAN is a Taoist inspired martial art developed within China, which aims to cultivate vital energy and economy of strength. T'ai Chi builds energy and reduces tension. It allows fuller breathing, which promotes body lightness.

TRAGER is an intuitive method of body-mind work. Practitioners use light, gentle, non-intrusive hand and mind movements to break up and release deep seated physical and mental patterns that restrict the muscles range of movement. Trager is practised in a relaxed meditative state. Tragering offers a feeling that the body and mind are integrated and together can effect positive changes in physical and other areas of life.

VOICEWORK is a term covering various ways of exploring oneself through listening and making vocal sound. It includes singing, chanting, improvisation, breathing techniques, bodywork, visualisation, ear training and other methods. Sound can help to rebalance the body and create exhilarating recharging effects.

YOGA originated in India where it was linked with philosophy and spirituality. The yoga student's aim is to reach harmony within their self, mind, body and spirit. Yoga is relaxing and reduces stress. It involves breathing and stretching exercises.

ZERO BALANCING is a hands on skill and a non-invasive means to restore and maintain wellbeing. Using held stretches and pressure from the fingers, tension is released from deep within.

Emotional Detox

By Louise Smart

Emotional detox is a healing process. It is about assisting people to recognise and release limiting negative beliefs about themselves. Negative beliefs are accompanied by painful emotions and fears.

The flawed self-concept is mirrored back to us in the outside world of relationships and materiality. We magnetise ourselves to people and circumstances that confirm what we believe about ourselves. If we want better lives we have to start changing from within.

We need to embrace the fact that we are a combination of masculine, feminine and childlike qualities. When any of these have been injured, abused or criticised we can unwittingly develop an unwhole concept of ourselves.

This can happen at any age but it often starts in childhood when we are more vulnerable due to obvious dependencies. We look to parents and parent figures for love, approval and protection. We often don't get what we need and start projecting that need in varying degrees onto our adult relationships and partners.

Although we want love, respect and approval, we subconsciously don't expect to get them, or can't accept or trust them when we do get them. So we keep re-running the cycle of pain. Because we lack trust due to mistreatment we sometimes mistreat others before they have the chance to do it to us. This is an abberated form of self protection.

People and events confirm our conscious and unconscious beliefs about ourselves, especially our sense of self worth. We tend to create circumstances or be attracted to people repeatedly that precipitate the same emotional pain. Even if we change jobs or move away from difficult situations or relationships we find that if we really look at our lives we see that situations get repeated, only with different people.

When we claim responsibility for what we create, we can see we have used our power against ourselves. This might annoy to begin with but, when we fully accept the situation, it can give the impetus to use our power positively and to cease seeing ourselves as victims of circumstances. We heal by changing our concept of ourselves to being loveable and valuable and worthy of respect. We have to learn how to love ourselves unconditionally. I do this by connecting people to the feeling of love, appreciation and adoration that they have for an animal, object, nature or person and direct that feeling back to their own heart centre and then the whole body. It starts as visualisation and turns into a real feeling of warmth and security. My healing process encourages the acknowledgement of anger, pain, grief, frustration and other emotions that have been repressed. Healing comes through a process of recognition, acceptance and release of pain and the release of the idea that love is something that has to come from someone. When we do this we become more energised, confident and powerful in creating the life we want. It creates an inner sense of self worth and emotional security.

Environmentally Friendly Products & Services

By M. Wilcocks Ph.D.

Why should we buy and use environmentally friendly products? The answer is best explained by describing the damage done to the ozone layer and acid rain. Governments, industry, transport and forestation management are aware of the damage pollutants cause to the density of the ozone layer and the devastating affects of polluted rain, but put profit before these considerations.

The ozone layer above us in the stratosphere protects the Earth from the harmful effects of ultra-violet radiation from space. Since 1984 scientists have been warning of the damage and the consequences to human life. It was in 1984 that a large hole was discovered in the ozone layer. For ten years afterwards the scientists stated that the use of chlorofluorocarbons (CFCs) in products discharged into the atmosphere could cause serious damage to the ozone layer, but it was difficult to prove.

The chemical companies which had most to lose if CFCs were banned mounted a strong denial of the suggestion and insisted that CFCs were quite safe, so little was done to reduce their use.

In October 1987 scientists were surprised again when the hole over Antarctica reached the same size as the USA. This increase in size led some scientists to demand immediate action to stop CFCs being used worldwide.

However, there is a long delay between CFCs being released into the air, and their arrival in the stratosphere. It can take many years for the gasses to reach the stratosphere, and hundreds of years before they are naturally destroyed. This means we may have to live with the consequences of past pollution for many years to come.

Apart from CFCs, which are now used far less frequently in the developed world than they used to be, two other 'greenhouse' gasses have a bad effect on ozone – nitrous oxide and methane.

Nitrous oxide breaks down and destroys ozone, while methane actually creates more ozone but in the wrong part of the atmosphere. The methane generates more ozone in the tropopause, which is below the stratosphere, and this layer can hide the holes in the stratosphere above it.

Why should we be bothered about the ozone layer anyway? Well, the importance of ozone is that it acts like a sun block, filtering out dangerous ultra-violet rays from the sun. Humans and animals exposed to excessive U.V light can develop cancers, their skin ages more quickly and their immune systems are impaired. Crops also seem to be damaged by extra U.V. Some forms of soya bean, an increasingly important crop, suffered a 25 per cent decrease in yield when their exposure to U.V. B rays was increased by 25 percent.

In the seas it has been found that phytoplankton, the foundation of the ocean food chain, are vulnerable to high exposure to U.V rays, as are some fish larvae. Since the human population acquires much of its food – especially protein from fish – from the oceans, damage to the phytoplankton might result in a massive reduction in fish stocks and the loss of an important food source.

Finally, and possibly most worrying is the possibility that in the future the ozone layer will start to let very harmful U.V-C rays reach the surface of the Earth. At the moment the layer stops all U.V-C from reaching us. We know that U.V-C can alter and destroy DNA and proteins. We can only guess at the consequences for the human race if our DNA was exposed to U.V-C for long periods.

Acid rain – the affects and causes

All rain is slightly acidic, but the term acid rain is used to describe rain that has mixed with a range of industrial pollutants and become far more acidic that normal.

Airborne pollutants such as sulphur dioxide, nitrogen oxides and assorted hydrocarbons react in the air with sunlight and water to form nitric acid, sulphuric acid and assorted other mineral acids and ammonium salts. The resultant acidic water can be carried thousands of miles by the wind before it falls to earth as rain, snow, fog or as dry particles which settle out due to gravity.

The biggest source of 'acid rain' chemicals that pollute the atmosphere is the burning of fossil fuels. Fossil fuels were created from organic (animal and plant) material that died millions of years ago. The original material was full of carbon, and its decay created sulphur; the coal, oil and gas we burn today is rich in hydrocarbons and sulphur. We burn these fuels in power stations to make electricity, in factories and oil refineries to make plastics and similar products, and in our vehicles which produce huge amounts of nitrogen and carbon gasses.

In recent years there have been some efforts to reduce the amount of pollutants that we pump into the air, but these efforts have been too small and too late to stop vast amounts of damage occurring across the world. Even though we know that acid rain is dangerous to us and the planet, we carry on producing the chemicals that cause it.

In some parts of the world scientists have recorded rain that is more acidic than vinegar. Animals, plants, and even some rocks cannot survive when they come into contact with something so acidic. In Greece, the famous Parthenon is being dissolved by the rain that lands on the rocks from which it is made. In India, the Taj Mahal is suffering the same problem.

In Sweden, over 18,000 lakes have become so acidic due to acid rain that all the fish have died. Some success has been achieved by dumping vast quantities of limestone into the lakes, because these rocks destroy the acid, but for most of the lakes it will be many years after we stop producing acid rain before the water returns to normal.

In what used to be called West Germany the government discovered that more than 70,000 square kilometres of forests had died because of acid rain. In the old East Germany, the damage was even worse due to factories creating much more pollution.

It is not always the country that produces the pollution that suffers from the aid rain. For example, industrial pollution from the UK is blown across the sea and falls as acid rain over Norway and Sweden.

Acid rain is not just a European problem; it occurs around the world. In North America thousands of lakes along the eastern coast are so acidic that fish cannot survive any longer, and at least ten percent of the lakes in the Adirondack region have a pH value of five or less – a pH of 7 is neutral, pure water. Lower values are acidic, higher values are alkaline.

In the Appalachian Mountains a World Resources Institute report in the late 1980s stated that the acidity of clouds on the mountains was 100 times greater than it would be if it wasn't polluted. In consequence, trees were dying.

With all this damage, why do we still produce so much pollution and continue to tolerate acid rain? Well, it's basically because governments don't consider it important enough. They believe that other things are more important, such as making sure that industry continues to grow and that the prices of goods are kept as low as possible.

Making factories cleaner costs money, and unless everyone does it, the clean factories won't be able to make goods as cheaply as the dirty ones, and will make less money. Developed countries also make huge profits from the exploitation and sale of the fuels that produce the pollution.

The technology exists to run all our cars and lorries on other 'cleaner' fuels, but the oil companies wouldn't want that to happen and neither would the governments which tax the oil companies!

I hope that this explanation will encourage you to think 'environment' when you next shop.

What should I buy to help the environment

GAS: Get professional advice on size and need. Size is one of the most important factors affecting efficiency. Too big a system wastes money and operates inefficiently.

WASHING MACHINES: Look for features that use less water, are front loading, have automatic water level and powder adjustments, and have a large capacity to minimise use.

WINDOWS: Lock windows that reduce heat loss in colder weather.

LIGHT BULBS: Buy the energy type; they cost a little more but save you money in the long run and are kinder to the environment.

DISHWASHERS: Look for features that will reduce water use.

REFRIGERATORS: Refrigerators with a freezer compartment on top are the most efficient.

INSULATION: Ceiling insulation alone can reduce heating costs by between 10-20 per cent.

NO OTHER ENVIRONMENTALLY FRIENDLY WASHING PRODUCTS ARE MORE EFFECTIVE & 'DOWN TO EARTH'.

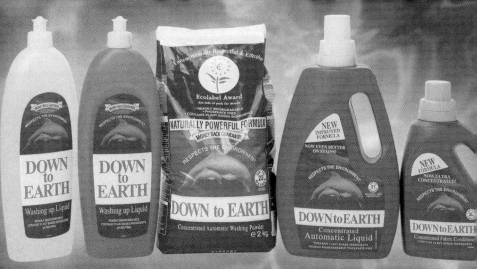

Phosphate-free and readily biodegradable, Down to Earth contains plant derived ingredients

help protect the environment, while optimising performance. It's therefore no surprise

we are the only washing powder to be independently judged and awarded the Eco label by

European Union. If you would like to find out more about how to help

environment, call the DOWN TO EARTH GREENLINE, FREEPHONE 0500 646645 (UK o

Equine Sports Massage

By Tina Ricketts, Dip Equine Sports Massage

The art of massage has been used for centuries, in more recent years much research has been carried out as to the benefits of massage for human athletes. As the horse is considered an athlete in the equine field, why should they not receive massage?

The horses muscle mass is 45 to 55 per cent of its body weight, these muscle undergo extreme work, and various muscle groups will be called into action depending on the disciple the horse is performing, this will also influence how the muscle is working. The dressage horse for example will be working with the muscle is a static formation, which is very exhausting for the muscle.

Some of the benefits therefore to the horse from massage are: Enhance circulation and lymphatic flow to the area of massage; Stretching of muscle fibres; To aid in the removal of waste products; Restore mobility between tissues; Increase or decrease muscle tone.

Massage for horses can be used both pre and post competition and as part of the horses training regime. It is important to ensure that your equine massage therapist is a member of a profession organisation, this offers the therapist, continual developmental training, insurance, and reassurance for the owner that this person has been professionally trained. Members will also work with permission of the animal's veterinary surgeon. Healthy muscles, allow the horse to perform at it's maximum potential with freedom of movement.

Facial Reflex Therapy

By Lorraine Myers

Facial Reflex Therapy has developed over a number of years, and combines techniques from several better known healing arts, such as reflexology, kinesiology, acupressure and ayurvedic face massage.

The result is an effective, relaxing method of stimulating healing on all levels. The person receiving FRT often sleeps or deeply relaxes during the treatment, and often reports feeling like they have had a total body massage. A further unexpected benefit of Facial Reflex Therapy is one of general anti-ageing. Aside from a relief of symptoms, clients have experienced improvements in skin texture and facial symmetry, with lines and wrinkles reducing, puffiness beneath the eyes lessening, and the face generally looking and feeling 'lifted'.

Facial Reflex Therapy balances mind, body and spirit by accessing the many different healing reflexes in the face neck and scalp. It has been developed over the last decade by fully qualified multi-skilled practitioners of the healing arts and combines theories from traditional healing such as acupressure, kinesiology and reflexology, as well as more recent discoveries within the realms of quantum healing, to bring you effective, enjoyable and visibly beneficial treatment.

In the same way that reflexology treats all levels of a person, by working on the feet, Facial Reflex Therapy effectively stimulates via the face, neck and scalp. It achieves this by using tiny massage like movements, acupressure, tension releasing techniques and other powerful reflexes that clear energy blocks and allow healing to take place. Specific health problems and emotional stresses can be eased, as well as relieving localised pain and tension locked into the neck, shoulders and jaw.

A typical course of treatments to treat a specific health disorder may take between two and six hourly sessions, although the beauty benefit of this soothing, relaxing therapy can be noticed in the face immediately. Each treatment can take many forms and, as with all truly holistic therapies, it tends to peel layers of stress, tension and ill health away. For example, the first session often works on releasing built-up layers in the neck and scalp, which instantly improves posture and wellbeing. Although this rejuvenating side effect can become apparent from the initial consultation, it can take several treatments to improve specific health problems.

During further treatments, a variety of other methods are employed to reactivate the body's healing ability, to improve not just symptomatic problems but the whole constitution. Throughout each session, it is common for the individual to feel either very energised or deeply relaxed. Although the anti-ageing benefits of Facial Reflex Therapy are highly desirable, any improvements in how a person appears is a visible sign that healing on a deeper level is taking place.

Fairbane's Holistic Approach

By Eileen Fairbane

Fairbane's Holistic Approach is truly effective in that it looks at all aspects of health whether it is the mind body or the spirit. The relationship between the mind, body and spirit is so intricate that no single treatment or formula focused only on one of those aspects can achieve balance between them.

Disharmony occurring in any one of these areas causes an upheaval in the body's systems and results in stressful symptoms.

Life is full of ups and downs, and many of the downs can be addressed if we first establish our foundations.

We are all different, as are our problems whether it be in family relations or marital issues, low self-esteem or physical conditions like migraine, hormonal imbalance, lack of sleep or the need for a better understanding of yourself.

It was for this reason that I established The Foundation for Living encompassing the following techniques, therapies and activities: Gold psychotherapeutic counselling therapy, breathing, exercise, movement and dance therapy classes, cookery classes, detox therapy, aromatherapy, pressure point, body alignment healing, meditation and retreats abroad.

How does the Foundation for Living operate?

Very simply! If you have a presenting challenge all you have to do is telephone to make an appointment for a consultation, which takes about 20 minutes to half an hour. At this point a suggested programme would be offered over a period of time which would normally involve one-hour sessions. During this time, an action plan would be discussed to cover the presenting challenge and progress will be monitored.

Training in the Foundation for Living method

Different levels of training are offered. Depending upon which area you are interested in, whether it be as a teacher, practitioner or both, there are training modules available. This could be anything from three months to two years. On completion of the training you will receive a diploma according to which module you have successfully completed.

Fairbane's Holistic approach is a gentle, but focused method which moves forward the ever presenting challenges of life. It is a positive approach which supports the client in making his or her own choices. It builds on rapport and individuals need. People who have used this method find it useful in everyday life. It allows the flexibility of stuck situations to arrive at a positive outcome. In discovering harmony you may find interesting and enjoyable paths on the way.

Eileen Fairbane

Cert. Ed Mifa., Dip NLP., Dip GPC

**FAIRBANE'S HOLISTIC APPROACH
A FOUNDATION FOR LIVING**

Offers Treatment Sessions in London.
Week-end Seminars, Seasonal & Wheat Free Cooking, Retreat Trips Abroad,
Training, Weekly Classes in Breathing, Exercise, Movement and Dance

Call **020 8450 2470** or **0956 553924**
Visit the website at **www.eileenfairbane.co.uk**
e-mail **eileen-fairbane@supanet.com**

Feet First

By M Willcocks PhD

Three out of four us experience foot problems. However, we think the pain and discomfort is normal and few of us actually believe it could be something serious.

Yet foot pain, infections, bunions and corns often mask more severe problems like diabetes, arthritis, gout, anaemia, or even heart problems.

Those darling feet of ours are the hardest working but most overlooked and undervalued parts of our bodies.

The average person walking a mile exerts the equivalent of 64 tons on each foot. And the average person will have walked 115,000 miles in their lifetime. That's four times the circumference of the earth. If you are an avid jogger or walker, you put even more stress on those tootsies of yours.

Yes, our feet bear a heavy burden. But what do they get for their toil? A footbath? A monthly pedicure? A massage? Most of us give foot maintenance short shrift. When was the last time you pampered those pedals?

The feet are akin to plumbing: you never think about them until something goes wrong. Ah, but when things do go wrong those pads may be trying to tell you something. No sensible person wants to spend a lifetime walking around in pain, saddled with corns, bunions and in-growing toenails. But that's just what many are doing – trying to look chic or suave while hobbling about like a child in his father's shoes. But those lovely, fashionable shoes just don't look the same with a bandage wrapped around your ankle. If you've been pestered by foot problems here are some things you can do.

CORNS AND CALLOUSES: Corns and callouses are caused by excessive pressure on the feet. One of the chief causes of corns and callouses is inappropriate footwear. This is especially true for women who wear heels.

Heels place additional pressure on the toes and can cause problems not only with your feet, but your back as well. Studies at Harvard even suggest that high heels may cause knee osteoarthritis. So stay away from heels if you can.

What's that you say? It's just not practical for you to go without heels? Then wear shoes with lower heels. Or, if you must! wear heels take along a pair of flat-soled shoes to wear en route to work or that formal event. Then switch back to heels once you get there. While at your desk or at a restaurant table you can always just slip the heels off. This little exercise could save your knees and back, and possibly a trip to the Chiropractor.

Also be sure to buy shoes that give your toes room. Snug, tight-fitting shoes cause corns and callouses. Buy shoes that breathe – those made of canvas and leather. Plastic and vinyl do not breathe and can cause feet to sweat, which creates a breeding ground for bacteria and fungi. Look for flat shoes with thick-cushioned soles that support the arch and have rounded tips. Podiatrists suggest buying shoes late in the day since that's when your feet are their largest.

Replace worn shoes as soon as possible and try not to wear the same shoes each day.

To get rid of corns and callouses gently exfoliate the soles of your feet by rubbing them with a foot file or pumice stone. Next, place your feet in four pints of warm water. Add three ounces of raw, unfiltered apple cider vinegar and soak for 20 minutes. Thoroughly dry your feet after soaking to help prevent fungal growth. Moisturise the tops and bottoms of your feet with eucalyptus, bergamot, or peppermint oil. Repeat this pampering treatment two times a week until the condition gets better.

If you have corns, you will also need to place several drops of tea tree oil (ten per cent concentrate) on the affected areas each night until better.

BUNIONS: Bunions are enlargements of the joint at the base of the big toe. They result when the bone or tissue of the joint in the big toe move out of place. Bunions are typically caused by tight shoes, poor foot mechanics (i.e., the way we walk), foot injuries, or neuromuscular disorders. Several therapies can be used to help treat bunions:

• Massage therapy by a trained specialist — chiropractor or podiatrist.

• Hot Epsom salt footbaths with whirlpool to aid circulation.

• Apple cider vinegar footbaths (mentioned previously).

• Foot exercises. To soothe aching feet, fill and freeze a plastic soda bottle with water. Then roll your foot backward and forward over the bottle. To add strength, tone and resiliency to your feet, try placing a pencil on the floor and with each foot pick it up 10-12 times. Do this once a day.

• Footwear. Make sure to wear shoes that give your feet plenty of breathing room.

• Walk erect using proper posture, since poor posture can cause poor foot mechanics.

If you experience severe pain from bunions you should see a licensed health practitioner right away.

ATHLETE'S FOOT: Athlete's foot is a skin disease usually caused by a fungus. It typically occurs between the toes. The foot fungus that causes athlete's foot just loves dark, damp and warm places. So the shoes make for an excellent breeding ground. Natural treatment of athlete's foot includes:

• Tea tree oil (ten per cent concentration) or calendula salve may be rubbed on the infected area daily until the problem disappears.

• Grapefruit seed extract powder can be sprinkled on feet and into shoes to kill and prevent fungal growth. Use ten per cent concentrated powder twice a day. Also use grapefruit seed liquid extract on socks and in the laundry to kill fungus (since fungi often survive regular wash cycles).

• Take footbaths in apple cider vinegar.

• Keep feet and socks dry.

IN-GROWN TOENAILS: In-grown toenails occur when the nail (usually the outside edge) of the big toe grows into the surrounding soft tissue.

In-grown toenails typically result from either trimming the toenails too close or wearing improper footwear. To ease in-grown toenails you can:

• Bathe your foot in an apple cider vinegar footbath for 20 minutes and then apply tea tree oil to the affected area, packing a little loose cotton under the toenail where it bites into the flesh. This will help to lift the edge of the toenail away from the surrounding skin as the nail begins to grow. You will need to get a feel for how much to use and how far to insert the cotton. This procedure should not hurt, if it does then you've inserted the cotton too far. You should check and replace the cotton each day.

• Trim toenails carefully. When trimming your toenails be careful not to cut them too short and do not cut into the corners of the nail, only cut across the front of the nail. After you've trimmed them, smooth out toenails with an emery board or nail file.

• Use proper footwear. Always buy shoes that give your toes plenty of foot room.

Finally, if you want to maintain beautiful, healthy feet remember to inspect them regularly for the warning signs of foot trouble. Look for swelling, sores, cuts, and changes in colour. Also look for signs of infection such as thick or discoloured toenails, peeling or scaling skin on the soles of your feet. If you have persistent foot pain, have it checked out by a chiropractor or podiatrist. And if you are a diabetic, be sure to have a foot exam performed at least once a year. Remember 'those feet were made for walking' so look after the only pair you will ever have.

GINSENG
It's a root... it's a herb ... and it's been curing people's ills for centuries

The root of the ginseng has for centuries been reputed to be a panacea for cancer, rheumatism, diabetes, sexual debility, and aging.

The claims date back to ancient China, and the root was long of great value there.

Europe did not hear of it until 1642, when the explorer Alvaro Samedo returned with a report of the restorative properties of Oriental ginseng, which he claimed was being sold for twice its weight in silver.

Ginseng is a perennial herb of the genus Panax, in the family Araliceae. Asiatic ginseng, P. pseudoginseng, is native to eastern Asia.

Wild American ginseng, P. quinquefolius, is native to eastern woodlands. It stands up to two feet tall, has leaves up to six inches long, and bears greenish white flowers. Dwarf ginseng, P. trifolus, is a smaller American species.

In 1713, Emile Jartoux, a Jesuit cartographer working in northern China, reported ginseng's effectiveness and power among the Chinese. Another Jesuit, Joseph Francois Lafiteau, read the report in Quebec, and after a diligent search found in the woods near his mission an almost identical species, American ginseng.

Demand for the American root grew in China, and many colonists and settlers, including Daniel Boone, hunted it avidly. Millions of pounds were uprooted, dried, and exported in the China trade.

Eventually the slow-maturing plant was almost extinct. Cultivation began in the late 19th century, but the Chinese market balked at the cultivated American product, and many investments were lost.

Today China and Korea export ginseng to the West, where its popularity has grown in recent years.

Russian scientists claim to have found substances in ginseng that stimulate endocrine secretions and act as a tonic to the cardiovascular system. Medical research in the West, however, has failed to substantiate these claims.

Feng Shui

By The Feng Shui Society

Feng shui is an ancient Chinese discipline dating back at least 3,000 years, although its philosophy can be traced back to the teachings of the I Ching – from 6,000 years ago.

Feng Shui was first used to determine the best sites for tombs. Later it was used to site palaces, government buildings and monuments, until finally whole cities were designed and built according to Feng Shui principles. Over time, the classical practice of Feng Shui developed to include detailed observation of the living world and the way in which the earth's energy affects our daily lives.

Feng Shui remained an integral part of Chinese culture until recent times when Western influences and Communism relegated Feng Shui to a more superstitious and mystical practice and the Chinese in Hong Kong reduced its essence to helping businesses thrive.

Feng Shui was devised through the cultural paradigms of China, with its unique geography and rather stable social structure, which varies little from generation to generation.

Despite these origins, however, its core truths are central to human awareness and experience. When it is stripped of culture and ritual, and synthesised with other bodies of knowledge to meet the specific requirements of culture, geography climate, and human uniqueness, the essence of Feng Shui can be applied to any space and time.

What Feng Shui Is

Feng Shui means 'wind and water' – the two most powerful forces of nature – and the fundamentals of life. The underlying principle of Feng Shui is to live in harmony with your environment so that the energy surrounding you works for you rather than against you.

Feng Shui is a complex art involving many disciplines from site planning to psychology, based on the Chinese understanding of the dynamic flow of energy throughout the universe.

Feng Shui explains how the environment in which people live affects their lives. Beyond this, it is the art of using the environment to influence the quality of a person's life.

Ultimately, Feng Shui is a sound and sensible way of living with a conscious connection between our outside environment and our inner world.

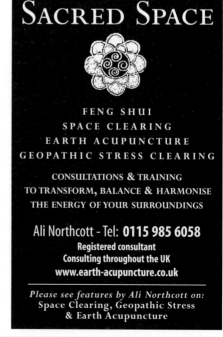

Feng Shui Today

Despite the fact that the Western World has not had the benefit of a consistent person-to-place philosophy through the ages, many people, on discovering Feng Shui, recognise things that they always knew deep down to be true. Many successful people practice some form of Feng Shui without realising it. The integration of the external world and our internal environment is a cornerstone of most traditional philosophies. Indigenous people all over the world have long understood that we are not separate from our planet, our homes, or one another.

In the West we have lost this connectedness with our earth and our environment and this lack of balance is a cause of much physical, mental, emotional and spiritual disease. Feng shui offers a means to reconnect and regain our balance, our health and our good fortune.

Feng Shui Principles

Here is a brief description of the essential principles at the heart of feng shui. In order to understand and practice feng shui, it is necessary to have a good understanding of these principles. These principles also underpin Chinese medicine, acupuncture, shiatsu, TCM (traditional Chinese medicine), herbalism – and philosophy. Any feng shui book will provide more detailed explanations. The most basic idea in Chinese philosophy, found in every one of its ancient arts and sciences, is the concept of yin and yang, the two opposing yet complementary cosmic forces that shape the universe and everything in it. Together yin and yang constitute a balanced whole known as Tao – or 'the way' – the eternal principle of heavenly and earthly harmony. Good, auspicious feng shui can only be created when there is balance and harmony between yin and yang.

YIN is dark, wet, quiet, soft, empty, cold, passive, moon, water, female, winter, night, and expanding, dispersing, delicate, vertical, thinner, bigger.

YANG is light, dry, loud, hard, full, hot, active, sun, fire, male, summer, day, contracting, gathering, durable, horizontal, thicker, smaller.

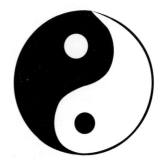

Everything in the universe contains varying degrees of yin and yang. Nothing is wholly yin or wholly yang. In the yin / yang symbol there is a seed of yang in the yin and a seed of yin in the yang. This symbolises the transient nature of yin and yang and emphasises that these two forces are always in a state of flux, thereby creating change, even as they interact.

The art of feng shui is the art of balancing these two energies within the landscape and interior environment

The Five Elements

The Feng Shui is greatly influenced by the theory of the five elements earth, wood, fire, metal, and water. These elements combine in different quantities to create all the permutations that are found in the forces of nature. A significant portion of feng shui practice is based on interpreting how these elements interact in the physical environment to create harmony or imbalance. The elements are involved in two kinds of cyclical relationship: the productive and the destructive cycles. In the productive cycle, fire produces earth, which produces metal, which produces water, which produces wood, which in turn produces fire. In the destructive cycle, wood breaks up earth, earth muddies water, water douses fire, fire melts metal and metal chops down wood. In interior decor, the elements are represented by colours, shapes and materials. When an environment needs balancing, one way to effect change is to add or subtract the colour, shape or material that each element expresses.

FIRE is red – pointed shapes, triangles, pyramids, diamonds, stars, zigzags, serrations and plastic.

EARTH is – yellow, brown – squares, squat, low, flat shapes, checks, horizontal shapes – clay, ceramics, plaster, china, bricks, fabrics, soft stone (e.g. limestone).

METAL is – white, gold, silver, spheres, circles, domes, arches, ovals, round shapes – stainless steel, brass, copper, bronze, iron, silver, gold, hard stone (e.g. marble, granite).

WATER is – black – wavy lines, amorphous, irregular or chaotic shapes – glass.

WOOD is – green, blue – rectangles, tall, thin, vertical shapes – wood, paper, wicker, bamboo, rush.

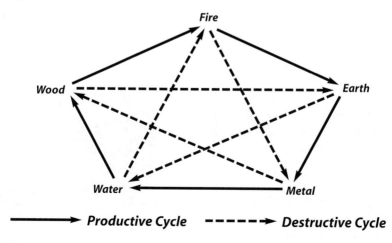

Therefore, understanding these two cyclical relationships and the symbolism of the elements enables feng shui practitioners to balance the elements within homes and workplaces.

For example, a metal wind chime in the west or northwest is auspicious, as these directions are associated with metal.

If you were born in a fire year, it is not advisable to have too much water in your home. Ponds, fountains, aquariums, and objects coloured black (the watercolour) should be avoided. This is because in the destructive cycle, water destroys fire. On the other hand, plants and green or blue objects, representing wood, are beneficial in the home, as in the creative cycle, wood creates fire. Also, your best bedroom location would be on the south side of the house – south being the fire direction.

Having too many plants in the home is not advisable if you were born in an earth year, because wood destroys earth. Instead, decorate with red objects and bright lights – fire energy – as fire produces earth. Since earth is the central element of the five, earth people can sleep in the centre of the home.

Chi

Chi is an energy that suffuses every particle of living and non-living matter. It is an energy that is finer and subtler than electric, magnetic or thermonuclear energies. In traditional Chinese culture, all matter is animated by and radiates chi.

The paths of chi flowing within the body are called meridians and manipulation of chi within these meridians forms the basis of acupuncture, acupressure and shiatsu. Practitioners of the Chinese martial arts such as chi kung or t'ai chi tap into the flow of chi within their bodies, rather than using aggressive force to overpower their opponents.

Feng shui is also concerned with harnessing chi and creating supportive environments by manipulating the chi within them. Chi can be stuck and stagnant or free flowing. It can be too fast or too slow. It can be too dispersed or too concentrated. A lot of the skill in feng shui depends on an ability to understand chi and perceive its effects within an environment.

Cutting Chi

As sharp edges and straight lines produce a harsh form of chi called cutting chi, feng shui creates ease and harmony by using flowing curves rather than geometric shapes, sharp angles and pointed objects or structures. There are, after all, no straight lines in nature.

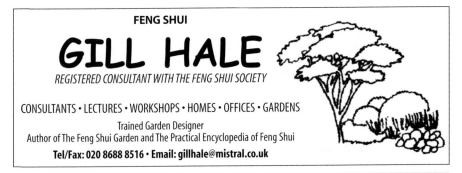

Cutting chi can be caused by straight roads, roofs, electricity pylons, the edges of furniture and buildings, crosses, protruding corners, overhead beams and so on.

An exercise to experience chi

Rub your palms together vigorously for about 15 seconds. As soon as you finish, place your hands six to ten inches apart, palm facing palm. Hold your hands at navel level and six to ten inches away from your body. Relax and you will feel a slightly magnetic pull of one palm toward the other.

If you have difficulty feeling this, slowly move your palms closer together and further apart until you do feel it. Play with that faint magnetic feeling for a while, first compressing it slightly, then pulling away. As you play with the magnetic feeling, the flow of chi will increase and become easier to sense.

Symbolism

Symbolism is very important in feng shui. Feng Shui is described in a completely allegorical manner using the symbolism of dragons, tigers, the elements of nature and so on. This makes it more widely accessible but, where the symbolism is culturally specific, it can also act as a barrier to understanding.

For example, the Chinese consider elephants to be wise, peaches to represent longevity and the colour white is associated with mourning. In Britain, elephants are more likely to be associated with long memory and white is the colour of purity and innocence.

We are surrounded by symbols. Everything in our homes says something about us and something to us. As these symbols can be very potent, it is important to use

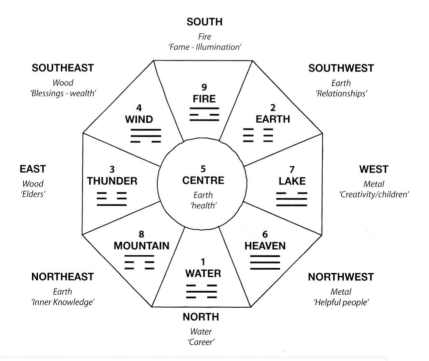

symbolism in a positive and life-enhancing way. Although symbolism acts at a subconscious level, we need to be aware of the messages our environments are giving us. In feng shui, it is important to understand which symbols are universal, which are cultural and which are particular to an individual, because they relate to some particular event in their past.

Feng shui uses pictures and ornaments in different areas of the pa kua to symbolise what is desirable in each aspect of your life.

Pa Kua

The pa kua is a grid which can be transported onto plans of your home, garden, workplace, and so on, to show which areas of the space under scrutiny relate to which aspects of your life.

There are two main ways to use the pa kua. It maybe placed onto floor plans by aligning it with the compass- north on the pa kua pointing to magnetic north on the plan.

An alternate method is the Three-Door Gate or Mouth of Chi. This takes the wall in which your front door is placed as a baseline. The pa kua is then positioned such that the side of the octagon that relates to the north is placed onto this baseline.

Change

Because the intangible forces that determine environmental balance are continually changing, practitioners of feng shui are constantly alert to change, whether man made or caused by natural phenomena. Feng shui is not static. It requires constant adaptation and to practice feng shui requires a good understanding of the cyclical nature of energetic change.

Types of Feng Shui

There are many different approaches to the practice of feng shui. Although the principles are the same, the applications of these principles can vary widely from one teacher or practitioner to another.

There are several reasons why feng shui practice varies so much. Firstly, feng shui developed over thousands of years and in several areas of the world. Many techniques were developed to deal with different situations and lifestyles. For example, feng shui as practised in rural China is different from the feng shui used in very densely populated Hong Kong. Also, as their skills and experience increased, feng shui masters developed their own techniques, based on their own observations. Today in the West, feng shui is still adapting and developing.

Traditional / classical / authentic feng shui

Form School and Compass School feng shui are two types of traditional feng shui. Form School examines shapes and symbolism in the environment without reference to compass directions. Compass School utilises the compass, pa kua, lo shu and feng shui formulae. Practitioners may consider this type of feng shui to be a science. Critics find it obscure, inappropriate or too literal.

Black Hat Sect Tantric Buddhist feng shui

Developed in the US 15 years ago by Thomas Lin Yun. It is a hybrid of Tibetan Buddhism, Taoism and feng shui, simplified for Western tastes. Has a huge cult following. Practitioners may be Buddhist or engage in Buddhist rituals and ceremonies.

Intuitive / modern / applied feng shui.

An interpretation of traditional feng shui adapted for the West. Can be practical and pragmatic but often has spiritual overtones. Most media coverage is of this type of feng shui. Criticism usually centres on the idea of feng shui as a new age religion.

So, to sum up, there is no such thing as generic feng shui. Although there are many similarities, everything you read or hear is coming from a particular style. These approaches aren't inherently right or wrong – good or bad – but some will be more appropriate for you and your circumstances.

Related Subjects

There are many disciplines that are similar or complementary to feng shui. It is often difficult to see clear distinctions between these subjects and in reality, the distinctions are not important. Feng shui is a small part of a much larger continuum concerning our health, our place in the universe and ultimately our evolution.

Feng Shui in Other Cultures

Feng shui is practised in many parts of the Chinese speaking world and many other cultures have their own equivalent of feng shui. Feng shui or something similar has traditionally been practised in China, Hong Kong, Singapore, Malaysia, Tibet, Vietnam, the Philippines, Indonesia, Bali, Japan, Hawaii and India and in Chinese-speaking communities all over the world.

Geomancy, which means 'to divine the earth spirit' is the science of putting man in harmony with nature and was widely practised in Europe until the late 1700s. The terms feng shui and geomancy are often used synonymously. Shamanism is also based on the ideal of living in

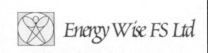

Energy Wise FS Ltd

Live in harmony with your environment and improve your health, wealth and happiness.

Private and Corporate Consultations
Feng Shui
Space Clearing
Energy Balancing

Registered Consultants
with the Feng Shui Society

Tel/Fax: 01344 752 633
01344 307 079
E-mail: energywisefs@hotmail.com
Website: www.energywisefs.com

harmony with nature. It states that all things in nature have a spirit with which shamans can communicate. This belief is common to many cultures including North American Indians, South American Indians, Tibetans, Indonesians, Australian Aborigines, Laplanders, Siberian Altai and many African tribes.

Astrology

There are many different types of Asian astrology from China, Japan, Tibet and India. Some systems, like feng shui, are based on the I Ching and are therefore naturally complementary to feng shui. Western astrology is based on charting the positions and movements of heavenly bodies. Chinese astrology tends to look to philosophy, the calendar, the cosmos and the rhythms of nature for its character descriptions and predictions for the future. Most people are familiar with popular Chinese astrology which uses a zodiac of 12 animals -rat, ox, tiger, rabbit, dragon, snake, horse, sheep, monkey, cock, dog, pig. As with Western astrology, the allocation of the zodiac animal is only the first step in a complex system of computations.

Space Clearing

The art of cleansing and consecrating buildings. Although this can mean physically removing dirt and clutter from our environments, it largely deals with clearing invisible energetic debris. Energy that is stuck, stagnant or left over from before and energetic entities such as ghosts.

Environmental Radiation

When considering feng shui placement, as well as chi energy, it is important to take into account the occurrence of natural and artificial electromagnetic energy, which can impact the health of those who encounter it. Unstable or disrupted naturally occurring electromagnetic radiation, emanating from the earth, can create harmful effects called geopathic stress. Man-made electromagnetic fields (EMFs) are generated by electrical equipment in our homes and offices, and sometimes need to be avoided.

Dowsing

Many feng shui practitioners use intuition during their feng shui analyses. Dowsing greatly enhances the understanding and effectiveness of feng shui because it allows dowers to gain access to their intuition. Meditation can also be used to enhance intuitive skills. Amongst other things, dowsing can be used to detect chi and earth energies and to help choose and devise feng shui cures.

Oriental Diagnosis, Physiognomy, Face-Reading, and Handwriting Analysis

These are techniques that examine the

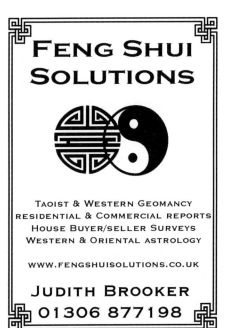

outward expression of our inner psyche by means of analysing our physical appearance, voice or handwriting. Some practitioners may use these techniques to support their feng shui analyses. These techniques are used in this supporting capacity as it is generally easier and more powerful, to change our environment than our handwriting.

Related Arts and Sciences

There are many other disciplines concerned with the larger environment and its affect on our biology. Some are concerned with ecological issues. These include environmental psychology and design; ergonomics; astronomy; Bau-Biologie; earth science; Gaja; natural or sustainable architecture and design and landscape /architecture.

Many of feng shui's most practical recommendations can be related back to the scientific principles underlying these subjects.

How Feng Shui Works

Often we are not consciously aware of the huge effect our home and work environments have on us. We think of buildings as being something in the background, unaware that they can substantially help or hinder our progress. We respond unconsciously without even knowing we are being affected.

When you look at your home, you are looking at an outer manifestation of your inner self. Everything in your outer life – especially your home environment – mirrors your inner self. Conversely, everything in your home has an effect on you, from the smallest ornament to the largest design structure.

It is all there in your home to be seen and felt. It couldn't not be there, because it all came from you in the first place. Consciously or unconsciously, you have chosen where you live, chosen everything in your home and positioned items wherever they are. It all has a significance and an effect. Your home is a living portrait of you and your life. So making changes in your home will create changes in your life.

Feng shui teaches you how to read the symbolism and energy of your home, and how to change it for the better. By adjusting and balancing the flow of energy within your home you can powerfully and effectively influence the course of your life.

Feng shui is a wonderful transformational tool that you can use to help you manifest the life you want. When you are clear about what you want, by consciously placing your desires and

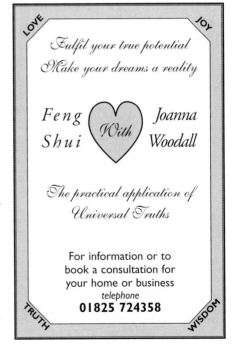

LOVE · JOY

Fulfil your true potential
Make your dreams a reality

Feng ♡ *With* *Joanna*
Shui ♡ *Woodall*

The practical application of
Universal Truths

For information or to
book a consultation for
your home or business
telephone
01825 724358

TRUTH · WISDOM

streetlights or telegraph poles, a church spire, or a long straight road aimed at your front door.

If any of these generators of cutting chi appear to be pointing at your front door, you should deflect their negative energy by placing a reflective object – such as a mirror -or other protective symbol, over the front door, facing outwards. Octagonal mirrors are used traditionally. Chinese people use eight-sided pa kua (or bagua) mirrors, which have the symbols of the I Ching around their perimeter.

STEP 2

Repeat the same process of checking for the back door and all your major windows. A word of warning – try not to energise too many sectors at once or you may find you are overwhelmed by change and you will be unable to see cause and effect.

STEP 3

Using a compass, and standing in your front door, determine the direction that your house faces. You can use an ordinary boy-scout compass. Ensure that you align the north pointing end of the needle with the northern point of the compass. (if you do not have a compass you may be able to work out the facing direction of your house from a street map.) Note this direction for later comparison with your personal best locations and directions.

STEP 4

If your home is neither square nor rectangular, check the outline of your home on your floor plan to see if there are any missing areas. This means an area on the pa kua, which does not correspond to a room or part of a room in your home.

This occurs when your home is L-shaped, for example. If you feel the missing life area is important to you then you should 'create' it by using mirrors. Mirrors placed on the walls of adjoining rooms will appear to 'fill in' the missing room space.

STEP 5

Place a pa kua diagram over a floor plan of each floor of your home using the compass directions to align it correctly. This indicates which areas of your home relate to which areas of the pa kua and of your life.

Check your kitchen. Make sure that your food preparation area does not involve you standing with your back to the door. If it does, try to reorganise the kitchen so that the door is visible from where you usually stand at the main food preparation area or use a mirror to reflect the door.

intention in your physical environment, your surroundings are able to support you rather than work against you.

How to Feng Shui Your Home

STEP 1

Stand at the front door and look outwards. See if you can identify any large structure or object pointing towards you, generating what feng shui refers to as cutting chi. These can be a neighbour's satellite dish, tall trees,

STEP 6

Ascertain which of the eight life areas you wish to improve or energise. To energise an area, use feng shui cures of the correct energetic type. For example, if you want to energise the wealth area, which is in the south east, and associated with the element wood, you need to place wood symbols, such as growing plants, in this area.

You can also use the element of water – which supports wood energy. You should avoid using metal energy – which destroys wood energy.

STEP 7

Ensure that there is no element conflict between the elements of fire and water in the kitchen. In other words, ensure that your stove (fire) is not directly facing or adjoining your sink, fridge, dishwasher or washing machine (water). If this occurs, try to relocate your appliances or use wood symbols between the fire and water energy

Step 8

Examine your entrance way and make sure that nothing blocks the smooth flow of chi through your front door and its accumulation immediately inside.

Any clutter and other obstructions immediately inside or outside your door should be removed. If possible the path from your gate to your front door should curve.

Finally check the direction of the 'mouth' of each of your cooking appliances – your oven, microwave, steamer, rice cooker, and so on to see that it faces ideally in one of your best directions. The 'mouth' of the appliance is at the front, for example, the oven door.

STEP 9

Check the lounge and dining room. Try to make sure that any mirrors in these rooms reflect the food on your table to 'double your prosperity'.

STEP 10

Check your bedroom. Make sure that nothing is suspended above your bed or threatens you subconsciously, such as overhead built-in cupboards or hefty pictures above the bed. Ensure that you can't see yourself in any mirror when you are in a sitting position in your bed.

If so, move the mirrors, cover them up, or angle them away from the bed. Make sure that the head of the bed has a solid support behind it, and is not located under a window. Arrange your bed so that your feet are not pointing out of the door of the bedroom.

STEP 11

Check the locations of your toilets and bathrooms. These are important areas because these rooms are where the most water exits from your home and as water is flushed out of the house, it tends to carry with it the beneficial chi energy. Ascertain if they are in any of the eight areas of the pa kua which you consider important. For example, a toilet in your Southwest sector will impact on your

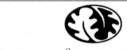

relationships. If one of these 'wet rooms' fall in a sector that is important to you try to keep the door closed the toilet seat down and the plug in the sink. Place a mirror on the outside of the door. These recommendations are doubly important if the room is en-suite to a bedroom.

STEP 12

Check your garden, if you have one, and apply the pa kua, using a compass, to a plan of your garden. Make sure that any paths are curved and do not lead straight to your doors. When you are a little more advanced with feng shui you might consider installing a pond or water feature, although the correct positioning of this is critical.

Having attended to the locations in your house and garden, you now need to look carefully at the locations and directions which are personally beneficial for you and should influence the precise positioning of moveable rooms and furniture within your home.

STEP 13

Calculate your kua number and, using the Pa Kua/Lo Shu Theory, ascertain your four best and worst locations and directions.

STEP 14

Orientate your bedhead to face your prime direction. If this is not possible then choose one of your other three best directions for your head to be pointing whilst sleeping.

If you have health problems for example you should orientate the head of the bed in your Heavenly Healing direction.

If you have a partner with different best directions, the rule is that for a happy marriage the woman's prime direction takes precedence, although you could agree with your partner which prime direction should be used.

STEP 15

Orientate your working direction. Try to make your desk chair face your prosperity direction if you have a home office. Extend this to your work environment if you can possibly manage it. But make sure that your working position does not leave your back to the door of your office. It is more important to have the door to your office where you can see it, rather than to be seated facing your Prosperity direction.

STEP 16

Orientate your eating direction or dining room seating to your prosperity or heavenly healing directions

Putting Feng Shui in Your Life

Finally, put feng shui into your life – don't put your life into feng shui. Let feng shui become part of the background of your life rather than it's primary focus.

Don't become religious or obsessive about feng shui. You do not want to be one of those people who cannot make the slightest change in their home without first checking with a feng shui consultant.

Feng shui tools are a means to an end, not the goal in itself. Integrate them into your life to empower yourself and to gain some measure of mastery over your future.

Flotation Therapy

An experience that is totally unique

Flotation therapy involves a series of visits to an enclosed space known as a float tank, which resembles a large enclosed bath containing a highly concentrated solution of warm water and salts, usually to a depth of about ten inches. A single 'float' will last anything from an hour upwards.

The environment that is created is one of sensory deprivation. There is no light in the tank, and no sound. Music may be used as a cue to leave the tank, but generally there is complete darkness and complete silence once you have settled into this unique space. Lying and floating on your back the usual sensory inputs disappear gradually. The water is skin temperature and it even becomes difficult to tell where you end and the water starts unless you wiggle your toes! The weight of the concentrated solution even removes the full effect of gravity. It is a strange feeling to be supported so firmly when you know that the floor of the tank is only a few inches below you.

You may think that this will be a relaxing experience, or perhaps a confusing time, where you would feel uncomfortably disorientated. All float experiences can be useful and there are many reactions, across a wide range. Physically and emotionally, floating is a unique experience, but also individual. Common reactions include feelings of calm, euphoria and occasionally, dream-like hallucinations are provoked. Floating can have intellectual and spiritual effects too.

The unique environment can offer deep relaxation to the organs of the body, triggering what is known as an 'automatic relaxation response'. Deep healing is helped in this way. This can act on a physical level. You will notice the gathering of soreness and sensation in areas of your body that are carrying stress. With other functions and sensory inputs absent the body can get down to dealing with any problems in a concentrated, effective way. This is the perfect chance to replenish and restore the body's healing systems. Insomnia, stress and anxiety can also be relieved. If you live with high levels of stress you may find that your float is a restless occasion, full of movement. These movements may start anxiously, but will often become liberating and relaxing in their own way.

Dr. John C. Lilly first developed the isolation/floatation tank in 1954 to explore the effects of sensory deprivation on the mind. When it became clear that there were also considerable health benefits this became known as Restricted Environmental Stimulation Therapy or REST. Over the last 45 years there has been much research to provide explanations for the wonders of floatation therapy.

One important factor is the absence of usual gravity, a state referred to as anti-gravity. It is believed that the effects of gravity take up as much as 90 per cent of all central nervous system activity. This helps to make gravity the single largest cause of many ailments, including bad backs, painful joints and muscular tensions. When floating, the body experiences total weightlessness. In theory, this means that the brain and musculo-skeletal system has vast amounts of energy, and large areas of the brain are liberated to experience other matters of mind, spirit and expanded awareness.

The brain also has a chance to relax during flotation. This means a change from the mentally busy fast brain waves known as beta to slower alpha and theta waves. Alpha waves are also generated in general moments of relaxation. Theta waves are associated with vivid memories, free association, sudden insights, creative inspiration, feelings of oneness with the universe. These will occur most frequently during dreams, sleep or trance like states. However, studies have shown that floaters often quickly enter theta states while remaining awake.

Research indicates that floating reduces the levels of stress-related neurochemicals such as adrenaline, norepinephrine, ACTH and cortisol. These are chemical substances associated with tension and anxiety. At the same time, tests show increases in the secretion of endorphins, the body's natural opiate that has an analgesic effect and often induce states of euphoria.

Stress management is vital in modern life. To keep a balanced, healthy body stress reduction and control has to be a part of an overall plan including a positive approach to nutrition and exercise. We all know that this is not as simple as it sounds. It is perhaps easier to do something about diet and exercise. There are definite, concrete steps that can be taken. The reduction and management of stress is less tangible, less straightforward. It is not easy to see that you are stressed. Do you know when you are truly relaxed? When accumulated stress is maintained without release for a prolonged period of time, the brain starts to accept this 'stressed-out' state normality. What you might see as an everyday state of mind could in fact be the result of a long term build of unhealthy levels of stress. In this situation it is very difficult for you to know your true homeostasis, or state of balance. You have forgotten what it means to have a relaxed body and mind.

If this has happened it becomes very difficult to learn ways of relaxing and returning to a healthier state of balance, or managed stress. Natural weapons, such as the automatic relaxation response, have been neglected. You may well have forgotten how to use them. However, there are natural ways of fighting stress and by removing stimuli and giving the body a chance to focus on any problem areas, what has been forgotten can eventually be remembered. During flotation therapy our naturally intelligent human system takes advantage of this new situation and automatically devotes all its energy to restoring itself.

The two sides, or hemispheres of our brain have different functions. The left hemisphere or neocortex operates analytically, processing information on a small-scale. The right hemisphere is intuitive and is able to absorb large scale information, putting all the pieces together in a bigger picture. In every day, modern life there is much more work for the left hemisphere than for the right.

We become used to this situation and it is easy to neglect the right side, or hemisphere, again leaving natural balance and function behind. Research shows that floating increases right brain function. This is because the lack of ordinary stimuli quietens the noisy chattering of the dominant analytical left brain. This is wonderful news as this literal peace and quiet give the chance for unlimited creative possibilities.

These are some of the benefits of flotation therapy. There is no medication to take, or complicated programme to follow. All you have to do is get in the tank and float! The effects can be immediate and dramatic, as well as effortless. For some situations it may take several floats to relax sufficiently and for long enough to make the difference. A clinic or natural health centre that contains a float tank will be able to give you the advice you need for your own situation.

Folk Medicine

By Louise O'Neill

The term folk medicine refers to the traditional beliefs, practices, and materials that people use to maintain health and cope with disease, outside of an organised relationship with academic, professionally recognised and established medical systems.

Non-European academic and professional systems, such as Ayurvedic, Chinese, and pre-conquest Aztec systems, are sometimes erroneously characterised as folk medicine. They are more correctly considered traditional medicines, however exotic they may appear to be. The beliefs and practices that make up folk medicine are systemically related to the history, traditions and life of a recognisable social group. They are reflected in the approaches taken to health maintenance and treatment of disease.

The practitioners of a folk medicine are in some way socially close to their clients and share their belief systems. Most practitioners are part-time specialists. Their training is informal or takes place through individual apprenticeship. Their validation is gradual and comes about through community recognition of success, rather than through documentation.

Whenever possible, a folk medicine is best understood in its historical context. Examination of the fate of Aztec medicine in Mexico provides an example. Before conquest by Spain, Aztec establishment (as opposed to folk) medicine was highly organised, with an herbarium, a zoo, an intellectual elite and a training and certification academy. It was based on a complex theoretical structure and experimental research. Some segments of the population, however, had only limited access to this medicine. They relied instead on traditional, non-academic medicine that would be best characterised as folk medicine. Aztec establishment medicine was eliminated when the Spanish conquerors killed the medical personnel and intruded their own medicine based on medieval Galenic (Greek) theory.

This intrusive medicine became the establishment medicine among the Aztecs. The system still offered limited access. Some elements of Galenic medicine, however, were compatible with the folk medical practice of the native Americans and were therefore incorporated into a new folk system. Mexican folk medicine thrived, albeit with regional differences, and continued to incorporate elements of the new medicine.

Academic and folk medicine have always coexisted. Plants found in a paleolithic burial in Turkey have been identified as modern folk herbal medicines, some of which in refined form have found their way into academic medicine. On the other hand, non-oral therapeutics developed in academic medicine have become part of folk practice in Mexico and South East Asia. Increasingly, the lines between 'folk' and 'academic' are becoming blurred.

Midwifery, for example, held an ambiguous status until the late 18th and early 19th century, when its functions were taken over by academic medicine and its practitioners were relegated to 'folk' and semilegal status. Not without conflict, this trend is now slowly being reversed. Practices and practitioners classified as 'folk' are now becoming professionalised and standardised.

Flower and Tree Essence Therapy

By Nicola Dunn

Flower and tree essences are the core energy of nature captured in a bottle. When we feel jaded and depleted it's the deep healing power of nature that we want, so we head for a meadow, a forest or even a garden, knowing that some how our balance will be restored.

Even though we can't always visit nature directly we can still connect with that same energy by taking the appropriate flower or tree essence. As soon as we take the essences they become personal energy catalysts because we are using their healing energy patterns as a stimulus to restore our own vibrations to a harmonious whole thereby revitalising our spirit, body and mind.

The healing power of the flower or tree is captured in water because liquids are considered one of the most sensitive carriers of vibrations. They have also been found to be effective in transferring subtle forms of energy into the body.

A flower/tree essence practitioner can diagnose or attune themselves to your energy imbalance in different ways. Some will work in a similar way to homeopaths, listening to the light and shadow of your words, observing how you present yourself and matching your energy patterns to those of the essences. Others will use muscle testing, a pendulum or flower/tree cards. If the issue is quite simple and occurred recently it should resolve itself fairly quickly with either one single essence or a small combination. On the other hand if the issue has been around for longer or is more complex it will require more time.

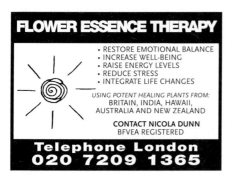

Several different combinations may be needed over quite a few months as the layers upon which the challenge is based are uncovered. The practitioner will prepare a treatment bottle to take away which will contain the essences preserved in spring water and alcohol. The essences can help you to be in tune with your life purpose and once this happens your life flows with greater dignity and grace.

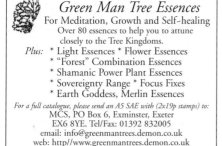

Geopathic Stress

By Ali Northcott

O ur health well being and vitality are strongly influenced by the nature and quality of our surroundings, which can either support and nurture us or deplete our energy. Geopathic stress is a kind of environmental disease, emitted from disruption in the earth's energy field.

There are a variety of sources such as streams, which are linked with underground watercourses, geo magnetic grid crossings and geological faults.

Buildings situated on geopathic stress tend to have a history of inhabitants who suffer from misfortune, ill health and problematic relationships. People and places do not tend prosper when situated on geopathic stress as it inhibits health, stability and growth. Especially when we sleep or spend long periods of time sitting where these energies cross our body, then we can become prone to disease. In such cases the locality of the lines are found to correspond with the symptoms and effected areas of the body. The effects vary according to the amount of time that we stay in these places, and the level of disruption.

When we are exposed to Geopathic stress it has a degenerative effect on our energy system, affecting the way in which we function on all levels; physically; mentally; emotionally and spiritually. It promotes negativity, affecting our ability to focus and relax properly, influencing the way that we relate to our selves and those around, encouraging tiredness, tension and irritability. Over a long period of time it brakes down the immune system and the human body becomes vulnerable to disease. Many disorders are linked with geopathic stress include candida, eczema, ME, insomnia, depression, infertility and in the worst cases wasting diseases such as cancer.

Detecting geopathic stress

Geopathic stress can be detected and cleared in a variety of ways, the traditional method is by dowsing to survey land and building. This will locate the various sources of earth energy including streams, ley lines, geomagnetic grid crossings, and indicate areas that are disrupted.

This can be done by map or site dowsing, practitioners who can provide this service includes dowsers, earth acupuncturists/earth healers, geomancers and some feng shui practitioners and space clearing consultants. Some natural health practitioners are aware of geopathic stress and will indicate when there is evidence that is effecting the health or recovery of their patient. A survey should include recommendations for correcting and balancing the energy wherever necessary; you should be advised on maintenance.

Correcting and balancing

If you find that your home or work place is located on geopathic stress there are many ways in which this can be resolved. Some work on a deeper level at the root of the problem, whilst others will alleviate the effects in that area. Corrective techniques include, transforming the energy, earth healing techniques, ceremony and ritual, corrective devices and a change in layout and use of space. Corrective devices include crystal, coils, metal, magnets, and protective symbols. Practitioners vary in their approach according to their background. It is important to find out if the practitioner is experienced in working with the various sources of geopathic stress.

Clearing geopathic stress relieves the symptoms associated with this environmental disorder and assists recovery from existing illnesses. Enabling the land and those living there may benefit from a more generative energy.

Creating a healthy environment that is able to ground us and nourishes us enabling our immune system to function properly and encourages a sense of well being and good health.

GEOPATHIC STRESS.

ALI NORTHCOTT for consultations Tel; 0115 9856058. For more information about energy transformation and training in Geomancy try our website; www.earth-healing.co.uk. Also see features written by Ali Northcott on Earth Acupuncture, Geopathic Stress and Space Clearing. Main advert in the Feng Shui section.

Helping the healers
By M Willcocks PhD

Mother Earth is making it clear we have the opportunity to help her heal. A number of people work to heal the land on a regular basis through interventions and ceremony.

This is non-violent, non-political, unobtrusive and direct healing activity. You can do this where you live, with contributions to environmentalists or by just getting out and walking the land. All that is required is your conscious and focused attention on healing. Your energy is needed! In complete reciprocity, the work you do with the earth mother enhances your own personal healing and the healing of those who live on the land. Perhaps you'd like to arrange a ceremony, a medicine wheel, a labyrinth, sweat lodge, drumming and solstice or prayer circle around earth healing. The options are endless; your intent to help is what's important.

Other ways to help: Walk on your own, in a park or city. Pay attention to areas that seem to need help. If you're so inclined, set healing crystals (clear quartz or amethyst are best) in 'trouble spots' with the intention that the crystals capture and focus healing energy sent to them. Discover sacred sites in your area. They are everywhere and are extremely empowering. Play healing music, the vibration of native and 'new age' music, sacred music and chants speeds the healing process of people, animals and other beings as well as the earth mother.

Hawaiian Huna

By Marcus West

Huna is an ancient system of self-development long practised on the islands of Hawaii. Many people believe it to be a direct descendent of an ancient shamanic system that once spanned the planet. Huna is a simple and effective system of knowledge and techniques to enable you to live more fully, encompassing emotional, mental and physical healing, connection with your spiritual side, and the realisation of your goals. It is not a dogmatic system demanding arbitrary beliefs, but is first and foremost practical

The starting point in Huna is its model of the three minds of humankind: the Unconscious Mind, the Conscious Mind and the Higher Conscious Mind or Higher Self. The Unconscious Mind governs emotions, memory, the physical body, and the senses, among other things.

The conscious mind is the one we are probably most familiar with. The higher self is considered to live in a realm of love, and generally is thought to intervene in our life only if we ask, though it will sometimes also intervene during emergencies. It crystallises our future according to the stream of ideas that drift up, or are sent up, from the Unconscious Mind.

The goal of Huna is the integration of these minds, so they function together. Such integration brings with it health, joy, happiness and spiritual connectedness. The absence of such integration can manifest in illnesses, and a lack of joy and vibrancy. To the extent that most people are only dimly aware of their unconscious mind and their higher self, they are firing on only one out of three cylinders.

So what stops the three minds functioning together? The Huna notion is that negative stuff lodges in the unconscious mind like intrusions of encysted energy, blocking the paths joining the three selves.

What kind of negative stuff? Things that block the paths between the three selves are unresolved emotions like guilt, grief, sadness, anger; and also unhelpful beliefs that limit or sabotage us, perhaps about our health or our abilities. Such beliefs are typically absorbed during childhood, or created during stressful events.

The Huna tradition likens these to 'black bags' into which the unresolved stuff is pushed, and which are then held in the unconscious mind, liable to be retriggered or reawakened by subsequent events, unless released.

These emotions or beliefs can become so familiar to us that we may come to think of them as being part of who we are. Huna processes help us to recognise these things as not 'us', but as things we created, and thus things we can 'uncreate' or let go of.

They are not 'us', they just overlay the magnificence that is 'us'. Even events we perceive as traumatic can ultimately be seen as just a bunch of things that happened, and be freed of any negative legacy.

Part of Huna is encouraging the unconscious mind to let go of this negative stuff. We can do this by learning how to cultivate rapport with our unconscious mind, becoming friends with it, and then communicating and negotiating with it. Some people can readily reach a state where they experience a valuable stream of images and information flowing between the conscious and unconscious minds.

Huna also uses processes that directly mobilise the higher self to assist in the process of releasing negative stuff from the unconscious mind. Such processes, when run well, are not some vague airy-fairy kind of thing, but are very powerful techniques for releasing powerful negative stuff, with potentially profound consequences.

Such processes frequently also give the client, as a by-product, a powerful sense of connection to the higher self, experienced as an all-loving, reassuring parental figure. And there are also other, more direct, techniques for inducing this experience of connection with the higher self breathing techniques and chant can also play a part in generating the requisite energy to assist these processes.

As well as clearing the 'vertical' connections between the three minds within the individual, Huna is also concerned with clearing the 'horizontal' connections between people. When we have upsets, whether as perpetrator or victim, we make an unhelpful energy connection with the other party.

If we hang on to grievances, our closeness to the divine is lessened, we attract further similar upsets, we waste energy, and our lives are diminished. So another Huna process, centred on an internal process of mutual forgiveness between ourselves and those we have upsets with, either cuts or cleans up these energetic connections.

By clearing up our internal state in this way, we free ourselves from the conditions which led us to manifest these things in the external world.

Huna holds that, in this magical universe we inhabit, the outer world is a reflection of the inner; thus the internal process of cleaning up these energy connections can have a magical effect on our relationship with the people in the world out there

Although Huna is not yet very widely known in its own right, there are individuals in the field of self-development who have been significantly influenced by it.

For example, Gill Edwards has incorporated many elements of Huna into her teachings (see for example her book 'Stepping into the Magic'). Indeed, she says: "The Huna wisdom is said by many to be the finest source of esoteric wisdom on the planet."

Practitioners of Huna see it not only as a set of therapeutic procedures, but also as a way of life why would something so valuable be left in the therapy room?

Words of Wisdom

"Formerly, when religion was strong and science weak, men mistook magic for medicine; now, when science is strong and religion weak, men mistake medicine for magic"

THOMAS SZASZ

Healing

By The World Federation of Healing

To many people who have received spiritual or divine healing, as it is sometimes called, it is a wonderful experience. Yet to many people it is still a mystery and they ask "what is spiritual healing?"

Although healing has been known and used for thousands of years it is even now not fully understood. It is an energy which flows between a healer and the patient but the precise nature of that energy is not yet known. It has been studied scientifically and is capable of being measured yet it does not conform to the generally accepted rules of physical science.

What can healing do for the patient?

It can assist the natural healing resources of the mind and body to recover their former functions. It should never be regarded as an alternative to normal medical treatments and patients should continue to consult their doctor. However, the medical or surgical treatments are often made much more effective if the healing is given side by side with the physical treatment. There is abundant evidence the healing quickly reduces the effect of shock whether the shock is due to accident or surgery. On occasions, these natural healing treatments produce unexpected beneficial results.

Can healing be guaranteed?

Healing, whether it is given once or many times, can never be guaranteed to produce either an improvement or cure. Nevertheless: healing given by a trained and experienced healer will never do harm but in most cases will produce a marked improvement.

What is felt during treatment?

Sometimes the person receiving the healing will experience a pleasant feeling of warmth. Others will only have a feeling of relaxation and comfort. Because healing has its origins in the divine,

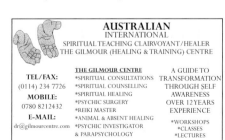

patients often experience a wonderful feeling of peace and spiritual upliftment.

Do I need to have faith in the healing for it to work?

Although undoubtedly faith does help, there are many examples of people being helped who do not have any faith in the healing. As the healing begins to work and the patient starts to feel better, the faith in the treatment grows naturally.

How often do I need to have healing?

There are no fixed rules concerning the number of treatments needed to improve a condition. Most healers work on the basis of giving one treatment per week... Where it is necessary- for example when a patient is in pain or the condition is chronic, treatment is twice or three times weekly. You cannot have too much treatment.

Does the healing given by one healer clash with one given by another?

Sometimes a patient is worried in case the benefits already received are lost by having healing from a second healer. The answer is no it does not. Healing should always benefit the patient. If your healer has helped you and for some reason cannot treat you more often or is away from home, ask if he or she is able to recommend someone to give you extra treatments between visits to them.

What can I do to help the healing?

During the actual healing session you can try to relax as much as possible and mentally open your mind to receiving the healing. Even if you do not have faith in it, by keeping an open or unbiased mind, it can assist the flow of healing energy.

Healing for Women

Living from the Heart

By Pratibha Castle

There are many misunderstandings in a woman's subconscious, both collective and personal; many experiences of pain in relation to living the feminine qualities. As a result, in striving for independence and recognition in the world of men in the last decades, women have tended to undervalue these qualities and to deny them.

They were associated with the pain of being dominated and undervalued as a woman, used traditionally in caring for others. But it is now time for women to heal these experiences and let them go, and be free to rediscover and reclaim their intrinsic qualities; to understand that these are indeed the source of nurturing and renewal, the source of women's empowerment.

As we look back down the road from where we come we see a world that has been dominated for over 2,000 years by the masculine principle – paying homage to a Divine Father and Son, honouring male values, political domination frequently supported by brute force, education that supported the intellectual, logical male mind, and was available until only recently to an almost exclusively male elite.

In the 1960s easy access to the contraceptive pill in the Western world enabled a greater number of women than ever before to step out of the traditional role of homemaker, to expand their education and step into positions of power and creativity in the world outside the home. This was undoubtedly a step forward.

However, there is another frontier waiting to be discovered and claimed that offers even greater possibilities for empowerment and fulfilment. This dimension connects women with their qualities of intuition, sensitivity, warmth, compassion, their source of nurturing and sense of contentment that arises naturally as each embraces her own inner space.

It is also an experience, which enables women to live these feminine qualities alongside the hard won masculine qualities, a dimension that offers an experience of wholeness that is inclusive, rather than exclusive. We are talking of the heart centre, which is the doorway that connects us with the feminine qualities. There is nothing complicated or difficult about the heart centre and it is an experience accessible to all.

You may like to explore for yourself with the following simple technique.

Putting on some gentle music, I sit back and allow my body to relax. Bringing my hand to the centre of the chest, I notice the physical sensation, the warmth, the weight of the hand, perhaps a little tingling or streaming of energy. The breathing becomes a little deeper and slower, allowing the awareness to rest in the space within the chest, beneath the hand.

Goddess Workshops
(A Healing for Women)

Dance/Sound/Heart Meditation

Shamanic Reiki Attunements

Aura-Soma Courses

Body/Mind/Energy Harmony Sessions

with

PRATIBHA CASTLE

01243 781 341

There may be some thoughts passing through the mind; simply take note of them, along with the movement of the breath – in, and out; up, and down – and the sounds of the music. Noticing, perhaps, that there is a letting go of tensions in the body, and that the feeling of relaxation is growing. Perhaps also a feeling of peace, or inner silence; maybe a sense of tears wanting to flow. Many different sensations, happening in this moment, now. All absorbed, without judgement, in the spaciousness of the heart.

Connecting with the heart literally means being present in the moment – to whatever that moment presents, unconditionally, unselectively. Whether it is sensations in the body, thoughts passing through the mind, emotional feelings, memories, external experiences, pleasure, pain or boredom.

Being in the heart means being present to these, without judgement, and simply experiencing them. And if you find yourself spacing out, or judging, the heart enables us to be present to that, as well. Nothing is excluded.

This means that since everything can be experienced, embraced, within the heart – there is nothing that life can send us which we have to fight or deny. We can 'go with the flow', be in a state of acceptance, and this attitude to life is how the strength, the power of the feminine expresses itself. Just like the willow tree, whose strength is in her flexibility, her capacity to bend in the wind, rather than standing rigid, and being battered, maybe broken.

Seen in the old way, to be in acceptance would look like being in the role of victim, or perhaps passive acquiescence rather than a quality. But this is not the case. There is a therapeutic model for consciousness which uses the symbols of the camel, lion and child. The camel is the victim, in collapse, powerless – woman before the 1960s.

IN THE CAMEL, I do whatever I'm told, whether it feels right or not

THE LION is in defiance. In the lion, I refuse to do what someone tells me, whether it feels right or not

IN THE CHILD, I respond, guided by my inner voice. For the word child, you could substitute the heart.

Another way to express this model is that we are moving from living our lives as victims in reaction, burdened by patterns from the past that repeat themselves endlessly, to living life from a place of empowerment, responding with freshness and creativity in the moment.

As we become more familiar with this space of the heart, we relax and experience greater ease within ourselves which affects every aspect of our daily life. We can discover who we are at a deeper level in each moment because we are more interested in experiencing what is true rather than in trying to be something that is false for others.

This is deeply relaxing on every level – physical, emotional, mental, spiritual. We may find an emerging quality of honesty, integrity and intimacy entering our relationships and our creativity flowing more freely in every situation as we respond to life's challenges from the space of the heart.

"Women want to be free to choose from the same range of options that men take for granted. In our quest for equal pay, equal access to education and opportunities, we have made great strides. But until women can move freely and think freely in their homes, on the streets, in the workplace without the fear of violence, there can be no real freedom" – **Anita Roddick**.

Healing with Angels

Our Guardian Angels are so easy to talk to. Just like any other old friend. And after all, who could possibly know you better than those who have been with you forever? Through practised guided visualisation you can meet your own Angel helpers and really open the channels of communication.

It is not difficult and luckily we don't have to be perfect, in fact we don't even have to be good. A genuine reason and an intention, which is pure of heart, are all you need.

Imagine allowing your angel to sow the seeds of love, joy, peace, and happiness deep within you then watching them blossom; I promise you will feel heavenly!

Many of us are searching. Some of us don't really know what it is we are searching for. Some for an inner peace and a return to the path of freedom perhaps?

Others would simply like to feel less stressed or have more peace of mind, or raise their self-esteem a few notches.

All of this comes when we learn whom we really are. For some the path seems easier and having seen the light at the end of their personal tunnel, bring them forward and radiate the light from within expressing a wonderful serenity and love, seemingly without even trying.

How is it that some people have this gift and where do they develop the knowledge? I believe that we all have the ability to find that space within ourselves to really connect to the memories of who and what we really are.

As busy people trying to juggle the many pressures of life above our heads we forget quite often that we cannot rest our bodies and forget the emotions and mind.

We cannot concentrate on educating the mind if it does not nourish the soul. We have a commitment to the care of our whole self… mind, body, heart, spirit and soul.

There are many teachers and interesting therapies on offer to start you off on the way to total nourishment. Many 'feel good' techniques will help you learn relaxation such as reflexology and aromatherapy. Then there are other skills and techniques which will de-stress and at the same time awaken spiritual awareness such as yoga, meditation and t'ai chi.

These are all of great value in nurturing our being but we still may find that in all our endeavours there is still a niggling something missing.

Ultimately our goal is one of reconnection and this is where our true happiness lies.

Each of us is unique, special and beautiful in our own right. We all have wonderful qualities. Notice how we reflect them in those aspects of our friends we so admire.

We all have an angel within, and many

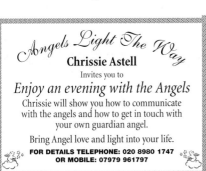

angels without, ready to help reduce our burdens in every way if only we would learn to ask! Did you think of the angels? People have been communicating with them, hearing their voices, feeling their presence since time began.

Angels don't have to prove their existence. There are billions more of them now than ever before, since the beginning of time. There is urgency in their work.

Many souls are awakening to the call of re-alignment, atonement and enlightenment. Now they are here in ever increasing numbers to help us do that very thing we crave – find ourselves and help us to return to a place of calm where the spirit can grow in peace and where we can reconnect with the spark of divinity within us all.

Getting in touch with the angels ignites the spark! Watch it fire up your enthusiasm. Imagine the security of knowing and believing that you are truly protected wherever you go.

Angels – winged messengers – beings of light – intermediaries between humankind and the divine – healers – protectors – sources of great inspiration – bringers of peace – bearers of joy – guardians of souls… the list goes on.

However you see them yourself they have been the inspiration for magnificent works of art since man learnt to hold a paintbrush. They appear in the great texts and daily teachings of all the major faiths and despite the seeming decline of mainstream religion, angels have taken a frontline in the rising interest of 'all things spiritual'.

Recently we have seen the media increase this awareness with films such as: *Michael*, *City of Angels*, *Dogma* and programmes on TV such as *Touched By An Angel*.

We have had documentary programmes investigating the belief in angels of 'ordinary' people, and post-graduate students enquiring through our major newspapers for people's genuine stories of 'real-life encounters of the angelic kind'.

And what about the books? You can buy books about connecting with angels in almost every high street store; in fact my poor bookcase is unable to take one more leaf on the subject!

I am tempted to say that my bookshelf is groaning under the weight of them all but as the angels' main task is to be a source of 'light' that would definitely not seem appropriate!

So there we are. The answers right in front of our very eyes if only we could see them for ourselves. Some people do, of course, but they are not the ones searching; they have already experienced the joy of reconnection.

Administering, guiding and protecting angels are with us all the time. Even on bad hair days! No judgement, no ifs and buts and no conditions. Only love, given as often as you need it.

You may ask again and again and, as long as it is within the best interest of your soul growth, you will be given the help you need.

All this sounds too easy, but believe me unconditional love comes your way in an instant once you open up to accepting that it is there for you.

HEALING WITH ANGELS

THE ANGEL CONNECTION Whitestone House, Grange Paddock, Mark, Somerset TA9 4RW. Send 2 x 1st class stamps for FREE catalogues full of beautiful Angel products. For yourself, Gifts – Angel Portraits, Cards, Ornaments, Stickers, Books, Candles and more.
Tel: 01278 641088
Angels4u@angelconnection.fsnet.co.uk

Health and Beauty

By Janet Mills and Lisa McLeod of Mills De-Win Studios

There are treatments available today to address the most common complaints that affect your body or face. Be it fatty areas, cellulite, muscle fatigue, sagging skin, lines and wrinkles or unwanted hair, there will be a solution to the problem.

Many beauty salons now offer holistic therapies such as the Bowen technique, aromatherapy, reflexology and reiki. Therapists will assess individual needs and offer advice on which treatment is best suited to meet those specific requirements. It is, of course, essential to support these treatments with the corresponding home care whether in the use of products, or in following a diet and nutrition program.

How many people do you know who visit a health and beauty salon regularly? The chances are you will know several who do.

Salons are a timeless business. There will always be a demand for beauty treatments and with more and more options offering quicker, more effective and less painful sessions you can even go for a treatment in your lunch hour.

What sort of people visits beauty salons? There are no specific types… whether it's temporary or permanent hair removal by waxing or electrolysis, a relaxing facial to unwind or a make-up application for a special occasion, there is something thing for everyone.

Salons are popular because every woman wants to look and feel her best. But it's not just women booking treatments… more and more men want to look and feel more positive about themselves.

There is no question that a massage or a facial makes you feel more relaxed, brings down stress levels, improves the appearance of the skin, unknots tight muscles and gives an overall feeling of wellbeing. This can be vital to someone with a stressful job; it can mean better performance at work and less tension at home.

For people with that little bit more time to spare why not consider a 'Pamper Day'. Most salons will have available full day treatments that will usually include spa baths, sauna or steam cabin followed by full body massage, facial, manicure, pedicure and make-up, where required. Since you are likely to be there the whole

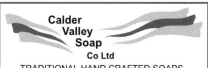

day, light lunches are often included. For beauty salons that offer combined hairdressing it would be usual to complete you day with a hair treatment and blow dry. Many people find their visit to a health and beauty salon essential because of the busy lives so many of us lead. For many, it will probably be the only time that you make for themselves.

Anyone who has never ventured through the door of a beauty salon should give it a try. You could even treat your nearest and dearest. Gift vouchers, available from most salons, make an excellent birthday or Christmas present.

Nature gives you the face you have at twenty. Life shapes the face you have at thirty. But at fifty you get the face you deserve.
Coco Chanel

Henna: Nature's hair product

Henna is a small, white and yellow, heavy, sweet-smelling flower. A distilled water prepared from it is used as a cosmetic, and the powdered leaves have been in use from the most ancient times in Eastern countries for dyeing the hair and nails.

Since 1890 it has been widely used in Europe for tinting the hair, usually in the form of a shampoo, many shades being obtainable by mixing with the leaves of other plants, such as indigo.

As a dye for the skin or nails the powder may be mixed with Catechu or Lucerne, made into a paste with hot water and spread on the part to be dyed.

Other uses

Henna has been found to also contain a brown substance of a resinoid fracture, having the chemical properties which characterise the tannins, and therefore named hennotannic acid. It has been employed both internally and locally in jaundice, leprosy, smallpox, and affections of the skin. The fruit is thought to have emmenagogue properties.

The Egyptians are said to have prepared both an oil and an ointment from the flowers for making the limbs supple.

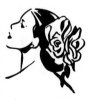

Herbal Medicine

By Trudy Norris BA, MNIMH, PGCE Information Officer

Herbal Medicine is the use of plants as medicines and thus encompasses many forms of practice. It is fundamental to primary health care worldwide.

Herbal practitioners see members by appointment, take a full medical history, make a physical examination as appropriate and discuss relevant factors such as diet, nutrition, exercise, home circumstances and emotional influences.

Prescriptions are usually made up at the consultation. Practitioners vary in the range of herbs used but, as a guide, I have over 150 in my dispensary made from European, North American, Chinese and some tropical plants.

Initial consultations usually last between 60 and 90 minutes. One of the practitioner's aims will be to enable the individual to become more involved in their health care and health promotion.

Herbalist and patient will try to identify underlying causes of illness thus working holistically and individually. Many people who seek help from practitioners have chronic (long term) and interconnected symptoms, may be taking pharmaceutical drugs and require careful monitoring and evaluation.

Following an initial visit the practitioner may see the patient two to three weeks afterwards depending upon the severity of their symptoms. Combinations of herbs in different forms are prescribed and as progress is made the prescription and outcomes are evaluated and the choice of herbs reviewed.

Herbalists may also make dietary recommendations to individuals where appropriate.

Can't I use herbal tea bags?

Many herbs can be used safely in the home for acute, self-limiting conditions or to enhance health and well-being. The

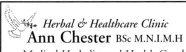
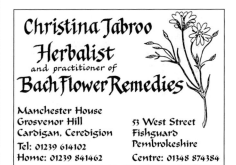

National Institute of Medical Herbalists recommends the following: if you have chronic health problems, are taking prescribed drugs from your doctor, are pregnant or breastfeeding, seek help from a qualified practitioner.

Can you give me examples of conditions that herbalists treat?

Herbalists treat people first! No one prescription will be the same for two people. Underlying causes of illness, resistance to stress, hereditary tendencies, medication all dictates an individual approach. However herbalists can and do treat a wide variety of people with conditions affecting all systems of the body – digestive problems, circulatory problems (such as high blood pressure), gynaecological problems (such as pre-menstrual or menopausal problems), emotional health symptoms such as depression, insomnia, panic attacks, conditions affecting the joints and the urinary system.

How do I identify a trained practitioner of herbal medicine?

Members of the National Institute of Medical Herbalists have trained for four years before becoming members of the Institute. Training involves western medical sciences such as anatomy and physiology, diagnosis, clinical methods, plant sciences such as pharmacology, botany and pharmacognosy, plant actions or material medical, philosophy and therapeutics and finally nutritional influences on health and illness.

Members of the National Institute of Medical Herbalists adhere to a strict professional code of ethics, have full professional insurance and programmed of continuing professional development.

The NIMH was founded in 1864 and membership has been by examination since 1902. It has departments for education, research, quality and safety, information dissemination, media relations, ethnobotany and clinical audit.

The use of herbs

If you are concerned about terminology and want to better understand the difference between intolerance, side-effects, adverse reactions and idiosyncratic reactions, this may help:

Intolerance is a low threshold to the normal pharmacological action of the herbs.

Side-effects are undesired but unavoidable effects which may occur. For example, long-term administration of some herbs may temporarily weaken internal organs and cause nasty things like frequent bowel movement etc. Most herbs are free of any adverse reaction. (Ask your herbalist for advice)

Idiosyncratic reactions are unexpected, undesired effects that are usually due to a genetic abnormality of the patient (an allergic reaction is a type of idiosyncratic reaction). Such a reaction is individual to a user and is not usually replicated in other people.

High Touch Jin Shin Acupressure
By the High Touch Network

High Touch Acupressure is based on recognisable Oriental traditions. Jiro Mural, its founder, came from a medical family and was an acupuncturist. During his work he collected the folk knowledge of his time but through his experience and study of western traditions when at the Japanese Imperial Archives he was able to incorporate a system of flows, which he presented in terms of a cabalistic understanding of numbers.

His works have been conveyed to us through Mary Burmeister, his first student, and later via Betsy Dayton, who has set up High Touch® as a network for training and support for practitioners.

The pulsing flow

The fundamental notions of the system are simple. When hands are placed lightly on two points on the body, they will initiate a flow of energy, which will travel through the known meridian paths to connect the two points. This transfer of energy from one hand to the other will help to balance energy and clear points that are blocked. When the energy has cleared the pathway, a gentle pulsing is felt and it is time to move on to the next series of points.

The language of the points

To explain in a simplistic manner one could say that between the point at the base of the skull and the forehead what is not conscious becomes conscious, and between the forehead and the cheekbone we take on the world as we see it. Through the chest and arms we are in a giving and receiving relationship, through the heart and digestion we formulate our inner response.

The creative nature of the body lies in the hips, we walk forward in life with lifting our knees, balancing fear and strength in the ankles, completing the cycle at the big toe where the energy begins to return up the back of the spine to the head.

The hands

Gestures conveyed by the fingers, the mudras, their positions and expressions have long had an important part to play in dance and ritual. Each of the 12 essential meridian lines can be accessed through the hands and fingers, thus it can be recognised that the holding of the fingers is of overall benefit to the body, particularly in the self-help work which is recommended as part of the treatment. The fingers are also cross-referenced to the toes to set up a complicated balancing system, which is particularly helpful for arthritis.

The treatment

It is not necessary to remove clothes. The 26 points are easy to find; each person is likely to find a certain sensitivity that will indicate a precise indication. Based on this simple alphabet of points, together with a procedure for taking pulses from the client, a clear treatment pattern can be planned. This will treat the body at all levels… spiritual, mental, emotional and physical.

The treatment pattern follows an immediate diagnosis of requirement and the effects are instantly noticeable and continue to work for 24 hours. There is a very specific index as to the range of flows suitable for most conditions.

The flows

The first flow pattern used in treatment, is usually a major energy balancing flow, removing energy balances to the left or right, centring energy that bounces from one side to the other (often causing sciatica), or deeply relieving an exhausted immune system. The most usual flow rebalances the Chakra system and brings energy to the central core of a persons being.

The second level of flow is to work on the life patterns and problems, including inherited and constitutional illness; these are chosen, as with all flows, from the pulses.

The third level of flow refers to the well known 'five element' theory in Oriental medicine, known as the five depths with their corresponding emotions of worry, fear, anger, grief and joy. The 'common' flows give attention to the mental, emotional, digestive or procreative sections of the body. Finally work may be done on the meridian lines themselves.

Jiro Mural took his healing to the poor people in Japan. Gathering sufferers of the same ailment together, he treated them and from his notes on each malady built up his knowledge. He called it Jin Shin Jyutsu, 'the art of the Creator, through the person with compassion'. In honour of his work, the Emperor gave him access to the Imperial Archives to further his study. As a young man he had taken to excesses to such an extent that he was warned that no-one could save him. He left for the mountains and began the meditative practices to release him from life. In and out of consciousness, he fasted and held the 'ritual of mudras' in profound meditation. He became so cold he wondered why he had not died. When healing came it was as rivers of fire and from then on he dedicated himself the knowledge of Jin Shin Jyutsu.

Jiro Murai's motto was: "First treat yourself, then your friends then anyone who comes through the door."

For all the tea in China...

Tea has been a daily necessity in China since time immemorial. Countless millions like to have their after-meal tea.

Medically, the tea leaf contains a number of chemicals, of which 20-30 per cent is tannic acid, known for its anti-inflammatory and germicidal properties.

It also contains an alkaloid (five per cent, mainly caffeine), a stimulant for the nerve centre and the metabolism.

Tea and the aromatics in it may help resolve meat and fat and thus promote digestion. It is, therefore, of special importance to people who live mainly on meat, like many of the ethnic minorities in China. A popular proverb among them says: "Rather go without salt for three days than without tea for a single day."

Tea is also rich in vitamins and, for smokers, helps to discharge nicotine from the system. After taking alcohol, strong tea may prove to be a sobering pick-me-up.

Holistic Retreats and Holidays

By M. Willcocks PhD

Relaxation and the chance to re-evaluate life in a quiet rural setting are invariably among the main reasons people choose an holistic break.

It can be one of the most beautiful, regenerating, life-changing experiences you will have had the opportunity to enjoy in a long time, allowing you to relax the body and mind, and to 'let go' with astonishing mental, emotional and physical benefits.

Venues for this kind of holistic break will usually offer facilities such as heated swimming pools, relaxing gardens, excellent gastronomic menus, well-stocked bars, carefully appointed rooms with aromatherapy candles, water, coffee, tea and herbal teas and lots of other creature comforts. Often, every conceivable therapy will also be at your disposal. Imagine being with a small group of people in a wonderful rural setting, away from your normal environment, relaxing and learning how to take control of your life's experiences and discovering how powerful you really are!

You will be able to talk freely with others and no doubt discover similar doubts, fears, stresses, hopes and dreams; listen to sound yet forward thinking knowledge from teachers who will also help everyone on an individual basis. Combined with all of this is the time to relax and explore the location on your own or with a group of your new found friends. Alternatively, you might choose a retreat where there is an opportunity to gain a greater sense of your inner reality and truth, and how it relates

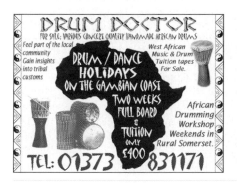

to the outside world. Where life may be seen as a learning experience, in a busy world actual reflective time is in short supply. The aim of this type of retreat is to create the context for reflective space. All activities allowing this to happen are seen as positive, be it hill walking, painting, dancing, singing, silence, working or studying holy texts.

These centres are an expression of a desire to realise the sacredness of all existence. At this end of the spectrum facilities can be basic, perhaps bare wooden floors, a horsehair mattress and plain cooking. It can take many years of workshops, books, meditation and so on to achieve self-understanding. How long has it taken you to achieve the level of understanding in your life now? At this type of retreat you will acquire much more knowledge of your true self in a controlled and helpful setting.

When considering your holistic break it is important to realise the purpose of these periods of solitude; this kind of holiday is not for the chatty or larger than life person. Retreats which offer the facilities of a four star hotel can be expensive, but with all the extras not found in a hotel, in relative terms the cost is justified.

The 'authentic' retreat is invariably devoutly religious and inexpensive, but as there are a variety of faiths and lifestyles offering 'holidays', and you will be expected to join in group therapy and respect the way of life. It is crucial to research your venue and to keep an open mind if you want to avoid a negative experience.

Whatever your choice, at the end of your of our holistic holiday you will have discovered how to create the experiences you want, unclouded by the fear and stress often associated with your normal holidays. You will find new possibilities and meaning for your life and a NEW YOU.

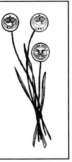
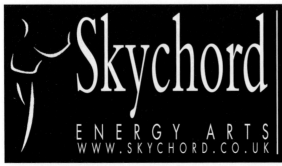

Holistic Design
by Suzy Chiazzari

Most homes use energy inefficiently and emit pollutants back into the atmosphere. Energy conservation in the home is still not taken seriously. Holistic design is concerned with educating everyone to put these essential ecological considerations into practice.

Not only will we benefit by living in a cleaner and healthier environment, a building which is ecologically friendly and energy efficient will need low maintenance, and the saving on energy costs can be substantial. With an ever more stressful lifestyles, the role our home plays in our physical and psychological health becomes ever more evident.

Holistic design recognises the profound effect that our living and working places have on us. Rather than creating buildings and interiors which are just pretty to look at or merely a fashion statement, holistic design focuses on creating healthy and harmonious interiors for comfortable living.

With the rapid increase in building on green sites, it is essential we create houses with a low visual impact. Your home should blend in as much as possible with the landscape and the architectural style and scale should be harmonious, too. Environmental concerns are a priority in holistic design, with a focus on the use of local and salvageable materials and other natural resources to enhance a building's aesthetic and sustainable qualities.

Often we are unable to build a house from scratch, but there is a great deal we can do to reduce environmental pollution by creating a healthy indoor environment. Our modem lifestyle has cut us off from the natural world, so much so, that we now live more than 80 per cent of our lives indoors. By making sure our homes are filled with natural light and air, we harmonise our biological clock with daily and seasonal rhythms, ensuring we get good sleep and keep our energy levels high. In this way our home can be our greatest ally in the fight against stress and control of viral infections.

With the increase in many physical and mental health problems related to environmental pollution, it is possible to alleviate many symptoms by using natural materials and furnishings free from chemicals and toxic pollutants. A growing number of people suffer from allergic reactions to petro-chemical vapours and this has led a number of manufacturers to produce natural paints made from sustainable ingredients such as plant oils, tree resins, beeswax and earth pigments. These can be used quite safely inside and outside and are especially useful in areas used by invalids, children and the elderly. In order to be healthy we require the energy from full-spectrum light, and the absence of sunlight can lead to Seasonal Affective Disorder (SAD). This problem affects thousands each year. Symptoms include depression, mood swings, headaches and general lethargy. The introduction of full spectrum lighting into home and work spaces has proved effective in minimising these problems.

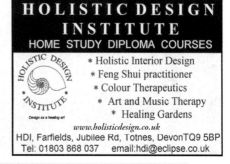

The home is a major culprit in pollution and energy waste. Homes can be substantially more polluted than the outside, especially if we seal doors and windows and centrally heat rooms without allowing air to circulate. The atmosphere in our home is just as important as the objects and furnishings in it, and this subtle environment makes all the difference. Light, colour, sound and aroma all play their part in creating the right sort of atmosphere, one where we can feel relaxed and at home. Certain colours and types of artificial lights have a direct influence on our moods, so natural interior design uses the therapeutic qualities of visible light and colours for their positive qualities.

Already a growing number of businesses are seeking out the advice of an holistic designer to help them improve the quality of the indoor environment. Sick Building Syndrome is well documented; buildings without a good circulation of fresh air and light or which are polluted by electrical smog cause untold misery to their occupants.

Absenteeism can be drastically reduced when the working environment is made healthy and uplifting. Thousands of man-hours are lost each week due to stress, backache, eyestrain and other similar ailments.

Hospitals and clinics which have employed the services of a holistic designer have found that by using natural cleaning products and by creating a less frightening and alienating interior the healing process and recuperation has been encouraged.

In schools, the use of colour and music has been found to be a positive aid to pupil concentration and learning.

It is unlikely the trend of information overload, long working hours and increasing noise and air pollution will abate within the foreseeable future. This means that more and more people will be retreating to their home as a sanctuary from the pressures outside.

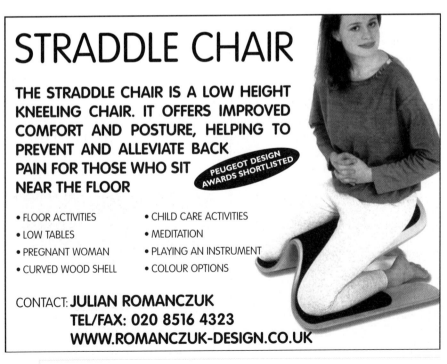

Holistic Products and Services

By M Willcocks PhD

I t is important that consumers know the policy of the shop or service provider but this is often difficult to achieve in practice. Professional shopkeepers, therapists and service providers will develop a relationship with their clients, thus creating a mutually beneficial scenario.

Effective two-way communication is essential to achieve a sound understanding with a chosen shop etc.

Keeping track of your progress is the main concern of any professional. They need to establish a rapport with you to ensure that processes are in place for monitoring and reviewing progress. Corrective action may be required to keep a programme moving in the right direction.

It should also be realised that to continue to improve your health and achieve goals, a pragmatic approach to change is needed to prepare you to accept failure or mistakes, to learn from experience and move on.

A major challenge for the health professions in the 21st century is to achieve the right balance between the short-term pressure for change in public demand and the longer-term development of natural health care.

This process requires the support of the public; hence you can help your favourite

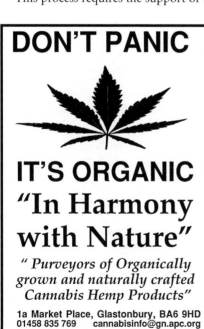
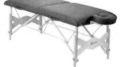

health shop or service provider by explaining your short-term requirements and ultimate goals in as much detail as possible.

This support may be an incentive to improve businesses, to enhance performance, or simply to ensure continued provision of services and products required by the customer. The solution may include the radical redesign of business processes, information needs and organisational structures. Change, whatever form it takes, needs to be managed, whatever the trigger. The approach to managing change should be holistic, and in the interest of the consumer.

Understanding the alternate health environment and by tracking this environment, with your help, shops and service providers can judge whether changes are likely to occur and can prepare contingency plans for likely scenarios. They need to be in a position to take advantage of the opportunities presented by change.

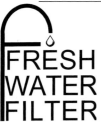

Holistic Therapists and Centres

By M Willcocks PhD

Various systems of health protection and restoration, both traditional and modern, that are reputedly based on the body's natural healing powers.

The notion of holistic medicine has been around for many years. But why, now, has interest in this area taken centre stage so to speak, and attracted so many new adherents and supporters?

The acceleration of interest in holistic medicine was probably commenced by the public rebelling against orthodox health care which is sometimes perceived as being high tech, unpersonal, authoritarian and increasingly bureaucratic and commercial.

A more caring, humanistic approach – encompassing the mind, body, emotions; to be nurtured and empowered, treated with respect, and made a partner in the healing process is the mood of today's public.

With the growing interest in holistic medicine, there has developed an increasing number of practicing holistic therapists who have followed public opinion and increasingly put into practice some of these sought-after ideals to treat the whole person as nature had intended.

They have preferred the safer, less costly, more effective and natural treatments, along with an emphasis on empowerment of the person, as a partner in their own

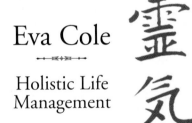

health care and healing. As more of the treatment benefits of holistic practitioners are getting reported in the scientific literature as showing efficacy, professionalism, safety, positive benefits and following the Government's code of CAM (Complementary Alternative Medicine, an initiative to regulate and license practitioners), a greater degree of acceptance and acknowledgment by conventional medicine is being seen.

There has been great reluctance to give full support, however, as much of the conventional health care establishment is historically attached to many approaches and technologies that have not proven their merit or superiority to holistic medicine practices.

Financial issues have also been a factor, as hospitals, for example, have become so heavily vested in certain technologies, such as bypass surgery and angioplasties for coronary artery therapies.

There is, however, a growing literature showing that, in many cases, more conservative management – especially holistic oriented approaches – work as well, with a tremendous added safety factor.

An example would be the impressive heart research study done, using a holistic approach and showed reversal of coronary artery blockage with arteriography studies, using a nutritional low fat diet, exercise, yoga, and group support.

There is also growing body of evidence that chelation therapy, which involves the administration in the vein of a medication called EDTA, improves symptoms associated with coronary artery disease and circulation problems, in a safe, and less costly way than traditional, invasive and surgical procedures for the same problems.

Informed members of the public requiring health care services have been seeking

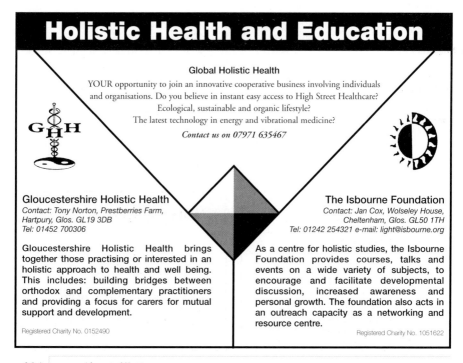

out and switching their health care to holistic therapists in greater numbers than ever before, because of several more recent factors. One has been the major shift in Government policy to move the NHS toward private medicine, or managed care, or PFIs – where to NHS rents the hospital from the private sector – with profits and cost saving being the bottom line.

These large-sized businesses were initially begun on an ethical basis. The goal was to match good patient care with cost effectiveness, monitored clinical outcomes, and collaborative relationships between the NHS and nursing homes, however this has often degenerated into unethical businesses, that lack clinical leadership.

They attempt to reduce cost by keeping out sicker patients, mixing medical care and clinical decision-making into a maze of bureaucratic red tape, and providing, in some cases, incentives to specialist clinicians to provide less care.

There have also been the large commercial drug companies that have developed and marketed drugs which are less safe and less effective than the more natural alternatives, such as botanical, nutritional, or other holistic approaches used by holistic therapists. These expensive drugs which are dispensed by GPs appear almost as a preference to accepting that there are less expensive natural cures available.

A recent positive trend has been in the medical colleges, which are beginning to invite holistic practitioners to lecture or to develop programs in the colleges to complement their more conventional curricula. Major companies are now supporting the NHS in the research of holistic and alternative medicine.

With these current trends, the changing needs and perceptions by a more informed public, and the increasing scientific validation of holistic approaches, the holistic method of treatment is coming of age and developing into a new frontier of health care and human awareness.

Holistic Retuning

By Jayne Williams

Holistic Retuning is a way for us to 'tune into and receive' what we want in our lives, rather than what we don't want. Sessions are gentle and informative yet fast acting and profound.

Information on how to retune is specific to each individual and is gathered by Kinesiology. The actual process of Retuning is truly holistic, and could be any one from about 400 ways, including flower essences, colour, sound, light, crystals to name but a few. Holistic Retuning can be used for anything physical, mental, emotional or spiritual, from allergy testing or asthma to emotional trauma and relationship issues. It can be carried out by someone else or learnt for use on yourself in your own home.

Our bodies are made purely from atoms that vibrate at a certain frequency. Our body can therefore be likened to a specific frequency. Depending what that frequency is, we will tune into and receive different things in our lives. These things are a bit like radio stations, so whatever we are tuned into we receive. With Holistic Retuning we find out what you're tuned into, and also what you would benefit from being tuned into. We find out how to get you from one to the other and then we check that you've really really changed. Holistic Retuning may be likened to removing a tree you no longer want. It does not remove leaves followed by branches, followed by trunk, followed by... it simply removes the roots and the tree can no longer exist. Holistic Retuning not only removes the tree you do not want it also plants a new flower or something else that you do want in its place!

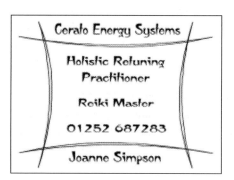

Holographic Repatterning

By the Holographic Repatterning Association

Holographic Repatterning (HR), developed by Chloe Faith Wordsworth, is an extraordinary and practical method that enables the HR practitioner to identify and transform the energy contradictions and unconscious patterns that underlie all problems.

New physics has proven that matter and energy are interchangeable and that the physical body, the emotional body and the mind are all frequencies of energy-knowledge that have been known and applied in China, Tibet and India for more than 5,000 years.

When frequencies move out of phase as a result of earlier painful experiences, it may manifest as health problems, unworkable relationships, depression, low confidence, issues concerning business and money or any daily distress we may be experiencing.

By receiving Holographic Repatterning sessions, the HR practitioner identifies the non coherent pattern so the client can experience positive change physically, emotionally or mentally.

Holographic Repatterning is an extraordinary step-by-step process of self-healing, which enables us to identify and transform the unconscious patterns that underlie our pain, sickness, unworkable relationships, career issues and other life problems.

Scientific research has shown that matter and energy are interchangeable and that all matter pulsates at different rates or frequencies. Our thoughts, feelings, organs and tissues all vibrate at their own unique frequency. When these frequencies are out of phase, we may find ourselves unconsciously resonating with poor health, unhappy relationships, failure, low confidence, depression and other life-depleting responses.

HR, based on the principle of resonance, facilitates a shift in our frequency wave patterns, similar to changing the waveband on the radio. The programme we experience depends on the wavelength we are tuned into, whether success or failure, joy or depression, health or sickness.

When we are in-phase with unconscious negative beliefs we create a reality based on limitation that prevents us from achieving our full potential in life. Only when we are in-phase with words and beliefs that empower and energise us can we achieve personal growth, fulfilment and thus happiness.

Through Holographic Repatterning these negative resonances can be transformed – repatterned – into positive ones, thus eliminating blockages that prevent us from reaching our full potential in life.

In Holographic Repatterning we use the strength or weakness of a muscle (muscle checking), as an indicator of the resonance of the body-mind frequency system.

Homeopathy

By M Willcocks PhD

Homeopathy, founded by German physician Samuel Hahnemann in the 1790s, is based on the idea that 'like cures like'; that is, substances that cause certain symptoms in a healthy person can also cure those same symptoms in someone who is sick.

This so-called 'law of similar' gives homeopathy its name: 'homeo' for similar, 'pathy' designating disease. In his experiments, Hahnemann developed a method of 'potentising' homeopathic remedies by diluting them in a water-alcohol solution and then vigorously shaking the mixtures.

His observations of patients convinced him that a high degree of dilution not only minimised the side effects of the remedies but also enhanced their medical efficacy.

Is Homeopathy safe?

Yes. Since the substances are given in minute doses unwanted side-effects are avoided, making them safe to use even in situations where conventional drugs would be dangerous or inadvisable, for example during pregnancy or when treating infants.

When should I consult a qualified Homeopath?

If you have a serious or recurring condition or you have had a number of acute illnesses recently, it is always best to see a qualified Homeopath. Remember

Homeopathy can be used to treat anything, even problems that have no clear diagnosis, because it treats the individual rather than the disease.

If you have a chronic, or frequently recurring, complaint the first consultation generally takes about one and a half hours. You begin by telling the Homeopath what is troubling you. It is helpful if you can give as much detail as possible about your symptoms, including anything that makes them better or worse. If you have noticed any other changes in yourself (mood, anxieties, sleep, dreams, appetite, thirst, temperature) since the symptoms started; these can also be very useful. The Homeopath will normally take a full medical case history from you and record details of any previous health problems in your family, going back to your grandparents. The aim of the consultation is to get an overview, not only of your complaint, but also of you as a person. Follow-up consultations usually last around 45 minutes. They help you and your Homeopath to assess your reaction to the previous remedy and decide how your treatment can best be continued. Sometimes, if the remedy is working well the Homeopath may wait and not prescribe anything, but the information gathered during the appointment may well be used later on, in selecting the next remedy.

How many consultations will I need to have?

This is a difficult question to answer and will depend on the individual. However, one can generalise a little. Acute cases and injuries tend to respond quickly once the correct remedy is found. The same is often true of more long-term problems which have a clear aetiology (i.e. if you have never been well since a particular event). For chronic illness there is a rule of thumb that it may take up to one consultation for every year that you have had the complaint.

Should I stop taking all other medication?

It is important to tell your Homoeopath about any medication you are taking. As a general rule, homoeopaths do not advise you to stop taking prescribed drugs suddenly, although hopefully the need for them will lessen as treatment progresses. Since each case is different this is something that should be discussed during your consultations.

How can I tell if the homeopathic medicine is working or not?

Reactions to Homoeopathic medicines vary with the individual. Some experience a clear improvement in symptoms early on. Others find symptoms worsening for a time before improving (this is known as an aggravation). Still others find that their general sense of well-being increases, but the symptoms they wanted cured stay the same. Perhaps surprisingly, this is a good sign as it shows the remedy is working at the most fundamental level and removing disease. Eventually the symptoms will disappear.

Apart from general improvements (in sleep, digestion, mood etc.) Homeopaths look for three particular things, which indicate a movement towards cure. The first is a shift in symptoms from above to below, that is from head to toe (for example, a rash moving down the body). The second is a shift from within to out, in other words from deeper parts of the body to the surface (asthma changing to eczema, for example). The third is that old symptoms start to appear in reverse order.

This is the equivalent of the body having a spring clean, clearing out old symptoms that have previously been suppressed. It will be a help to your Homeopath if you can mention any changes that you have noticed since taking the remedy.

HOMEOPATHY

CHELTENHAM HOMEOPATHIC CLINIC is Gloucestershire's longest established homeopathic clinic. We can provide the best in homeopathic care for all ages, from pre-conceptual treatment, through pregnancy, birth, childhood and adulthood to old age. Just 'phone 01242 520704

DO SOMETHING GOOD for your body and your soul. Beautiful and tranquil surroundings. Bed and breakfast offered. Homoeopathy, Soft Tissue Massage, Kinesiology, Spinal Touch. Barbara Baylis, Two Oaks, Mynd, Bucknell, Shrops SY7 0BD. Tel: 01547 530712

ANNE ELAND LCPH, MHMA. Homoeopathy at home in West and Central London. Home visits by qualified and experienced homoeopath. Gentle healing for mind and body, female problems a speciality. Tel 020 8995 8108 after 6pm for appointments.

DOROTHY MCLAUGHLIN, LCCH., Homoeopath, Healer & Kinesiologist. Shrops/Wales, Midlands (Market Drayton) Tel 01630 657642 Mob. 07989 318209.

HOMEOPATHY

DOY DALLING: RSHom. 126, Hanworth Road, Hampton, Middlesex TW12 3EY. 0181 979 049. TRIO CLINIC: Trio Pharmacy, 21 High Street, Shepperton Surrey TW17 9AJ. Tel: 0181 979 0497. Ashford Osteopathic Clinic, 23 Feltham Road, Ashford, Middlesex TW15 1DQ. Tel: 01784 255535 or 0181 979 0497.

WANDA WHITING LCH. MCH. R. S. Hom. 5, Priory Avenue, Hastings, East Sussex, TN34 1UQ. Tel: 01421 421438. 6, Springfield Road, St Leonards on Sea, TN38 0TU. Tel: 01424 7136433. Registered Homoeopath. Effective, gentle, treatment for general health problems.

MRS R DURSTON, The Bees, Beaworthy, Devon, EX21 5AN. 01837 871276

MRS H CONWAY, 4 Fore Street, Bishopsteignton, Devon, TQ14 9QP. 01626 779054

MRS S CREATON, Verona, 1 New Street, Paignton, Devon, TQ3 3HL. 01803 557635

MR Y P MAINI, 21 Latham Road, Bexley Heath, Kent, DA6 7NW. 01322 521334

Hypnotherapy

By the National Register of Hypnotherapists and Psychotherapists

In the right hands, hypnotherapy is a safe and beneficial therapy. A properly qualified practitioner will take a client's full medical, emotional and social history before deciding on a treatment strategy.

Unlike most comparable therapies, hypnotherapy measures its history not in years or decades but in centuries. The usually acknowledged forerunner of modern hypnotherapy, Franz Mesmer (1734-1815), believed in the existence of a universal fluid, an imbalance of which caused illness.

However, Mesmer's contemporaries attributed his undoubted success to his manipulation of a patient's imagination. During the 19th century, this theme was followed by several doctors who used hypnosis successfully, not only to treat psychological illness but also as an anaesthetic for surgical operations.

Although the development of chemical anaesthetics displaced the use of hypnosis in surgery, and Freud's use of psychoanalysis began to displace it in psychotherapy, the benefits and uses of hypnotherapy are such that it remains a popular and adaptive form of therapy.

Hypnotherapy may be used on its own, as a simple relaxation therapy, or it may be integrated with any of the great schools of psychological thought. This integrative approach, termed hypno-psychotherapy, has very wide therapeutic applications.

In addition to treating emotional, neurotic and some psychiatric disorders such as smoking, overeating and insomnia, to social difficulties such as lack of confidence, examination or driving test nerves, phobias, panic attacks and depression, it is also widely used for enhancing sporting performance, creativity, memory and concentration.

Hypno-psychotherapy also has other clinical and medical applications including pre- or post-operative treatments, anaesthesia and pain relief strategies. Many stress related physical problems such as skin disorders, migraine and irritable bowel syndrome also respond well to hypno-psychotherapy.

Only a small selection of the many problems posed by our society and the way we live are mentioned above. There are many others which may be alleviated by hypnotherapy and they can be discussed in total confidence with a qualified hypno-psychotherapist. There are some instances where the use of hypnosis is not recommended, or where it should be used only with care.

These include epilepsy, recent electro-convulsive therapy, drug or alcohol intoxication and heart or breathing problems. In these cases, other forms of psychotherapy may be more appropriate.

If only simple relaxation therapy is required, then someone with basic hypnotherapy training should be able to help. However, more complex emotional, psychological or physical problems require the help of a fully qualified hypno-psychotherapist who will have skills to recognise and treat a wide range of disorders and conditions.

People looking for a reputable hypno-psychotherapist should ensure that the practitioner has completed an accredited training and belongs to a recognised professional association which requires members to adhere to a code of ethics and carry appropriate insurance.

A well-regulated professional body should also have a complaint procedure and will require members to submit to ongoing peer supervision and to undertake continuing professional development.

HYPNOTHERAPY

A & F HORMASJI [Established 1972.] MNCP CMH MUKGHE MNCP (Acc) C.Hyp NRHP DHP UKCP Registered. Essex [Romford] 01708 764740, London [Hale Clinic] 020 7637 3377. Specialisation: Smoking, Slimming & Phobias E.mail: fhormasji@talk21.com

HYPNO-PSYCHOTHERAPY
At Optimum Health: 0115 914 3311

For Stress, Smoking and Weight Loss

Jennifer Craven-Griffiths
CHP (NC) MRHP (ASSOC)

58 Edward Road, West Bridgford, Notts NG2 5GB

TEL: **0115 914 0622** • FAX: **0115 914 0623**

REMEMBER

Check that the therapist is registered with a recognized professional association, which holds a public register, code of conduct, effective disciplinary procedure and complaints mechanism.

Get the address of the organization and contact them for information on their training criteria and practice standards.

Indian Head Massage

If you want to get ahead – get a head massage

By Narendra Mehta

As a child my mother and local barber used to give me a head massage. I came to Britain in 1973 and a few weeks after my arrival I was very stressed out and needed a relaxing head massage.

I searched high and low but found that no-one had even heard of this therapy. So a few years later I decided to go to India specifically to learn the technique. On my return I then adapted it to meet the needs of a highly stressed Western culture.

Few people remain unaffected by the stresses and strains of modern living; in fact a high proportion of modern illnesses can be attributed to it.

Those of us who suffer often complain that we feel tense in the shoulders and neck areas and these can lead to tension headaches. Indian champissage, also known as head massage, is guaranteed to put a stop to those feelings.

The technique is based on the ancient Ayurvedic healing system. It has been practised in India for over a thousand years originally by women who believed that massaging their heads with natural vegetable or Ayurvedic oils kept their hair long and lustrous. This is one of the reasons why so many Indian women have such beautiful, thick locks.

Men also receive this massage when they go to the barbershop or on the beach from

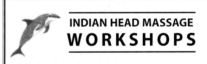

a champiwallah. The word 'champi' means massage of the head and the word shampoo is a derivative of it.

There is a sound scientific reason why massaging the scalp is good for your hair. It stimulates the flow of blood to the hair follicles, improving the supply of nutrients needed for healthy hair growth.

Nowadays the most common cause of poor blood flow is stress generated muscle tension. By relieving this tension, champissage not only improves the condition of your hair, but also provides an invaluable treatment for stress-related problems like eye strain, headaches, insomnia, lack of concentration, tense muscles in the neck and shoulders and feeling lethargic.

In addition to traditional head massage, I incorporated the massage of the shoulders, upper arm and neck as these are the areas which are vulnerable to the build up of stress.

Gradually I also included the massage of the face and ears and at a later date added chakra energy balancing. This massage stimulates blood and lymphatic circulation, breaks down knots and nodules, disperses toxins and improves joint mobility. Energy balancing leaves you with a deep sense of peace, calm and tranquillity.

The beauty of this massage is that you don't need to undress to enjoy it, no oils or creams are used and so it can be carried out in the workplace. Right now there are many qualified therapists who make their living by visiting offices and giving head massages.

The therapy became so popular that Thorsons approached me to write a book on Indian Head Massage, which was published last year. This clearly illustrated book gives step by step instructions of the massage technique. It also looks at the history of Champissage and introduces you to the importance and power of touch.

It teaches you how to manage stress, how to look after your hair and how to improve your relationship with your partner through the practice of Champissage.

I have travelled throughout Europe, the Unites States and Australia where Champissage has really taken off.

Indian Head Massage – Discover the Power of Touch – paperback £12.99 Published by Thorsons, ISBN 0 7225 3940 1; www.indianchampissage.com

Courses
Running for 8 years
all year round

Professional training – so you can practice right away **or**

Interest – you can treat friends and family

For information pack contact
Penny Upchurch-Davies LicAc, MBAcC, Itec
Belmore Centre, Lower Stoke Manderville Road,
Bucks HP21 9DR

01296 612361

Words of **Wisdom**

"There are worse occupations in this world than feeling a woman's pulse"

LAURENCE STERNE

Iridology

A Major Analytical Tool Using the Iris of the Eye
By Angela Bradbury, Vice President of the
Guild of Naturopathic Iridologists

The Iris, the coloured part of the eye surrounding the pupil, is made up of thousands of nerve endings, all of which are connected to the brain. At the foetus stage of our existence, the Iris is part of the brain.

As we develop, the Iris Stalk extends these nerve endings outwards, providing a God-given, exposed, microchip of information. The Iris is referred to by the German Medicos and Heilpractikers as an 'optic-neuro-reflex' of information. It is also well established in France, being part of their medical curriculum.

Iridology is an ancient science which has gained more recent resurrection through scientific and medical research, particularly in Germany, Russia and America. In 1000 BC the Chaldeans of Babylonia were carving depications of the Iris topography into stone slabs, along with the reflex zones to human anatomy.

More recently, the writings of physicians such as Philippus Meyen's *Chiromatica Medica* published in Dresden in 1670, Dr. Ignatz von Pecsely's *Discoveries in the Realms of Nature* and *Arts of Healing* published in Budapest in 1880, Dr. Haskel Kritzer's *The Book of Iris diagnosis* published in the early 1900s and soon to be re-published by The Holistic Health College, London UK, and Dr. V.L. Fernandiz's *Iris diagnosis* published in Spain in 1970, to name but a few, record extensive research corroborated by surgical, autopsy, X-ray and other modern pathology techniques.

A professionally trained Iridologist is merely map reading. Providing they have a good grounding in Anatomy and Physiology, they can give the patient a very thorough breakdown on their genetic strengths and weaknesses, precisely localised congestive and irritative conditions, and the inter-reactions of various conditions throughout their system, hormonally, toxically, neurologically and systemically.

Most Iridologists use a medical torch and a magnifier. These allow an unobtrusive surveillance, to include a manipulation of the torch, so enabling the light to reveal the three-dimensional aspects of the Iris. A hand-written record is taken, sometimes along with photographs, if the practitioner has the necessary equipment.

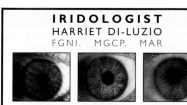
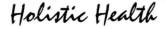

The latter is more for record purposes rather than being diagnostic, as photographs can mislead, being one-dimensional and reflective of light and shadow variations.

Certain markings reveal various conditions. For example, a lesion, or lacuna, which appears as a closed hole in the uppermost surface layer of the Iris, means a weakness exists in that zone. Which particular zone is involved is easily revealed from the corresponding zone in Iris map or chart.

The Iris charts used today are based upon those put together by medically trained physicians such as Dr. Ignatz von Peczely, whose research was recorded in the 19th century, and, more recently, by Bernard Jensen, D.C., Ph.D., who studied initially under Dr. Henry Lane, M.D., and Dr. Henry Lindlahr, MD. Other medicos such as Dr. Haskel Kritzer and Dr. D.L. Ferrandiz also used autopsy and surgical corroborations to verify their findings, to mention but a few.

Those who understand the mechanics of Reflexology will quickly grasp those of Iridology. The difference between these two sciences is that the Reflexologist provides a therapy by stimulating the nerve endings which pronounce themselves, whereas the Iridologist is purely a diagnostician, able to pin-point the root cause, or causes of problems and also provide a personalised analysis for preventative medicine measures. Iridologists are not classified as therapists as such, unless additionally trained to prescribe or administer treatments.

The genetic Constitution is immediately apparent in the Iris. The three main Iris colours are Blue, Brown and mixed Hazel, or brown/green, Iris, the last being a combination of the former two which has developed through the generations.

Although there are 25 Constitutions to be analysed from the Irides, there are only three basic Constitutions, the TRUE BROWN, or Haematogenic Constitution, the BLUE, or Pure Lymphatic Constitution, and the MIXED, or Biliary Constitution.

Although the BLUE EYES are subdivided into several sub groupings, they predominantly reflect what is known medically and naturopathically as a LYMPHATIC CONSTITUTION. This means that such people have a predisposition towards a re-activity of the Lymphatic system.

They will be prone to swollen lymph glands, coughs, bronchitis, asthma, sinusitis, catarrh, diarrhoea, arthritis, vaginal discharges, eye irritations, eczema, acne, flaky dry skin, dandruff, fluid retention, splenitis etc. In other words, should conditions exist which exacerbate anything to do with the lymphatic system, this group will be more re-active or vulnerable.

The true BROWN eye reflects the HAEMATOGENIC CONSTITUTION and there are no underlying green or blue nerve fibres to be found. This type is prone to blood disorders such as auto-intoxication; anaemia; lack of catalysts such as gold, copper, zinc, iodine, arsenic, gold and iron; blood diseases such as hepatitis or jaundice; arthritis; endocrine disorders usual stemming from thyroid, adrenal or pituitary irregularities; poor lymphatic drainage; flatulence; constipation; digestive insufficiencies and poor enzymatic production to include a cow's milk intolerance; ulcers; liver, gall-bladder and pancreatic malfunctions to include Diabetes; and circulatory disorders.

The MIXED, or BILIARY IRIS has a basic background of blue with a brown overlay, giving the appearance of what is often called a Hazel Eye. These Irides reflect a combination of the Haematogenic tendencies as well as the Blue Eyed traits.

Thus such people are prone to flatulence; constipation; colitis; Diabetes; hypoglycaemia; blood diseases; gall-stones; liver, gall-bladder, bile duct and pancreatic disorders; gastro-intestinal weakness with spasm as well as the lymphatic reactivies which can manifest in many ways such as allergic, arthritic or irritative skin disorders.

Just because we are all born with various genetic traits, manifesting as both strengths and weaknesses, it does not mean we will be subjected to all, or even several of the problems that could afflict us.

Self-abuse, environmental influences and neglect could stimulate these tendencies to manifest but the value of fore-knowledge is that we can avoid provoking such inherent weaknesses.

On the basis of 'Man Know Thyself', we can reverse congestive and irritative conditions within if we know their true source, or 'Root Cause'. We cannot change to any great degree, our inherent weaknesses, but we can adapt our life styles in order to meet our highly individualised needs and wants.

For example, if three patients visiting a Practitioner who was also an Iridologist, in one day, all suffering from Chronic Fatigue Syndrome, it is quite common for each to go away with a totally different programme to reverse their problems.

With one, the Iridologist might find that spinal impingements are limiting the nerve impulses to various organs and especially to the brain and/or pituitary. With another, their Irides may reveal chronic toxicity of the intestinal tract causing an overload onto the liver which explains why, despite eight hours of uninterrupted sleep, they wake feeling 'hung over'.

With the third patient, one or two food intolerances due to inadequacies of their stomach and/or pancreatic secretions could be found creating allergic and hypoglycaemic conditions which can be quickly reversed.

Some, poor unfortunates may even have a combination of one or more of the above disorders. However, their Irides will reflect the conditions within. Once these are known, the areas for attention are revealed.

It is then up to the appropriate therapist to reverse the abnormalities and educate the patient as to what has been happening, in order to restore GOOD HEALTH. Iridology has cut out the guesswork.

Where to find a qualified Iridologist

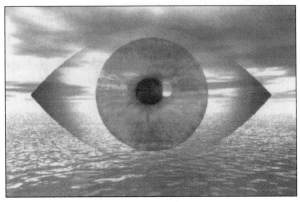

Send SAE to, or phone:

The Guild of Naturopathic Iridologists International
94 Grosvenor Road, London SW1V 3LF
Tel/Fax: 020 7821 0255
Further information: www.gni-international.org

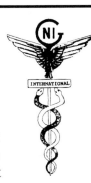

Iridology with Equines

By Ellen Collinson

Iridology is a recognised tool of diagnosis in humans and has been around since the ancient Egyptians and in the later part of the 19th century it was more scientifically chronicled by German Doctor Ignats von Peczeley.

It is not widely known or practised on horses, however there was a man named Syd Mercer who used to diagnose through the eye, he lived in England.

Syd Mercer worked in the remount services on the south coast of England during the First World War and handled a large number of injured, dying and dead horses.

He noticed the different markings in the Iris and noted the connection due to the origins of the body. He helped a lot of horses to win races, including Barona to win two Scottish Nationals, and also Rheingold to win the Arc de Triomphe.

There are also at least two equine iridologists working in Australia. Three years ago I visited them, and had the opportunity to work with them. It was of great benefit to us all as the Australian horses are on the whole much healthier than the English or Irish due to diet and climate, but they have a lot more injuries due to their racing, so I learnt more about injuries and they learnt more about internal problems.

I have recently been asked by several Veterinary surgeons in Ireland to help both with diagnosis and also with herbal treatment, when the conventional medicine has not worked, the horses always respond very quickly to the herbs.

Once I have detected a problem I then recommend a course of treatment, this can be herbal remedies which I make up specifically for that horse, or it can simply be dietary changes or it can be massage, laser, nerve stimulation or Shiatsu.

The system of herbal medicine I use includes the traditions of the Native Americans and several Chinese herbs and formulas.

The remedies are made from powders and tinctures, which are extremely potent and the formulas can include up to 20 different herbs.

Even though the remedies are for specific ailments, each remedy works in a holistic way, cleansing and detoxifying the whole system.

There is a combination of herbs suitable for the majority of problems.

Jin Shin Jyutsu

*By David Burmeister, Michou Landon
and Compiled by Editha Campbell*

Jin Shin Jyutsu, physio-philosophy, involves the application of the hands or fingers for gently balancing the flow of life energy in the body. More generally, it is the awakening to awareness of complete harmony within the self and the universe.

It is an ancient Japanese art of harmonising life energy within the body. Our bodies contain energy pathways that feed life info all of our cells. When one or more of these paths become blocked, this damning effect may lead to discomfort or even pain. This blockage, stagnation or deviation will not only disrupt the local area, but also will continue and eventually disharmonise the complete path or paths of the energy flow.

Jin Shin Jyutsu releases tensions which are the causes to various symptoms in the body. It is a helpful complement to western medicine and other complementary modalities. According to ancient written records, which remain in the archives of the Imperial Palace in Japan, Jin Shin Jyutsu is said to predate Buddha and Moses. It is an innate part of man's inner wisdom, simplifying the complexities of existence – an art of living.

This art was passed down from generation to generation by word of mouth and had fallen into relative obscurity when it was dramatically revived it in the early 1900s by Master Jiro Murai in Japan.

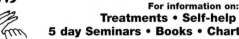

After recovering from a life-threatening illness, Master Murai devoted the rest of his life to the research, development and revival of the Art. He gathered insight from a range of experiences and resources including the Kojiki (Record of Ancient Things). In the late 1940s Master Murai gave a talk in a house where a young Japanese American happened to be giving English lessons. It was a life-changing encounter. He approached her and asked if she would take a gift from Japan to America.

Mary Burmeister, not fully understanding the meaning of this offer, was open to it and said yes. She became a student of Master Murai for the next 12 years until Master Murai's death in 1961. She returned to the United States in 1954 but it was not until 1963 that Mary Burmeister began teaching and sharing the art actively. She stopped teaching the five-day seminars in 1990. These seminars are now taught throughout the US, and in Canada, Brazil, New Zealand and in Europe by associate teachers.

Learning Jin Shin Jyutsu engages one in self-study and self-help. Through the process of 'now know myself', we recognise the wisdom of the body and we learn to interpret the messages provided and utilise them to restore balance. We learn from the body through daily applications. We begin to 'listen and talk' to our bodies in the most universal of languages – that of energy.

There are two important distinctions between Jin Shin Jyutsu and many other massage and oriental healing modalities to which it is often compared. First, Jin Shin Jyutsu is an art as opposed to a technique. It is a skillful creation. Second, Jin Shin Jyutsu does not involve massage, or physical manipulation of tissue or muscles or use of drugs or substances and uses only minimal pressure. The hands or fingertips are placed, over clothing, on designated sites, called 'safety energy locks' to harmonise, unblock or restore the energy flow along its pathways.

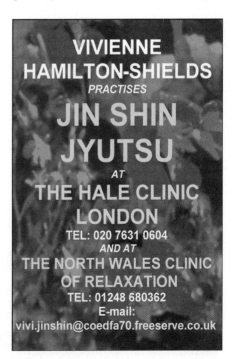

So we see that Jin Shin Jyutsu can be applied as self-help and also by a trained practitioner. A practitioner of Jin Shin Jyutsu is not the 'do-er'; he or she simply assists in the flow of an infinite supply of universal energy.

This process does not affect the practitioner's personal supply of energy. In fact the person applying or 'jumper cabling' often benefits as well. In a typical session, which lasts about one hour, the receiver lies face up, fully clothed, on a couch or cushioned surface. After 'listening' to the energy pulses in the wrists, the practitioner employs a harmonising sequence or 'flow', appropriate for unblocking and restoring the circulation of energy along the pathways.

This facilitates the reduction of tension and stress, which accumulate through normal daily living. To a certain extent the experience of a session is unique to each person at each session. However, the most common effect is that of deep relaxation.

For those of us addressing existing stress or health disharmonies, or for those simply wishing to participate actively in maintaining health, harmony and well-being, the art of Jin Shin Jyutsu is a simple and powerful tool available to all.

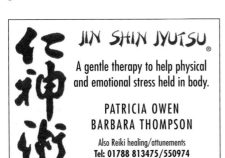
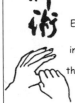
JIN SHIN JYUTSU

HELENA HERRING, Duxhurst Place, Duxhurst Lane, Duxhurst, Nr Reigate, Surrey. Tel: 01293 862045. Jin Shin Jyutsu Practitioner. Also practising part time in Appledore, Devon.

JIN SHIN JYUTSU. Physio-philosophy, an ancient Japanese art of harmonising and balancing life energy within the body. Individual appointments and Self Help groups contact Stephanie Stevenson. Tel/fax: 01344 776926.

MS D MCCARTHY, 63 Turtle Gate Avenue, Withywood, Bristol, BS13 8NN. 0117 964 7763

MR & MRS R MCCATHIE, 9 Gressenham Court, Aran Drive, Stanmore, Middlesex, HA7 4LZ. 020 8954 5157

MS E MANSFIELD, 23 Harmans Mead, East Grinstead, Sussex, RH19 3XX. 01342 300988

Journey Work

A journey into wholeness

Since the publication of her book,'The Journey – An Extraordinary Guide For Healing Your Life & Setting Yourself Free', the demand for places on Brandon Bays' weekends has rocketed! So what is it that draws people so strongly to this work?

Brandon Bays has been described as one of the most dynamic and innovative teachers in the personal growth field today and has appeared on stage with Anthony Robbins, Wayne Dyer and other leading personal development teachers.

'The Journey' processes, which she now teaches in her seminars, were born out of dramatic personal experience. In 1992 Brandon was diagnosed with a basketball size tumour. At the time she received this terrifying news she'd been at the forefront of the alternative healthcare field for over 12 years.

The tumour forced her to go beyond everything she had learned in the alternative field. She was driven to look beneath the surface for something deeper. In a profound process of introspection she discovered that stored inside the tumour was an old unresolved traumatic memory from her childhood. Through a powerful process, she was able to finally face, resolve, forgive and complete that old issue. When it was complete her body went about the natural process of healing on its own. Only six weeks later, she was pronounced perfectly clear – without medicine or surgery!

What Brandon experienced was the effect of cell memory. Dr. Deepak Chopra in his book Quantum Healing teaches that trauma and suppressed negative emotions are often stored as 'phantom memories' in our cells. He argues that these cellular memories act subtly over long periods of time, and can cause disease and illness many years after they have first been put in place. What Brandon discovered was how to access specific cell memories and, more important, how to actively resolve and let go of the stored issues.

The impressive results from The Journey are a testimony to how effectively it enables people to access their own natural healing potential. Emotional issues evaporate, unresourceful behaviour disappears and physical conditions resolve and heal. Brandon's landmark book is now available in all major bookshops.

So what is it about The Journey that evokes such profound and lasting success where many other approaches fail? Brandon attributes all 'curative' success to the part of us that is already whole, pointing out that all Journey work is carried out 'at the deepest level'. This 'deepest level' has many names. Athletes call it the zone, scholars call it universal intelligence or Soul and quantum physicists call it quantum soup. The Journey offers a way to connect with this – your true nature and your own highest wisdom. Beyond the excellent presentation and the learning of life transforming skills – it is the remarkable awakening to who we really are, with the deepest recognition of our own Body-Mind's natural healing genius, that is the greatest gift of the Journey Intensive Weekend.

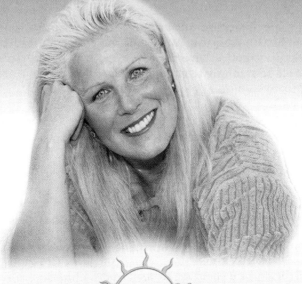

Kinesiology

By Brian H. Butler

In 1964, an American chiropractor, Dr George Goodheart D.C, discovered that specific muscles when gently tested could reveal a great deal about the state of health of the body not possible by other means. He called this new science 'applied Kinesiology'. 'Kinetics' relates to energy and movement.

Muscle responses, a sort of bio-feedback, are affected by our thoughts and emotions, foods and chemicals, and the ways we use the muscles and bones. Small differences in strength can show up undesirable 'imbalances'.

The idea

The body can cope with the effect of most minor stresses. It has amazing self-healing powers. Excess stresses are not handled so well. They may cause slight imbalances which may give rise to the need for the body to make compensations. Such compensations, if ignored, can lead to impairment of function. If these symptoms are not resolved they may produce distressing symptoms. Muscle response testing correction procedures of Kinesiology can detect and resolve these minor imbalances, even before we are aware of them. Each muscle relies on a nerve to activate it and blood supply to oxygenate it. They also need lymph, which feeds and cleans them.

Meridians, or energy lines of acupuncture, have energy connections all up and down the spine. These electrical energy 'circuits', largely ignored by conventional approaches, link muscles to organs, to our mental activity and nutritional factors. Almost all disease is the result of stressing the body to a greater extent than it can adapt to. If enough stresses remain unresolved, they cause changes in function. These functional changes, in time, may give rise to symptoms, which if still unresolved lead to the onset of disease, and ultimately death.

If Kinesiological 'balancing' of imbalanced 'circuits' is performed on a regular basis, aches, pains and other minor symptoms are usually relieved. Everyday small imbalances are resolved as they occur. The accumulation of functional changes is addressed and effective steps taken to prevent a recurrence. Kinesiological balancing not only solves the ailment but raises general health levels. The soundest protection against any form of discomfort or disease is radiant health. The most powerful function of Kinesiology is prevention.

The interaction with a Kinesiologist

A Kinesiologist will listen carefully to the reasons that made the person seek help. He or she will ask whether the individual has consulted a medical practitioner, and whether other forms of therapy have been tried. The practitioner, without prying, will encourage the client to give as much background information about home life, work, food intake, sleep, rest and exercise patterns, as is necessary to form a picture of possible lifestyle causes.

Then follows the muscle testing analysis procedure, which is gentle and non-intrusive. Any muscle weaknesses or energy imbalances are recorded, and structural compensations noted. Kinesiological muscle test responses tell the practitioner what needs correcting. A great advantage of Kinesiology is that the muscle tests can reveal

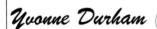

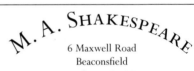

the order in which the body prefers corrections to be made. Corrections not made in priority order may help for a short while, but the problem usually returns quickly. This may account for why many people who seek help from various therapies and get relief find the beneficial effect is only short lived.

In practice, priority testing means that the Kinesiologist does not have to guess at the diagnosis, or form an opinion as to what treatment is required. They merely make the detailed specific corrections dictated by the results of the muscle tests. Everyone gets a different, individual treatment. Corrections are made in a number of ways. Sometimes firm massage on specific reflexes is also used to restore balance to muscles which have tested weak. This can be a little uncomfortable for a few seconds but this quickly passes and full muscle power is quickly restored.

Treatment usually take between 15 and 40 minutes. Research shows that it is unwise and unnecessary to give prolonged treatments. Treatments often promote profound changes in bodily functions, which may have been impaired for years. It is wise to allow the body to adjust to these changes before more corrections are made.

What illnesses?

Kinesiologists do not address disease unless they are professionally and medically trained to do so. Kinesiology is effective with many health problems that are not identifiable diseases. Most things people suffer from cannot be diagnosed as named illness, nor effectively treated by orthodox means. Kinesiology is helpful with general aches and pains, stiffness, pre-menstrual and digestive problems, food sensitivities, backache, sore shoulders, headaches; wrist, elbow, knee and ankle problems, sprains, stresses and strains of everyday life, depression, anxiety, fears and even phobias.

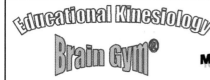

Kinesiology promotes a strengthening and balancing of the structure, the immune system, the endocrine and digestive systems. The whole bio-chemical and bio-energetic systems benefit. Kinesiology also promotes mental strength, positivity and emotional balance. 'Rebalancing' empowers the bodies' own self-healing resources to deal more effectively with any long-term stresses.

Benefits

Kinesiology does not offer 'cures'. However, remarkable and sometimes seemingly miraculous results do occur from appropriate regular Kinesiological 'balancing'. Kinesiology has helped many people who had 'tried everything', sometimes over many years, to resolve problems they had been told they had to live with. Kinesiology is used by professionals in all branches of health care. The American Olympics teams use Kinesiologists to tune athletes for peak performance.

LaStone Therapy

By Debbie Thomas at the British School of Complementary Therapy

The brainchild of Arizona-based Mary Hannigan, LaStone Therapy is sweeping across the oceans with its amazing therapeutic effects. LaStone Therapy involves the use of warmed basalt lava stones, providing soothing deep relaxation, effleurage, toxin clearing and energy balancing qualities.

Chilled marble stones are integrated into the treatment accelerating the flow of blood and lymph, and healing.

The stones, of all shapes and sizes, are used warmed and chilled depending on the needs and pains of the client, thus experiencing deep levels of sensation in response to the alternating temperatures, providing therapeutic, deeper stress-relieving benefits, enabling the therapist to assist the client in healing on all levels.

LaStone Therapy truly is a complete body, mind and soul treatment enabling the client to reach a state of relaxation within minutes of using these fascinating stones, something not normally associated with traditional massage.

Covered with a towel or sheet, the stones that address different healing aspects are then placed under the body, either side of the spine and a pillow stone. The therapist will then place more stones on the topside of the client, typically following the chakra positions, under the palms and in between the toes.

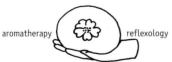

Next comes the massage itself, which can involve a variety of treatments including deep tissue, Shiatsu and basic Swedish. The therapist applies oil to the body and puts the stones to work.

Each of the 54 warm stones each have a role in the session; some are for trigger-point work, effleurage and some specifically for energy balancing. Each stone, once put to work in massage form, holds its heat for approximately three minutes.

As the stones lose their heat, the therapist quietly exchanges them for newly warmed ones. Working over the whole body this treatment lasts for about 75 minutes in total.

Finally the session ends with the removal of stones and energy balancing and a resting period for the client to absorb the work. While not tools, the stones are conduits to all levels of experience – physical, emotional and spiritual.

On the physical level, if the therapist uses the full concept of LaStone – incorporating hot and cold – there will be a chemical reaction to the client's tissues described by Mary Hannigan as 'a vascular gymnastics going on in the body'.

When you apply heat to the body, it pulls blood to the area. When you pull blood to an area, it moves through the heart and lungs to be oxygenated. Nutrition (of the blood) starts to take place, all pulling to the affected area.

This allows you to work at a deeper level, to realign muscle fibre and to facilitate relaxation of that muscle fibre.

When applying the cold stones, it lessens the inflammation in the muscle fibre. For a short time you push the blood away; then, if the cold stone stays on for more than four minutes, it starts pulling blood again to warm back up and the gymnastics

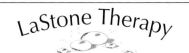
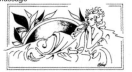

begins. It is the balance of yin and yang (hot and cold), which allows for healing to begin.

This treatment is also very beneficial to the therapist. It's meditative and also opens up doors if the therapist wishes to explore working with the energy fields, it also assists the therapist from a self-care perspective, and it gives your fingers a break!

You use a lot of intended energy and power coming from your arms and fingers however using the stones is like having an assistant in the treatment room.

Utilising the warming stones on a client helps with the often-fatigued wrists and thumbs of therapists, as they can apply more pressure with the hard stones, requiring less effort from their own body. The hot and cold stones therapists hold in their hands start to facilitate their own healing and slows down the possibility of injuring themselves any further.

Aside from the physical relief as a massage therapist, it most definitely has an emotional and spiritual impact. The more you work with the stones, the more they seem to work with you.

What the stars say about LaStone Therapy

"This is like nothing I've ever experienced before!" – *Barbara Windsor*

"The LaStone Massage is wonderfully warm and nurturing and is very effective in melting away knots and stress in the body." – *Wendy Craig*

"It's luxurious and powerful, causing great relief of tension and pressures." – *Paul Mount*

"Some of my favourite placements of the stones are the ones that go between my toes, the one that cradles my neck, and the ones that I hold in my hands." – *Wayne Sleep*

I can't imagine a massage without the warmth and healing power of the stones. You don't feel uncomfortable lumps on your back when lying on them, you don't feel the weight from them resting on top of you either. You just feel absolutely balanced, comforted, cradled in all the right places. They seem to absorb all the aches and pains and you become one with the stones, you just don't know they are there. I have to examine them afterwards just so I know what size stone was placed and where it was. My body craves the warmth I get from the stones, which is as important as is the massage. They are magical! – *Dennis Waterman*

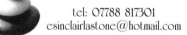
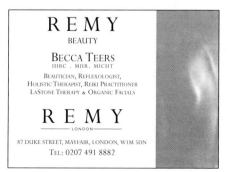

Light Therapy

By Pauline Allen

Light has been used as a healing remedy as far back as ancient times. The Egyptians were amongst the first to recognise the enormous therapeutic benefits of the various colours of light in the spectrum.

But it wasn't until 1903, when Niels Finsen M.D. of Denmark was awarded the Nobel Prize for using light to treat tuberculosis, that light therapy was officially recognised as a valid health remedy. Today, light therapy is used in a number of ways to promote healing. These range from the use of lasers in surgery, through to full spectrum light boxes to treat Seasonal Affective Disorder (SAD).

Lightwave stimulation

Latest scientific findings have shown that a revolutionary new light therapy technique called Lightwave Stimulation is effective in treating a wide range of conditions including attention deficit disorder, cerebral palsy, dyspraxia, dyslexia, depression, ME, addictions, eating disorders (anorexia and bulimia) and obsessive compulsive disorder. It has also been shown to promote improvements in learning ability, concentration, memory, co-ordination, athletic performance, self-esteem and mood.

The treatment was originally developed in the US by Dr. John Downing OD, PhD, an internationally acclaimed optometrist and neuroscientist, and is based on 25 years of research and clinical observation in the study of neuro sensory stimulation. During this time Downing identified the many effects light has on different types of brain function, and applied these findings to create this unique, therapeutic system of light therapy.

How does it work?

Lightwave Stimulation is a neuro-sensory development programme. It increases a person's ability to absorb light energy so that the brain and body can function more efficiently. This leads to improved mental, emotional and physical well-being. Humans just like plants are photo-biotic and need to absorb a certain amount of sunlight to stay healthy. Sunlight controls the body's circadian rhythms (internal body clock) and this in turn influences many important biological functions, including sleep patterns, hormone production, body temperature, breathing, digestion, sexual function, mood, the immune system and the ageing process. Without sufficient light the body cannot carry out these physiological functions as effectively.

When light enters through the eyes it is converted into a series of photo-electric nerve impulses called photo-current. This passes through the optic nerve and associated pathways into key areas of the brain, each of which governs specific mind-body functions.

What happens during treatment

Lightwave Stimulation can help to redress physiological imbalances that arise as a result of insufficient light energy. The technique improves brain energy, opens up neural pathways and balances biological rhythms. Treatment involves the use of a specially designed piece of equipment – the Lumatron machine – which breaks down broad spectrum light into 11 different colour bands.

The narrow bands of coloured light are used to enhance the light receptor cells (called rods and cones) at the back of the eyes, in order to rebalance the autonomic nervous system. These wavelengths of visible light vary in colour – from violet through to indigo, blue, green, yellow, orange and red. Each colour vibrates at a different frequency and affects different processes within the body.

To work out which colour or colours a person may benefit from, the practitioner first carries out a visual field of awareness test. This helps to assess to what extent the cells at the back of the eye are taking in enough light for proper brain function.

The test shows up where there is a decrease in the flow of photo-current to specific areas of the brain, or whether a problem has arisen through an imbalance of Biological Rhythms (caused by an imbalance of the hypothalamus gland).

When Biological Rhythms are disrupted by a malfunctioning of the hypothalamus gland, this can lead to all sorts of emotional disturbances. Further visual awareness tests are carried out in order to measure progress.

Treatment involves sitting comfortably in a darkened room, listening to music, in front of a Lumatron machine which has been set to the appropriate colours and flicker rate, as indicated by the initial assessment. The therapy works, because light energy is taken in by the eyes and converted to photo-current. This reaches the pineal and hypothalamus glands, and influences the endocrine systems and circadian rhythms as well as hormonal and emotional balance, bringing varying degrees of relief to many different conditions.

LIGHT THERAPY

MR B PAYNE, Kaizen Lifestyle Ltd, 18 Redgrave Place, Marlow, Buckinghamshire, SL7 1JZ. 01628 481336

Magnetic Therapy

By the British Biomagnetic Association

Biomagnetic Therapy combines the two ancient and proven healing systems of magnets and acupuncture. It uses small dot magnets, about the size of the end of a pencil and only 400 gauss, on the master points of the acupuncture eight extra-ordinary meridians to achieve better, safer and longer lasting results than with acupuncture alone.

Magnets can be used to promote better health, as a self-help aid, like bracelets or pads, and as part of a clinical treatment by a practitioner. People fitted with pacemakers should NOT use self-help aids without seeking professional advice.

Generally speaking, North Pole magnets are thought of as negative and are used to sedate, fight infection, promote sleep and reduce acidity, inflammation and pain.

South Pole magnets are positive, stimulating growth and endorphin production but should not be used at powers above 1000 gauss for long periods of time.

Bi-polar magnets – with both north and south poles – such as in bracelets, improve circulation with increased oxygenation and are used to help those with stiffness in muscles and joints.

Practitioners themselves use widely different systems, from high-powered mains electro-magnets to light application of low gauss-rate earth-fixed magnets.

They generally use the principle that ionisation of blood cells makes the flow better and the increased circulation aids the recovery. However the magnetic field can also be used to stimulate acupuncture points to give 'acupuncture without needles' or biomagnetic therapy as it is called in the UK.

The magnets are attached with sticky tape to various parts of the body, mainly the hands and feet, and act as acupuncture needles. As they have a polarity, they tone or sedate automatically, all without puncturing the skin. As the primary diagnosis is determined by the physical differences in body alignment – the length of arms, legs and any other structural abnormalities – the effectiveness of the treatment is equally measurable, often within minutes of application.

Treatment is usually quick, about 20-25 minutes, and is quite painless. Some patients find it difficult to accept the simplicity of the treatment but most experience a feeling of great relaxation and some even fall asleep during treatment.

Since it uses an alternative approach to medicine, based on a physical, energy and mineral balance, biomagnetic therapy is effective on a wide range of conditions, but is especially suitable for structural problems such as bad backs, whiplash and sports injuries. One could call it 'acupuncture without needles' or 'osteopathy without manipulation'.

Case history

"I had severe tennis elbow and a frozen shoulder, which I believed to have been caused by my work with horses. I had this condition acutely for eight months back in June 1997.

"It was sufficiently bad for me to not be able to sleep on my right side, nor could I hold my right arm up in the horizontal position. I could not lift or pull anything without suffering severe discomfort.

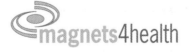

"My doctor gave me a course of tablets, saying that if they did not help she would have to give me an injection into the elbow joint. Needless to say the injection was necessary. We planned the injection for a Friday so that I could completely rest the arm over the weekend.

"The injection straight into the joint was extremely painful. It improved the condition of my shoulder by 60 per cent and that in the elbow by 40 per cent, by my estimation.

"However, this improvement only lasted for three weeks, after which time the effects seemed to wear off. Within six weeks the percentage improvement had gone down to between ten and 15.

"A friend of mine had tried a magnetic wristband for her arthritis and was overjoyed with the result. She had been unable to climb over a stile outside her house without lifting her leg over with her hands. Within four days of wearing the magnetic wristband she could walk over the stile unaided.

"She persuaded me to try a wristband for my condition. Within four days of wearing the band on the pulse of my wrist, I noticed a decided improvement – the pain in my shoulder had completely gone and my elbow was 60 per cent better.

"Another two weeks and I was able to sleep on my right side for the first time in nine months, and the elbow had was, by my estimation. 85 per cent better and the shoulder 100 per cent better. Seven months later and the improvement has been maintained."

Magnetic therapy for pets

ACCORDING to information now available on how magnetic therapy works, the magnetic field produced by magnets stimulates the vascular supply in the targeted area and improves blood oxygen levels.

This, in turn, stimulates the healing process, promotes health at the cellular level and decreases pain. In many cases, if magnets are used in conjunction with prescription medication, as the medication runs out it has been found that the magnets alone continue the anti-inflammatory effect and pain alleviation.

In this day and age many people are looking for alternative forms of therapy for themselves and their pets. Magnetic mats have proven to be extremely successful in relieving arthritic pain for older pets. Perhaps there is a message here?

Manual Lymphatic Drainage

By Geraldine Sherborne

Manual Lymph Drainage has been used for many years by the nursing profession and lymph massage practitioners for post chemotherapy and lymphoedema and other lymph conditions very successfully. As a massage it can contribute as a major aid to health maintenance.

The main function of MLD is to encourage the return of plasma, life giving nutrients and blood protein to the systemic circulation. The lymphatic system consists of a series of vessels and glands throughout the body that transports waist products, plasma, proteins, fats and leukocytes.

The glands or nodes filter and breakdown bacteria and harmful substances and the vessels return 'lymph' to the blood. Lymph is a transparent fluid that flows through its own system of vessels. This fluid is filtered and passed through the lymph nodes situated all over the body. A network of fibres in the nodes traps the harmful substances, and lymphocytes, macrophages and antibodies attempt to destroy and detoxify them. The main function of the nodes apart from the filtration of lymph and phagocytosis of toxins and bacteria etc. by macrophages, is the antibody production of B lymphocytes, and to aid the increase of varied activities by T lymphocytes, lymphocyte mitosis (division of cells) and to help increase the concentration of lymph by re-absorption of some fluid. The nodes direct the lymph into appropriate drainage pathways, and store foreign particles out of harms way, that cannot be phagocytosed.

Most white blood cells 'live' in lymphatic tissue and go foraging in blood vessels and tissues when necessary. The lymph system acts as a quick transport system for many white blood cells; its walls allow cells to move in and out easily and aids balance in the bodies fluid and electrolyte levels.

MLD is a series of light, precise movements applied to the whole surface, or part of the body to stimulate movement of lymph circulation. This slow massage sends soothing messages to the central nervous system, returning proteins to the circulation when they have leaked out, flushing the tissues with fresh blood and lymph fluid.

The treatment is helpful in reducing the perception of pain by inhibiting the nerve muscles. The rhythmical strokes encourage activity of the parasympathetic system, which will often help the body to regain overall homeostatis. Areas of the body no longer able to function due to node removal can successfully be retained to accept a new pathway with consent MLD over a period of months. This can be achieved by encouraging the lymph fluid away from the missing node, with the reflex action of the motoricity of MLD emulating the natural motoricity of the lymphangions, i.e. their ability to contract spontaneously at an even rhythm. This occurs naturally, with the bodies' continual movement.

Tension interferes with production, distribution and function of lymph, and the toxic build up is partially created by this tension. It is believed that the electrical impulses triggered by light pressure massage, stimulates the subtle energy flow which can bring that remarkable return to vitality of the patient even whilst receiving the treatment. This in turn may be the springboard needed to help the client tap into his or her own resources for the natural process to occur.

Why do I need MLD?

By M. Willcocks PhD

Manual Lymphatic Drainage can be a valuable addition to treatment regimes for Hodgkin's disease (HD) and non-Hodgkin's lymphomas (NHL) – together called lymphomas – which are types of cancer.

Cancer is a word applied to many different diseases with diverse causes and a wide range of treatments. The cells which make up our bodies normally divide in an orderly fashion so they can repair our tissues. This process sometimes goes wrong and there is an uncontrolled growth of cells.

A characteristic of all cancers is this disorderly formation of body cells, causing swellings or tumours. A tumour is referred to as benign when it remains contained in a localised area of the body and, on removal by surgery, does not recur.

The term cancer is used when the tumours are malignant, that is they spread and invade healthy tissue.

When the natural division of cells in the tissues of the lymphatic system become disrupted, tumours called lymphomas occur. In common with other cancers, lymphomas are not infectious and cannot be passed on to other people.

The causes of lymphomas are uncertain but, in some types of lymphoma research points to a connection with particular viruses.

About 8,000 new cases of lymphomas are diagnosed in Britain each year. Less than a fifth are cases of Hodgkin's disease, the greater number being non-Hodgkin's lymphomas.

Many people feel helpless when they are diagnosed with cancer and it is easy to become isolated from the mainstream of life. Armed with the right information, however, there are many things you can do to help yourself.

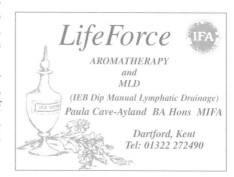

LifeForce IFA

AROMATHERAPY
and
MLD

(IEB Dip Manual Lymphatic Drainage)

Paula Cave-Ayland BA Hons MIFA

Dartford, Kent
Tel: 01322 272490

Massage

By Clare Maxwell-Hudson

Massage has profound effects on the health of the person being massaged. It improves circulation, relaxes muscles, aids digestion and, by stimulating the lymphatic system, speeds up the elimination of waste products.

These direct benefits, combined with the psychological benefits of feeling comforted and cared for, can produce a feeling of wellbeing that cannot be matched by modern drugs. Hippocrates said: "The Physician must be experienced in many things but above all he must be a good rubber. For rubbing can bind a joint that is too loose and loosen a joint that is too rigid."

Touch can play an indispensable part in healing as can be shown in many recent studies. Professor James Lynch of the University of Maryland confirmed the importance of touch between patients and nurses. The heart rates of critically ill patients were monitored during the simple act of pulse taking. A significant slowing of the heart rate was noted as soon as the nurse picked up the hand. This even applied to a patient in a coma.

Touch is so natural to us that without it we fail to thrive. Experiments have shown that children brought up in families that touch each other are healthier and more able to withstand pain and infection than children deprived of touch. They sleep better, are more sociable and generally happier. The French Obstetrician, Fredrick le Boyer said: "Being touched, massaged, is food to the infant. Food every bit as necessary as minerals, vitamins and proteins."

Touch and massage not only comforts the baby but can actually increase the weight of premature babies and decrease medical costs. In one study, underweight premature babies were given three ten-minute massages daily for ten days. Warm hands stroked the babies from head to toe. These massaged babies thrived, compared to the other premature babies who were left in their incubators. Even though they had the same number of feeds, the massaged babies gained nearly 50 per cent more weight per day than the control group. The massaged babies were sent home from the hospital six days earlier. The massage also had lasting benefits; eight to 12 months later the stroked babies maintained their advantage and had better psychical and mental abilities. All this for just a few minutes of massage a day.

But our need for touch does not stop at childhood. We all need it to give us a feeling of warmth and security. In fact, Relate, the marriage guidance society advises couples to touch each other more. It goes as far as to say that the rising rate of divorce could be due to a lack of physical contact within families. Perhaps just a few minutes massaging each other could prevent numerous physical and mental ills.

Yet with all this evidence to show the benefits of touch we are still hesitant about touching each other. This may be due to the Victorian idea that if it feels good it must be bad. But the sheer pleasure of massage is therapeutic.

In more research at Harvard Medical School, psychologists asked volunteers to visualise receiving tender loving care and their immunoglobulin levels, which fight viruses, rose sharply.

We need to be encouraged to touch each other more and massage is the perfect way of doing this in a non-aggressive, non-sexual way. Massage is formalised touch and therefore gives you a licence to touch; it can remove the taboos of touching and allow people to touch in a positive way.

Massage is a truly complementary therapy that can benefit us all. Whether we are old or young, ill and hospitalised or fit and healthy massage can be of help.

We all ought to learn to massage so that we can help each other and ourselves to lead healthy and more stress free lives. Life takes it out of us, but massage puts it back.

MASSAGE

MRS J KAY, 119 Thatch Leach Lane, Whitefield, Greater Manchester, M45 6FN. 0161 796 5092

Megavitamin Therapy

Megavitamin therapy is a controversial mode of nutrient therapy that involves the ingestion of large doses of vitamins.

A sub-category of Orthomolecular Medicine, megavitamin therapy was introduced in 1952 as a term by psychiatrists Humphrey Osmond and Abram Hoffer, who used it to describe the prescription of large doses of niacin in the treatment of schizophrenia.

In fact, large doses of niacin and several other vitamins can have very serious side effects, and the medical community as a whole has not endorsed the theories of megavitamin therapy.

In some rare disorders, however, certain selected megadoses of vitamins may be employed therapeutically.

McTimoney Chiropractic

By Linda Feeley

McTimoney Chiropractic is a straightforward method of adjusting the bones of the body using a variety of techniques and no instruments other than the hands of the practitioner.

McTimoney chiropractic was developed almost 30 years ago and is named after its originator, John McTimoney. His whole-body style of treatment offers a refined, effective and safe treatment developed from mainstream chiropractic and is based on the sound chiropractic principles as originally taught at the first chiropractic college, The Palmer College in the US.

At every treatment the skeletal system is assessed as a whole and adjustments are made to the limbs and head, as well as to the pelvis and spine. To the observer, and usually the receiver, McTimoney chiropractic seems, and is, extremely light, with rarely any cavitation or 'popping' of the joints. The key to the success of the adjustments is the speed, dexterity and accuracy with which they are performed.

The gentle nature of the treatment makes McTimoney chiropractic especially suitable for people of all ages, including; babies, young children, pregnant women, those with osteoporosis and the elderly. The treatment is beneficial for a wide range of complaints ranging from back, neck and shoulder pain, stiffness and pain in joints and bones, tension headaches and migraines, to whiplash and sports injuries and general muscular aches and pains.

Chiropractic the McTimoney way – case histories

For the last almost 30 years McTimoney chiropractors have treated thousands of people across the UK using the chiropractic treatment developed by John McTimoney. John's philosophy was based on DD Palmer's original discoveries and Dr Walker's teaching that the main cause of disease and pain is the misalignment of bones, chiefly in the spine, which in turn interrupts the functioning of the nervous system and affects our general health.

Today, as chiropractic treatment continues to gain ever-growing approval from the medical profession, still more and more people are discovering the many benefits treatment can bring. Back pain, migraines, sciatica and more severe problems are just some of the symptoms regularly seen by McTimoney chiropractors. The following case histories will demonstrate the success of the treatment and show some of the many varied conditions for which treatment can be beneficial.

Back pain

With over 85 per cent of the population likely to experience back pain at some stage in their lives, it is no surprise that the popular notion is that chiropractic is for back problems. The first case history shows the success of the treatment after a fall, which left the patient in great pain.

An active 76-year-old widow slipped when standing on a chair trying to open a jammed window in the bathroom. She fell backwards across the edge of the bath. When she came for McTimoney treatment, some six months after the accident, she was in continual, very severe pain and almost unable to walk. She was considering using a wheelchair. Chiropractic examination showed a right-hand curve in her thoraco-lumbar junction, which in six months had become fairly immovable with adhesions and muscle spasm. Progress was slow at first, but after two months she was able to move more freely. A month later this delightful elderly lady, whose favourite activity was ballroom dancing, came in to say she had done two waltzes and a foxtrot. In all over a period of nearly four months and 23 treatments, she had made a full recovery.

Such simple accidents either in the home or at work can have devastating effects, leaving people not only in pain but unable to work and unsure as to their future. While it is always best to seek treatment as soon as possible, both these cases show that treatment is still possible even after six months.

A 36-year-old mechanic wrenched the middle of his back while lifting an engine out of a car. He was off work for six months with excruciating knife-like pain on the left of his mid-spine. When he came for McTimoney treatment he had tried all the conventional treatment routes and was very distressed that, at his fairly young age, he might be an invalid for the rest of his life, especially as he had three young children to support. This previously fit man used to work out at a gym three nights a week; now he had lost three stone in weight and was emaciated. The weight loss was consistent with the area of the spine from which the pain came because the nerves from that area also serve the stomach.

Every meal he had eaten for the past six months had passed through his system almost undigested, accounting for the weight loss. The chiropractic findings included two jammed mid-thoracic vertebrae and a lot of local muscle spasm. After the first treatment, he gained 7lbs in weight and the pain was reduced by half. When he came for the second treatment a week later, he had gained a stone in weight and was virtually pain free. After the third treatment he went back to work totally recovered.

Headaches, migraines and facial problems

Millions of pounds each year are spent on painkillers for headaches but, while these may remove the symptoms, they do not treat the cause. As these case histories show, chiropractic treatment can be very beneficial in the treatment of headaches and migraines, the causes of which range from tension and stress, physical stresses, to visual or dental problems. One study revealed that of 6,000 long-term headaches, neck injury, (whiplash, falls) was the most important factor causing headaches and should be suspected in every non-specific case of headache. The next case history shows that chiropractic treatment is not just for adults:

A 12-year-old schoolgirl who usually enjoyed good health was taken to her doctor with an extremely severe headache – so bad that her parents feared she had meningitis. Her doctor diagnosed migraine and gave her medication. Forty-eight hours later, and after a good sleep, she felt better and was able to go to school. Three weeks later she became ill again with the same type of headache. The medication was repeated and again she recovered. This pattern was repeated twice more, so her parents decided to try McTimoney chiropractic. After two treatments she is headache free.

Facial pain can be excruciating, however, McTimoney chiropractic can help. Because the bones of the face are adjusted as necessary in each treatment, it can be extremely effective in reducing pain as this case study shows.

A 28-year-old woman suffered excruciating facial pain for three years. After five consecutive nights when she could neither sleep nor lie horizontally she went to her doctor who prescribed Ibuprofen and told her to see a dentist. The dentist diagnosed the problem as trigeminal neuralgia – an extremely painful form of facial neuralgia which is quite difficult to treat. The dentist prescribed Tergatol, which allowed her to sleep but produced unwanted serious side effects. She decided to visit a McTimoney chiropractor. Since her first treatment, she has only had three mild attacks in three months – all treatable with over the counter painkillers.

Children and chiropractic

The gentle nature of McTimoney chiropractic means even young children and babies can receive treatment. Many McTimoney chiropractors treat children and believe that treatment should ideally be given as soon after birth as possible to correct any misalignments at the start and lay the foundations for the development of a healthy spine and nervous system. Although the bones are not properly formed at birth, stresses in the soft tissue, perhaps from a difficult birth process, can develop into spinal problems as the baby grows. For older children chiropractic can be particularly useful when problems arise after falls, bumps or from incorrect posture, carrying heavy school bags and sitting slumped over desks.

Chiropractic can relieve a surprisingly wide range of childhood conditions, from colic to rheumatic diseases and even behavioural difficulties and hyperactivity. The following case studies describe a wide variety of conditions and how chiropractic treatment benefited the child.

A remarkable case is that of a boy of 15 whose bone growth was delayed by two years. He came to the chiropractor with a fractured right hand; on assessment, the chiropractor learned that he had been delivered face up, and deduced that the resulting misalignments of his skull and facial bones could be affecting his pituitary gland. After six treatments he had grown two and a half inches and his face had noticeably changed shape for the better.

If a happy child below the age of speech suddenly becomes fractious and difficult, this may be his only way of telling you that he has pain or headache. A spinal examination may well be worthwhile, particularly if the child has had a fall before the change in behaviour. Falls can also lead to altered behaviour and uncharacteristic aggressiveness in older children, especially if the neck has been affected.

A seven-year old girl suffered from stomach aches and headaches on walking most weekdays, together with pins and needles in her hands. She had suffered these symptoms for about a year. Her mother had recently remarried and had a new baby, and thought the cause was emotional. On the point of taking her to the psychiatrist, she decides to see a McTimoney chiropractor first. The history taking revealed that at the age of 18 months the girl had fallen, hitting her head.

Examination showed subluxations of all the neck vertebrae, and the left jaw-joint was misaligned, as was the right lachrymal bone at the inner corner of her eye. The girl had four treatments and at the final consultation had experienced only two headaches and one episode of stomach ache in the previous two months. For the mother, the realisation that the problem was physical, not emotional, was a great relief.

These case histories have been reproduced with kind permission from the book, The Essentials of McTimoney Chiropractic, Courtney & Andrews, ISDN 0722537476.

Meditation

By M Willcocks PhD

The mind is normally busy jumping from one thing to the next as our attention is attracted by this and that, here and there. Meditation is an activity where the mind is quieted so that deeper levels can be experienced.

Our basic state is one of purity and awareness. As a baby you were in a virginal, joyous condition. The events of your life have caused you to add layers of negativity around this state to such a degree that now you suffer more and more and experience the best in life too rarely. Yet, ecstasy might be said to be your birthright and the first step towards recovering this state of perfection is to discard your tension.

Relax and feel your breath as it comes and goes. With every exhale, send out a negative thought that has caused you to be blind to your true self. With every inhale, bring into your body something positive and feel yourself relaxing.

Negative thoughts occur when you put yourself down, criticise yourself for errors, doubt your abilities, expect failure. Negative thinking is the negative side of suggestion – it damages confidence, harms performance and paralyses mental skills. Positive thoughts; you may find it useful to counter negative thoughts with positive affirmations. You can use affirmations to build confidence and change negative behaviour patterns into positive ones.

You can base affirmations on clear, rational assessments of fact and use them to undo the damage that negative thinking may have done to your self-confidence. For instance, say to yourself 'I can do this', or 'I can achieve my goals', 'I am completely myself and people will like me for myself', 'I am completely in control of my life', 'I learn from my mistakes, they increase the basis of experience on which I can draw', 'I am a good valued person in my own right'.

Traditionally people have advocated positive thinking almost recklessly, as if it is a solution to everything. It should be used with common sense. No amount of positive thinking will make everyone who applies it an Olympic champion marathon runner – though an Olympic marathon runner is unlikely to have reached this level without being pretty good at positive thinking. Firstly decide rationally what goals you can realistically attain with hard work and then use positive thinking to reinforce these.

Thought awareness

Thought awareness is the process by which you observe your thoughts for a time, perhaps when under stress, and become aware of what is going through your head. It is best not to suppress any thoughts – just let them run their course while you observe them.

Watch for negative thoughts while you observe your 'stream of consciousness'.

Normally these appear and disappear

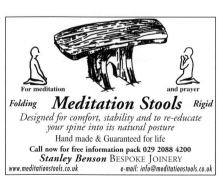

being barely noticed. Normally you will not know that they exist. Examples of common negative thoughts are: worries about how you appear to other people, a preoccupation with the symptoms of stress, dwelling on consequences of poor performance, self-criticism, feelings of inadequacy.

Make a note of the thought and then let the stream of consciousness run on. Thought awareness is the first step in the process of eliminating negative thoughts – you cannot counter thoughts you do not know you think.

Rational thinking

Once you are aware of your negative thoughts, write them down and review them rationally. See whether the thoughts have any basis in reality. Often you find that when you properly challenge negative thoughts they are obviously wrong. Often they persist only because they escape notice.

Stress reduction

In choosing methods to combat stress, it is worth asking yourself where the stress comes from. If outside factors such as important events or relationship difficulties are causing stress, then a positive thinking or imagery based technique may be effective.

Where stress and fatigue are long term, then lifestyle and organisational changes may be appropriate. If the feeling of stress comes from adrenaline in your body, then it may be effective to relax the body and slow the flow of adrenaline.

What is imagery?

Remember that your brain is a mass of nerve cells. Your sense organs convert signals from your environment into nerve impulses. These feed into the areas of your brain that interpret that environment. Imagery seeks to create a similar set of nerve impulses that can feed into those areas of the brain that provide you with your experience of the outside world.

This can be illustrated effectively if you have access to equipment that measures body stress – this functions by measuring, for example, muscle electrical activity, electrical conductivity through skin sweat, and so on.

By imagining a pleasant scene, which reduces stress, you can cause a needle on the machine to move in one direction. By imagining an unpleasant and stressful situation, you can move it in the opposite direction. This can be quite alarming when you see it happen the first time!

Imagery in stress reduction

You can use imagery in the following ways to reduce stress: One common use of imagery in relaxation is to imagine a scene, place or event that you remember as peaceful, restful, beautiful and happy.

You can bring all your senses into the image, with sounds of running water and birds, the smell of cut grass, the taste of cool white wine, the warmth of sun, etc. Use the imagined place as a retreat from stress and pressure.

Scenes can involve complex images such as lying on a beach in a deserted cove. You may 'see' cliffs, sea and sand around you, 'hear' the waves crashing against rocks, 'smell' the salt in the air, and feeling the warmth of the sun and a gently breeze on your body.

Other images might include looking at a mountain view, swimming in a tropical pool, or whatever – you will be able to come up with the most effective images for yourself. Other uses of imagery in relaxation involve mental pictures of stress flowing out of the body; or of stress, distractions and everyday concerns being folded away and locked in a suitcase.

Imagery in preparation and rehearsal

You can also use imagery in rehearsal before a big event, allowing you to run through it in your mind. It allows you to practise in advance for anything unusual that might occur, so that you are prepared and already practised in handling it. Imagery also allows you to pre-experience achievement of your goals. This help to give you the self-confidence you need to do something well.

Unsure

Uncertainty can cause high levels of stress. Causes of uncertainty can be: Not having a clear idea of what the future holds or will be wanted from you in the future. Not knowing what your boss or colleagues think of your abilities. Receiving vague or inconsistent instructions.

In these cases, lack of information or the actions of other people are negatively affecting your ability to perform. The most effective way of countering this is to ask for the information you need. If you ask in a positive way, then people are usually quite happy to help.

Confidence gaining.

A number of factors can make an event take on a high level of significance and cause stress as a result: The importance and size of the event, the prospect of a large financial reward, of promotion, or of personal advancement, the presence of family, friends or important people. Where stress is a problem under these circumstances, then think carefully about the event – take every opportunity to reduce its importance in your eyes.

If the event seems big, put it in its place along the path to your goals. Compare it in your mind with bigger events you might know of or might have attended.

If there is a financial reward, remind yourself that there may be other opportunities for reward later. This will not be the only chance you have. Focus on the quality of your performance. Focusing on the rewards will only damage your concentration and raise stress.

If members of your family are watching, remind yourself that they love you anyway. If friends are real friends, they will continue to like you whether you win or lose.

If people who are important to your goals are watching then remind yourself that you may well have other chances to impress them.

If you focus on the correct performance of your tasks, then the importance of the event will dwindle into the background.

More tips

By anticipating stress you can prepare for it and work out how to control it when it happens. This can be can be carried out in a number of ways:

Rehearsal: By running through a stressful event, such as a job interview or your first public speech, several times in advance you can polish your performance and build confidence.

Planning: By analysing the likely causes of stress, you will be able to plan your responses to likely forms of stress. These might be actions to alleviate the situation or may be stress management techniques that you will use. It is important that you formally plan for this – it is little use just worrying in an undisciplined way; that would be counter-productive.

Avoidance: Where a situation is likely to be unpleasant, and will not yield any benefit to you, it may be one you can just avoid. You should be certain in your own mind, however, that this is the case.

Psyching Up

Where you are not feeling motivated towards a task, either because you are bored by it or because you are tired, then you may need to psych yourself up. This will increase your arousal so that you can perform effectively.

You can use the following techniques to psych up:

Set yourself a challenge – for example, to do the job in a particular time or to do it to a particularly high standard Break the job down into small parts; do each part between more enjoyable work; take satisfaction from the successful completion of each element.

Action Plan

Once you understand the level of stress under which you work most effectively, and know precisely what is causing you stress, the next stage is to work out how to manage stress effectively.

The best way of doing this will probably be to make an action plan of things you are going to do to manage stress. Some elements of this plan will be actions you intend to take to contain, control or eliminate the problems that are causing the stress.

Other elements may be health related, such as taking more exercise, changing your diet or improving the quality of your environment. Another part of the plan may cover stress management techniques you will employ when stress levels begin to build.

Different techniques will be effective for different situations and causes of stress. The contents and structure of your plan are for you to devise – it will depend entirely on your circumstances.

Exercise

Taking frequent effective exercise is probably one of the best physical stress-reduction techniques available. Exercise not only improves your health and reduces stress caused by unfitness but also relaxes tense muscles and helps you to sleep.

Exercise has a number of other positive benefits you may not be aware of:

It improves blood flow to your brain, bringing additional sugars and oxygen which may be needed; when you are thinking intensely hard, the neurones of your brain function more intensely. As they do this they build up toxic waste products that cause foggy thinking in the short term, and can damage the brain in the long term.

By exercising you speed the flow of blood through your brain, moving these waste products faster. You also improve this blood flow so that even when you are not exercising, waste is eliminated more efficiently.

It can cause release of chemicals called endorphins into your blood stream. These give you a feeling of happiness and well-being.

There are a lot of wrong approaches to exercise. Many traditionally recommended forms of exercise actually damage your body over the medium or long term. It is worth finding reputable and up-to-date sources of advice on exercise, possibly from your doctor, and then having a customised exercise plan drawn up for you.

An important thing to remember is that exercise should be fun – if you do not enjoy it, then you will probably not keep doing it.

Never give up!

Sir Winston Churchill took three years getting through eighth grade (nowadays GCSE exams) because he had trouble learning English. It seems ironic that years later Oxford University asked him to address its commencement exercises.

He arrived with his usual props. A cigar, a cane and a top hat accompanied Churchill wherever he went. As Churchill approached the podium, the crowd rose in appreciative applause.

With unmatched dignity, he settled the crowd and stood confident before his admirers. Removing the cigar and carefully placing the top hat on the podium, Churchill gazed at his waiting audience.

Authority rang in Churchill's voice as he shouted, "Never give up!" Several seconds passed before he rose to his toes and repeated: "Never give up!"

His words thundered in their ears. There was a deafening silence as Churchill reached for his hat and cigar, steadied himself with his cane and left the platform. His commencement address was finished.

Peeling away the layers

Television star Oprah Winfrey says: "As I peeled away the layers of my life, I realised that all my craziness, all my pain and difficulties, stemmed from me not valuing myself. And what I now know is that every single bit of pain I have experienced in my life was a result of me worrying about what another person was going to think of me.

"Here is one way to look at your life: Every day you are creating a masterpiece. As you create you take the feedback from it, so you see how you can change what you create tomorrow. And you have to be willing to delve very deeply and very honestly into yourself in order to do that. You have to take that reflection and see what it is really teaching you about yourself.

"Where are you really expressing yourself in a way that feels full and right to you? Where are you holding yourself back? Where is there distortion? How can you heal that? Where is not truth in this creation, and how can you allow that truth to come forth?

"I am learning daily from my own creation."

Meridian Therapies

Mind and Body Healing for the New Millennium

By Chrissie Hardisty and Silvia Hartmann-Kent,
Directors, the Association For Meridian Therapies AMT

All meridian based therapies are gentle, rapid and startlingly effective. It is not uncommon for long-standing or chronic pain to be released entirely in less than half an hour. Similarly, psychological pain such as anxiety, depression and addictions, caused by traumatic incidents or childhood memories, can often be relieved fully in minutes.

The basic ideas and approaches involved in Meridian Therapies are stunningly simple, and the techniques lend themselves perfectly to be used by professional therapists in combination with their existing mind-body healing modalities.

Thousands of professional therapists testify to Gary Craig's Emotional Freedom Techniques' (EFTTM) unique ability to bring rapid and permanent relief from:

Addictive cravings, allergies, anxiety and panic attacks, anger, compulsions and obsessions, depression and sadness, dyslexia, fears and phobias, grief and loss, guilt, insomnia, negative memories, nightmares, pain management, physical conditions and healing, peak performance, post traumatic stress disorder (PTSD), self-image, sexual abuse issues and many more.

EFTTM, the 'ambassador of meridian therapies', has one further and most remarkable aspect. It is designed so that once you have learned this simple technique; you can easily use it at home at any time, in any place, in any situation. This means that you can use it on any problem you wish to apply it to, without any further training or many years of study. In spite of its apparent simplicity and ease of use, EFTTM produces highly beneficial, lasting results in 85-95 per cent of cases.

In 1976 a remarkably well-preserved body, approximately 6,000 years old, was discovered in a glacier. It bore tattoos marking the major meridian treatment points. When this discovery became public, everyone was astonished – apart from the acupuncturist communities around the world, whose classic textbook on the subject was by then just under 4,500 years old.

Acupuncture, the ancient Chinese health care system that works by stimulating these mysterious meridian points with tiny needles, was already well on the way to becoming acceptable practice in the field of alternative health care.

But there were others investigating how to stimulate and balance the meridians, and to find further ways that meridian based treatments could bring positive benefits to health in body and in mind.

In 1964, chiropractor George Goodheart began to pursue links between muscle strength, organs, glands and meridians and developed diagnostic muscle testing, later naming it Applied Kinesiology. One of his students, John Diamond, saw the potential for using the balancing effect of meridian work for psychotherapy, and another then student, psychologist Dr Roger Callahan, discovered a whole new approach to working with mental health and meridians.

One of Dr Callahan's long-term patients at that time was a woman called Mary, who suffered from a water phobia. Dr Callahan later explained: "Her fear of water was so severe that she could not go out when it rained, would have panic attacks at the sight of bodies of water and could not stand more than an inch of water in her bath. I treated her weekly for two years, using every approach I could think of, and all I had achieved in that time was to have taught her that she could stand more fear than she previously thought possible. I would have her sit by the side of a swimming pool and she was absolutely terrified in spite of everything we did."

Dr Callahan asked Mary to 'tap' with her fingers under her eye – an important meridian point. She did, looked up and 'the fear had disappeared' – just like that, in an instant, and it never came back.

Dr Callahan devoted his life and practice from that moment onwards to develop a treatment approach to help people overcome crippling fears, phobias and mental problems of all kinds. His approach is called TFT or Thought Field Therapy and is still in use today. TFT uses just 14 basic meridian points, and the order and sequence of how they are stimulated by lightly tapping upon them is diagnosed through muscle testing for individual problems.

In 1996, Gary Craig, a Stanford

Engineer and a student of Dr. Callahan's had the brilliant idea of creating a simple technique that would cover all the 14 points by default – thus either reducing or eliminating the need for extensive muscle testing and diagnostic training and providing a comprehensive therapeutic tool that is unprecedented in its ease of use and in its astonishing effectiveness.

Gary Craig's Emotional Freedom Techniques, EFTTM, is one of the easiest and most effective and efficient therapeutic approach imaginable, providing fast and usually permanent relief from psychological, physical and neuro-physiological problems. These techniques have been described as one of the most important breakthroughs in the area of mind-body healing in the last hundred years.

Already thousands upon thousands of people all over the world have benefited from using EFTTM and it is rapidly becoming known as a modern day miracle being capable of dramatically relieving emotional disturbances and physical problems.

Since Thought Field Therapy revolutionised the way psychological and neuropsychological problems are being treated, with its unprecedented success rate, many other forms of meridian based healing have proved to be highly effective. As more and more innovative therapists move into the rapidly expanding field of meridian therapies, new and different approaches are being developed.

Other Meridian Therapies include: BSFF – BE SET FREE FAST; TAB – Touch and Breathe; TAT – Tapas Acupressure Technique; AFT – Attractor Field Therapy.

The Association for Meridian Therapies (AMT) was established in 1998 to provide insight and training in the new meridian therapies.

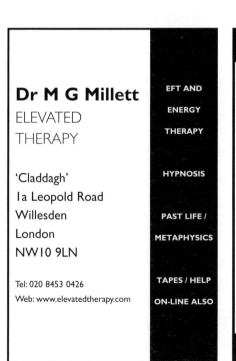

The Metamorphic Technique

By The Metamorphic Association

The Metamorphic Technique is a simple approach to self-healing and personal development. We all have great potential, but due to limiting beliefs that we hold about ourselves and our lives we tend to get ourselves stuck in particular patterns that keep us from fully realising that potential.

These patterns can show up in various ways – physical or mental illness, emotional problems, limiting attitudes or repeating patterns of behaviour. Beneath these external symptoms are corresponding patterns of energy. The Metamorphic Technique acts as a catalyst to this energy, also known as the life force, gently enabling you to transform your patterns and begin to move from who you are, to who you can be.

The Metamorphic practitioner uses a light touch on points known as the spinal reflexes in the feet, hands and head. At the same time, he or she remains detached from the achievement of specific results. This allows your energy to be guided by your own innate intelligence – the 'wise guide within' – transforming your patterns in whatever ways are right for you.

The Metamorphic Technique has its origins in the work of Robert St. John, a British naturopath and reflexologist. During the 1960s he discovered that he could bring about significant changes by applying a light touch to particular points on the feet that reflexologists call the spinal reflexes. Later, he realised that everyone has their own capacity for self-healing and that, if he allowed it to become fully active whilst practising, then his patients would be empowered to be their own healers in a truly effective way.

Gaston Saint-Pierre, who studied extensively with Robert St. John during the 1970s, went on to further develop the work and created the term 'The Metamorphic Technique' to differentiate the new direction the work was now taking.

The Metamorphic Technique is based on a new way of looking at energy patterns. While other approaches often focus on removing energy blockages, the Metamorphic Technique looks at transforming energy patterns.

It does not consider people to be 'blocked' or 'broken' and in need of being 'fixed'. Instead, it simply notices that you may have patterns that no longer serve you and that you wish to transform. The energy that was involved in creating the old patterns is released and can be used to create new patterns. The Metamorphic Technique is not a therapy or a treatment, as it is not concerned with addressing specific symptoms or problems. There is no need for practitioners to know about your personal or medical history. The technique is gentle, non-invasive and completely safe. It can be used on its own or alongside conventional medicine or alternative and complementary therapies.

It is easy to learn and, since no special abilities or background are needed, it is accessible to everyone. Many people take short courses so they can use the technique with family and friends. Parents are especially encouraged to learn, so they can give the technique to their children.

The Metamorphic Technique is suitable for anyone who wishes to make changes that will enhance their quality of life. Change and transformation can occur on a number of levels – physical, mental, emotional and behavioural.

While practitioners cannot predict the outcome, as each person's life force is unique, the majority of people who have experienced the technique do report benefits – it is unusual for the technique not to be helpful in some way.

People are often drawn to the Metamorphic Technique at difficult times such as illness, bereavement, divorce and so on, or because they feel at a crossroads or 'stuck' in their lives. They find that it can help them to cope better in these difficult or transitional times. Many people are drawn to the technique because it allows them to deal with emotional issues and make deep inner changes without having to discuss their problems or delve into their past.

On a physical level, people come with a variety of conditions from cancer to chronic fatigue. The technique does not seek to address these conditions or their symptoms; however in many cases people find that symptoms diminish over time, or that they respond better to other treatments they have been following.

The Metamorphic Technique has been used a great deal in work with physical and mental disabilities, as well as in schools for children with learning difficulties, in hospitals, in prisons, and in helping people overcome addictions, eating disorders and stress-related conditions. It is also used by pregnant women and midwives, as it can allow an easier pregnancy and birth.

Whereas people may seek medicine or therapy because they want to be healed of something, they come to the Metamorphic Technique because they want to transform their patterns. It is an empowering tool for enabling people to 'get out of their own way', let go of past limitations and move forward in their lives.

Metamorphic for Mums

In the Metamorphic Technique we are getting in touch with the principles of life itself. We find ourselves embarked on a most exciting, a most rewarding adventure. The potential help that people can receive through this work, like the life principle with which we are working, is limitless.

The principle we are working with is life itself. The Metamorphic Technique is directed towards all those persons who are anxious to change themselves for the better. The changes come about through our own power to heal ourselves.

The most important time of our lives, is the pre-natal period. From the moment of conception, every cell in the body fits the individual, and for real changes to happen we have to go back to this pattern. Life patterns are stored, like bits of information on a computer, from the moment of conception until birth and they remain with us always.

All of this is reflected in the feet. For instance, the point of conception is reflected in the joint of the big toe. The whole of the big toe embodies the cerebral faculty and there are strong associations with authority and inner decision to be who you are.

The heel area corresponds to the base of the spine and the genitals, which reflects maternal, loving and caring qualities. Between the two points, lies an energy pathway which has the power to bring about profound changes in the body and psyche.

No claims or predictions are made as to what will happen after Metamorphic treatment because the practitioner does not know. Results are determined by the individual's innate response. People who have experienced the Metamorphic Technique find positive changes in the majority of cases – ranging from outstanding improvement in physical and emotional well-being to rehabilitation after chronic drug abuse.

You do not have to be ill to benefit from a Metamorphic session. Children respond naturally to this foot massage because they do not have the same fixed patterns as adults. Much work is being done in schools and institutions with mentally handicapped and emotionally disturbed people with surprising results.

During pregnancy the Metamorphic Technique is especially beneficial because the unborn child is, through the mother, being enabled to emerge into the world and able to cope more readily with the birth process. It is said that a difficult birth is more often due to resistance in the child than to any weakness in the mother.

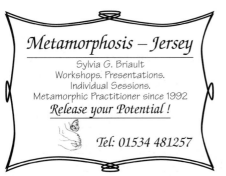

Metamorphosis – Jersey

Sylvia G. Briault
Workshops. Presentations.
Individual Sessions.
Metamorphic Practitioner since 1992
Release your Potential !

Tel: 01534 481257

Music Therapy

By Louise O'Neill

Music has become one of the best ways to combat stress either on its own or to complement various therapies. We all know how music can effect our mood whether it be a love song, rock, pop or classical; but how many of us have actually tried listening to relaxation music after a hard days work?

What we really need at this point is music to slow down our mental clatter in order to slow our heart rate and thus reach a point of ultimate peace and tranquillity. On the other hand if you are feeling at a low ebb or need a boost, uplifting tones will encourage mind body and soul. Research suggests that music can have profound effects for the relief of anxiety – and even physical pain. Certain types of sound, such as a bird or the natural sounds of the sea, release endorphins from the brain to combat pain or discomfort.

Many therapists are now turning to music to assist them during practice, such as aromatherapists, masseurs, reiki healers and so on. The specific music may be chosen by the therapist or the patient for its positive associations or its nostalgic, calming influence. Music as a therapy is for everyone; if you're a parent why not try playing some womb music for your baby, she will remember the sound and will undoubtedly relax if not sleep more comfortably.

Children and young adults can benefit from listening to relaxation music during study; pre-exam nerves are hard to combat but research has shown that playing therapeutic music whilst revising releases stress and aids concentration.

If you work in the city and invariably face traffic jams every evening listening to the bad news on the radio is not going to make the ride home any more pleasant; consume some relaxation music instead!

So if your having a bad time, or you can't sleep don't turn to tranquillisers use music as your natural alternative. Come home, run a hot bath, light some candles, turn on your favourite CD and chill out; you'll love it!

 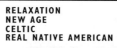
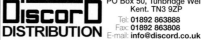

Natural Weight Loss

by John Vernon

Having been an alternative therapist for many years I can definitely say that weight has been the most intriguing condition that I have treated. Years ago, when people had time to relax and listen to their audio tape every day, good results were achieved using hypnotherapy.

So many times we've uncovered subconscious programmes where, in childhood, the client was torn between eating what they needed – and so being the correct weight – and eating more to please mum or dad so they'd grow big and strong – which they unfortunately did – or not to leave food because of guilt about the starving people in the third world. Emotional pressure meant they so often chose the unhealthy way. This along with other things that affect a persons self image and self confidence means that people often revert to eating for comfort when under stress.

Nowadays people so often don't have the time, or have even forgotten how, to relax and also they want what they're used to – instant results. Hypnotherapy combined with assisting the body's natural chemistry is now much more successful and for many people because they have a strong desire to be slim, therapy is not needed and natural supplements alone will create results. Above all, the emotional desire for a successful outcome is essential.

Exercise is also needed and it starts with just a little extra each day. Starting earlier and walking the children to school or walking to the shops or whatever can be fitted in without causing too much extra pressure. This can be increased as you become slimmer and start to feel more energetic.

The amount of food you eat is of great importance. There is lots of evidence that diets don't work. An experiment with people who couldn't put weight on, who were put on a diet provided amazing results. Having previously not put on weight whatever they ate, when put on a diet their weight increased until they even developed a weight problem! When measuring our client's body fat percentage, it is fairly common nowadays to get percentages twice what they should be.

Many independent sources are of the opinion that dieting causes loss of lean muscle mass. Most people who have dieted report that each time they start eating again they end up heavier than they started. This is also partly due to the fact that, not unreasonably, the mind thinks that during dieting there must be a famine so when food is available again more should be stored in the body in case there is another famine!

We are constantly aware of the vast number of different chocolate products and fast foods. Not only are we exposed to the high sugar content but also to foods made from refined ingredients. People get used to the quick energy fix which plays havoc with the body's blood sugar levels. Much is written about how this leads to carbohydrate intolerance and then to type 2 adult onset diabetes. However you view this, the fact is that every 30 seconds somewhere in the world one person is being newly diagnosed with this condition.

Reverting back to how people ate in times gone by seems to make a lot of sense, starting the day with a really good breakfast, a reasonable lunch and a light, early evening meal. Incorporating fresh vegetables, fruit, protein and complex carbohydrates etc will allow the body to take in and use nutrients to create energy and maintain optimum health.

Common sense should, of course, prevail regarding eating before going to bed. Three hours without eating/drinking except water is considered ideal and gives the body a chance to achieve its alkaline state ready for the night time repair/maintenance activity. Taking a collagen supplement just before sleep has been shown to achieve an improvement in body fat percentage and weight/inch loss. Products are also available that 'absorb' fat whilst different herbal mixes can help the body to metabolise fat in a better way. High protein meal replacement drinks are yet another protocol which some people prefer.

An important point to consider is that whilst dieting people restrict the foods they eat and they can suffer a shortage of minerals/vitamins, which in turn affects how they feel and so detracts from the enthusiasm of continuing the diet. This deficiency needs to be addressed for optimum results.

By chance when performing renal dialysis it was found that fat dissolved around the insertion points of the needles. Technology has now developed this phenomena to achieve weight loss but uses pads rather than needles! All of these approaches have been reported in many magazine and newspaper articles. Reporters have researched or tried them out and found them all to perform well but different approaches are appropriate for different people

Most people really need to take some action. Our current lifestyle must be somehow to blame as the average weight is increasing year by year. It's far easier to address the problem of a few pounds. rather than postpone action until it's many stones. We saw adults being pushed around in wheelchairs at the Epcot Centre in Florida because they were too huge to walk around! They'd left it too late.

If you'd like to share in our expertise in this essential field of health and well-being or have any other need for a natural approach, please call John or Linda on 0800 316 6944.

Is this you the typical YOU

"I have been exercising for the last year and I have lost 20lbs – not enough! I know what my problem is I do not eat healthily. How do I eat healthily without dieting? I do not like foods with fancy names. I like to keep it simple: chicken, beef (occasionally), rice, vegetables, green salads and SWEETS! I want to do better. How many grams of calories and fats should I consume per day to lose weight? Also, I do not understand the nutrition labels on foods. There are low fat, saturated fat, low sugar, low salt etc. how much of each should I consume per day? I am more serious now about my weight. I have to lose 60 lbs for my doctor to consider taking me off my blood pressure medication.

Losing 20 lbs in a year is actually enough to have a positive effect on your blood pressure, cholesterol and many other measures of health. When you lose weight that slowly you have put yourself in an elite category: People who are more likely to maintain the weight loss. Be patient. Take the focus off of your weight and soak up your success at exercising.

Continue to work on healthy eating. Measure your success by your healthy living, not by your weight. If you focus on your weight, you will get frustrated and give up. If you focus on your successes, you will stay motivated and change for a lifetime.

Naturism

By Brian Gibbons

Dare to go bare? Naturism is the ultimate freedom movement

If you enjoy the caress of warm breezes on your bare skin, or the exhilarating freedom of nakedness in the bath or if your body cries out to escape from the constrictions and encumbrances of unnecessary clothing, then you are already three quarters of the way to becoming a naturist.

Nudity is one of the most natural, most pleasurable and relaxing of human experiences – a feeling of being at one with nature. Another strong desire by most humans is to be part of a loving family and of a wider circle of like-minded friends. Naturism encompasses all of these joys and more. Social nudity in the safe and carefully regulated environment of bona fide naturist club offers therapeutic stress free feeling of freedom and peace. It is very much a family way of life – membership units of three generations are not uncommon – and, as such, the highest standards of moral and social behaviour are expected

Naturists come in all shapes and sizes and from all walks of life. Without our clothes, who is to know what background we come from? The only shared characteristic is enjoying the freedom that nakedness brings. Children can play in a completely safe environment where every member of their extended 'family' looks out for their welfare and they grow up without many of the 'hang-ups' of their non-naturist friends.

Most other European countries have a more enlightened attitude to nude bathing so, for many British, their first exposure to, or experience of this is on a foreign holiday beach. When everyone else is *'au naturel'* and you feel conspicuous in your completely unnecessary swimwear it becomes very easy to strip off, merge into the crowd and enjoy that first indescribable feeling of physical freedom.

Daring to go bare back at home is often another matter however. Thanks to years of lobbying by the movement's parent body, the Central Council for British Naturism (CCBN) there are now more than a dozen designated naturist beaches in this country and many more enjoying council 'blind eye' consent. From the number of enquiries to CCBN it is obvious that there is a huge growth in beach nudity.

More easily accessible are the many naturist clubs and centres, far removed from the so called 'nudist colonies' ' immortalised by seaside postcards. They vary from simple clubs with only basic facilities to sophisticated resorts offering package holidays and a huge range of things to do. Most are in beautiful countryside where nature and naturists exist side-by-side and all are full of friendly people who will make you feel welcome and not at all self-conscious.

Families and couples – only a small quota of 'singles' is normally allowed – typically have their own touring caravans or sited mobile homes. Around 120 clubs and 30,000 individuals belong to CCBN (Tel: 01604 620361), which will be happy to put you in touch with those nearest to you. Because of the rising cost of land for new clubs, many local authorities have been persuaded to regularly hire public swimming pools and leisure centres to naturists. There are now about as many naturist swimming clubs as there are outdoor sites.

Typical of the best of CCBN sites is Croft Country Club in East Anglia. Facilities include a well-appointed clubhouse, covered and open patios with barbecues, large kitchen, sauna, heated swimming pool, shower and toilet blocks, electricity hook-ups to all caravan pitches, tree-lined dog walks and superb gardens and flower beds. For the sporting minded there is petanque, mini-tennis, 18-hole putting green, volleyball, table tennis, pool, shuffleboard and even clay pigeon shooting. The social life is also richly varied.

The modern naturist movement is well aware to the harmful effects of too much sun on the skin. CCBN members are regularly reminded to take sensible precautions and hats and T-shirts are much more in evidence. Being nude all the time is certainly not compulsory, especially if it's too hot or cold. The object is to be relaxed and comfortable among friends at all times. That's the whole essence of naturism.

Author and journalist BRIAN GIBBONS has enjoyed naturism with his family for more than 30 years and has penned award-winning articles about the exhilarating freedom it offers.

Naturism promotes general health
by M Willcocks PhD

An obsessive sense of modesty often correlates to a reluctance to share healthy forms of touch with others. Research has increasingly linked touch-deprivation, especially during childhood and adolescence, to depression, violence, sexual inhibition and other anti-social behaviour. Research has also shown that people who are physically cold towards adolescents produce hostile, aggressive and often violent offspring.

Exposure to the sun, without going overboard, promotes general health. Research suggests that solar exposure triggers the body's synthesis of Vitamin D, vital for, among other things, calcium absorption and a strong immune system. Exposure to the sun is especially essential for the growth of strong bones in young children

Clothing limits or defeats many of the natural purposes of skin: for example, repelling moisture, breathing, protecting without impeding performance, and especially sensing one's environment. In the words of Michaelangelo: "What spirit is so empty and blind, that it cannot grasp the fact that the human foot is more noble than the shoe, and human skin more beautiful than the garment with which it is clothed?"

It is a noticeable fact that clothing makes people look older, and emphasizes rather than hides unflattering body characteristics. Nude, older people look younger, especially when tanned, and younger people look even younger… in addition fat people look far less offensive naked than clothed. The first-time Naturist doesn't take long to master the paradox that it is stockings that make varicose veins noticeable, belts that call attention to 48-inch waists, brassieres that emphasise sagging breasts.

Naturopathy

By Nina Victoria Gallagher

Naturopathy is a multi-disciplinary approach to healthcare that recognises the body's innate power to heal itself, if given the chance – vis medicatrix naturae (only nature heals).

There are three main principles of Naturopathy-

• The body has the power to heal itself if given the right conditions. Treatment should be given to support the healing mechanism as it works to restore the whole person to health.

• The symptoms of disease are a sign that the body is striving to restore its natural state of balance (homeostasis). They should not be suppressed.

• Treatment should be natural and given to support the Triad of Health. The Triad refers to our three constitutional elements of structure, biochemistry and emotions. The aim is to maintain a healthy balance among all three factors.

Naturopathy aims to strengthen your immune system so as to decrease your risk of infection and improve your health generally. It is primarily concerned with prevention, but it can benefit a wide range of problems including allergies, candida, constipation, irritable bowel syndrome, sinus problems and many others.

Naturopathy can assist you in finding the root causes of your problems, stimulate your own natural healing ability, increase your energy levels and vitality, teach you about your own body, advise and inform you on a healthy lifestyle, and put you back in charge of your own health. Naturopaths believe that the body has the power to heal itself and that prevention and cure of disease depends on strengthening the healing mechanism. They are skilled in tailoring natural health programmes to your individual requirements to assist you in creating a healthier diet and lifestyle and they use a variety of natural tools to do so.

These include: the correct nutrients, fasting where appropriate, clean water, fresh air, sunlight, adequate rest and relaxation, regular exercise, in addition disciplines such as Osteopathy, Herbalism, Homeopathy and Acupuncture are often used.

Naturopaths undergo four years of full time training. They study the same basic medical sciences as doctors – anatomy, physiology, pathology and pharmacology. In addition they study nutrition and detoxification methods and the influence of the emotions on health and disease.

Many Naturopaths are qualified osteopaths, some are also trained in herbal medicine, acupuncture, homeopathy or other natural therapies.

When you consult a Naturopath for the first time, the initial appointment may last approximately an hour. The practitioner will spend time finding out as much as possible about you, asking detailed questions about your illness, past

Nina Victoria Gallagher
BSc (Hons.) Ost. Med. DO. ND. MRN
Registered Osteopath & Registered Naturopath

THE FIXBY OSTEOPATHIC PRACTICE
1 GLENEAGLES WAY
FIXBY PARK
HUDDERSFIELD
WEST YORKSHIRE HD2 2NH
TEL: 01484 454845

medical history, diet, job, family, exercise, lifestyle and emotional status. Stress levels and bio-mechanical factors are also taken into account.

The Naturopath may use various ways to assess your health, including a full physical examination, where necessary refer you for X-rays and blood tests. Many Naturopaths use alternative forms of diagnosis which include: iridology (iris diagnosis), applied kinesiology (muscle testing), allergy testing and laboratory tests. Your treatment programme will be based on the elements mentioned above together with your Naturopaths own areas of expertise.

A typical naturopathic treatment might involve the use of a variety of treatments. These include: nutritional advice, supplementation, detoxification, hydrotherapy, hands-on work (such as Osteopathy and massage), herbal medicine, homeopathic remedies and acupuncture. Stress management, counselling, relaxation and meditation techniques complete the holistic package.

Rate of improvement will depend on the illness, how long you've had it, whether or not it has been suppressed, your age and general health. Treatment can sometimes provoke a healing crises, a period where your symptoms get worse before they get better. This is a sign that your body is beginning to respond to treatment.

Diet and Dietary change
By M Willcocks PhD

While diet is a cornerstone of naturopathic practice, the diet is usually worked out to be as easy as possible. It will take into account your previous lifestyle so the transition is easier; after all you would not put a tiger on raw carrots! In the same way, someone doing a heavy industrial job would not be placed on a fast – it wouldn't be practical.

Great emphasis is placed on the quality of foods. Often we seek to do the best for ourselves and family by changing our diets unaided. Many people use margarine in place of butter, yet margarine is a man-made product containing hydrogenated fat which is difficult for the system to break down properly and utilise. Olestra is a similar product which also has the ability to strip the digestive tract of fats, oils and fat soluble vitamins. Olestra is also known to cause digestive disorders in some people (IBS like symptoms).

We often turn to these synthetic products because of advertising, peer pressure and a desire for better health. Butter is a natural product containing vitamins, enzymes, fats and minerals needed for good health.

White refined sugar and white bleached flour and products that contain either, have no value, except to provide energy (refined carbohydrates); most substances useful as building blocks have been refined out and, ironically, often repackaged as a health giving bran cereal. Systematic over-use of this type of energy source can, eventually, result in metabolic disturbances, such as reactive hypoglycaemia, environmental sensitivities and/or digestive dysfunctions. Man in the 21st century consumes in two weeks the same amount of sugar as 18th century man did in a year. The impact of this 2600 per cent increase of sugar intake on our biochemistry is enormous and far reaching, we are not designed for such a toxic load.

It is a curious fact that most of the diseases we now accept as 'common' were unknown to our ancestors. They have only begun to emerge in our society with the increase of refined and processed foods being eaten on a daily basis.

Neuro-Linguistic Programming

By Ron Bowles

Neuro-Linguistic Programming (NLP) was initially developed from therapy, but it also offers communication and educational opportunities. Communication starts with thoughts and we use language, spoken and body, to convey these thoughts to others. When we think about the things we see, hear or feel we recreate those sights, sounds or feelings in our minds. If you think about an elephant, you will probably recreate your personal experience of an elephant from your memory.

If that experience was pleasant, say, during an enjoyable trip to a circus or safari park, then the feeling that is recreated will be pleasant. If you were practically trampled to death in the dark by an evil-smelling rogue, then clearly the recreated feeling will carry overtones of panic, revulsion and fear.

Thus, all memory is affected by the feelings related to the original experience, which created it. A simple example, which many people will identify with, is associated with shortened names. I am called Ron. I dislike being called Ronald, and this is caused by my memory of being called Ronald by my parents – only when I had done something wrong! Many Mikes, Daves, Sues and Gills will have the same feelings, and for the same reasons.

One of the many uses of NLP is to 'adjust' individual memories by dissociating them from the feelings they are 'attached' to. This is often done by encouraging the subject to create a picture in his or her mind which has pleasant associations; in the elephant example above, this might be to picture yourself on a tropical beach, playing with a friendly baby elephant in the warm sun.

NLP can also be used to change unwanted behaviour patterns such as nail biting or overeating, to improve sporting performance such as tennis, golf, or skiing; to improve co-ordination, to dispel phobias such as fear of spiders or flying; it can enhance the skills of counsellors, help build or repair relationships, remove blocks to personal growth and development, build confidence and reduce stress.

In a business context it is used in creativity training, sales and negotiating training, accelerated learning, stress management, and time management programmes.

NLP, a relatively recent development of Behavioural Psychology, was developed in the US in 1975 by Richard Bandler, a mathematician researching into Cybernetic Theory, and John Grinder, an associate professor of Linguistics, following detailed studies of the work of three outstandingly successful psychotherapists, Fritz Pens, Virginia Satir and Milton Erickson.

"Arguments are to be avoided, they are always vulgar and often convincing" – **Oscar Wilde.**

New Age

By M Willcocks PhD

New Age is a modern term for 'metaphysics'. Meta means change, transformation, and beyond; physics is the science dealing with the properties, changes and interactions, of matter and energy. So, New Age explores the nature of being, reality and so forth.

It's not a religion as such – there is no set dogma – yet it is spiritual because most New Ager's believe in the continuous existence, or experience, of the entity, soul or spirit.

New Age also includes studies or practices associated with, but not limited to, any of the following: Tarot, runes, crystals, herbs, aromatherapy and psychic phenomena, dream work, auras, spirit guides, reincarnation, channelling, meditation, alternative healing, etc. Of course, not everyone who has New Age interests believes, studies or practises all the above.

There are three qualities which are vital to all of us for life in the New Age, the Age of Aquarius. These qualities have always been important, yet they have sometimes eluded us as we searched for them with hearts too anchored in the third dimension.

New insight will help us to recognise and fully use these qualities as we look inward for solutions to the challenges we face every day. The qualities are truth, trust, and passion.

In this era of computers, networking, and the information explosion, truth often seems further away than ever before. We are desperately seeking for the ultimate truth, the one piece of information which will make the pieces of the universal puzzle fall into place.

And yet we find that truth is something which cannot be set down on paper; it can't be crystallised and bottled like some rare fragrance. It is a quality which begins in the heart of each person and radiates outward to envelope everyone that person touches.

It is an experience which is different for each person, changing from minute to minute – chameleon-like – as we all redefine our personal realities. It grows and evolves as each of us does.

So the truth which shaped the reality of our world even a few years ago are no longer adequate for the present moment, let alone the future. Trust is a quality born of the child in each of us. It is the small voice that says "go ahead, take a chance".

It is the foot which dares to step on the path of life, knowing that the way ahead may not always be easy. Yet the only way to reach the end of any journey

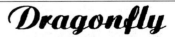

is to always move forward. It is the heart which continually opens itself to the world in innocence and wonder, no matter how many times it has known pain in the past. It is the quality which gives birth to hope.

Passion is that emotion we give to things that we care about very much, to those people or things which are very near to our hearts. The heart essence is at the centre of all life; it brings to each of us the passion which helps us live each day to the fullest, not merely exist.

To exist is to be static. To live is to learn and grow every day on our paths and to take great joy in the things we experience along the way. Vincent van Gogh said: "The best way to know life is to love many things."

When we feel joy or great excitement for something in our lives, we know that what is causing that feeling is something which is very important to the essence of our being.

It is something that comes directly from our Creative Source, which is the same as our source of life. There is no separation between the two. So it is vital for each of us to do the things we love... and to love the things we do. Passion is the spark of the soul; it is the sacred fire which touches every living being

The Capital of New Age

By M Willcocks PhD

Glastonbury is a fairly ordinary town at first sight; mostly brick-built with little grandeur or style. But one can't walk very far along its streets without becoming aware that this isn't an average English country town.

Bookshops, tea-rooms, souvenir stalls with Arthurian, Arimathean or New Age themes abound. Even the postcard advertisements in newsagents' windows tell of a different world to the usual run of second-hand prams, settees and bicycles – here you'll find Tarot-readers, crystal-healers, Shiatsu masseuses, astrologers and the like. There are shops full of pottery, hand-knit woollens, 'smokers' requisites' (mostly with little relevance to tobacco) and trippy posters. In short – Hippy Heaven.

These aren't just targeted at day-trippers (if you see what I mean). There is plainly a substantial local population buying into this. Because, for decades now, artists, musicians, writers and advertising executives have 'escaped' the metropolitan rat-race, and have established themselves here. Many of them arrived with a tidy little fortune – earned in some youth culture fad – so they didn't need serious work. But they wanted something to do – so they threw pots, learned some mystic art or wrote guide-books to the soul. The real surprise has been that some of them have managed to turn their little jobs into thriving careers – with business plans, accountants and the whole bit.

The so-called 'New Age' culture turned out to be rather more than a few fey optimists with warm hearts and no brains. It's become an industry. Glastonbury must be the world capital of that industry – in the Western world, at least. It's easy to sneer, but as industries go this one has one advantage over most of the others – it's mostly harmless. There are times when these New Agers fit rather uncomfortably into a conservative agricultural community, but Vegans and beef farmers are never going to see eye to eye on everything.

Numerology

By Trisha Morgan

Numerology shows your motivation, the occurrences which have formed your belief system, can explain why you do not always get what you want and the adjustments which are necessary for you to achieve understanding and ultimately success in your chosen path.

The world works in an orderly fashion based on cycles that form part of our understanding and common knowledge. Without these cycles we would be in suspended animation in which space and time were continuous and unidentifiable.

Can you imagine a world without day or night? A world where the seasons did not change? We accept these patterns, for instance the lunar cycle – where we know that the moon will be full at one point in the cycle, it will diminish and become a new moon in a regular pattern.

The natural order of death and rebirth is constantly around us. We do not give any conscious thought to these patterns or cycles, we accept that the sequence will stretch into the future ad infinitum. Astrologers can tell us what the placement of the stars in the skies will be in a week, a month, ten years or even thousands of years from now.

So what has this got to do with numerology you may ask? Well numerology constitutes part of the sense of order that exists. Numerology is a metaphysical, divining science that allows us to tune into the deeper meanings of our lives through the vibration of numbers. Through numerology we can understand the practical and spiritual significance of orderly progression of all manifestation.

Numerology is based on the study of the quality of numbers. The Universe is founded on numbers; certain numbers are mentioned in religious writings and have special significance in many ancient writings. Letters can also be reduced to numbers, thus allowing every word or name to relate to a number and each number has its inner meaning. The letter and number code when rightly understood and applied brings us into a direct and close relationship with the underlying intelligence of the Universe.

Numerology, like astrology, is an ancient art. Pythagorus is just one of many sages who have discovered the significance of numbers. He lived in the sixth century and believed that 'all things are numbers'. He introduced the mystical significance of numbers noting that the numbers 1 through to 9 stand for universal principles and these were subject to predictable progressive cycles.

Pythagorus was not the only person to understand the significance of numbers; the Chinese, Egyptians, Greeks and Romans have all used types of numerology systems. The significance of Pythagorus is that as a mathematician he used the numbers as figures, which represent quantities, but also unleashed the deeper meanings to be found in the numbers, that represent qualities, as a practical, spiritual and divining tool. In bygone days there was not the divide that we experience today between the logical processes and spiritual understanding.

Numbers by themselves represent Universal Principles through which all things evolve and continue to grow in a cyclical fashion. The digits 1 through to 9 symbolise the stages through which an idea must pass before it becomes reality. The way that these numbers can be related to the individual is through data that is processed by the numerologist. This information is then read to give indications of the experiences that will be presented in the life, the type of personality and how the individual will respond. The plan or chart can explain the past, identify the challenges of the present and look into the future, allowing the positive to be enhanced and the negative to be identified and dealt with in a positive manner.

Numerology works because it is unique to you; you alone possess two pieces of information that no other person possesses. Your date of birth and your full name at birth (usually the one on your birth certificate) is the basic information that a numerologist will require from you and, although you may share the same name with someone or the same birthday, the combination make you unique and original.

The numbers encapsulated within your date of birth will give the life path or destiny number and the sub-pathways that are individual to you which remain constant throughout the life.

The life path number will reveal the experiences that will be presented in the life and the sub-pathways give added lessons and experiences, both positive and negative, that will be encountered.

From your full name, a numerologist can derive elements of your personality, abilities and responses, talents that are inherent to you and talents that you will seek to expand in your life.

In numerology, numbers are reduced to a single digit from 1 to 9. Your life will be governed by a certain life path that will present you with the experiences that you are required to pass through, likewise each year will denote a personal year energy which will give guidance as to the optimum time for certain tasks or actions.

To gain even more detailed information the cycles can be applied to 9 monthly cycles, 9 day cycles and even down to 9 hour cycles, giving detailed data of the experiences and challenges presented within those time elements.

The life path will denote the pathway that you as the individual will walk down in this life and the type of experiences that will be encountered. Understanding of the meanings and properties of this number will give clarity of your motivation and your drives as an individual.

The life path number is found very simply by adding together the digits of the date of birth, so for someone born on the 13th October 1973 the process is as follows: –

$1 + 3 + 1 + 0 + 1 + 9 + 7 + 3 = 25$

then $2 + 5 = 7.$

Thus the life path number of someone born on 13-10-1973 will be 7.

Each number 1 to 9 as it relates to the life path will exhibit the following characteristics throughout the life.

1 The adventurer, is ambitious, original, full of action, independent, works best alone. Prefers to take the lead. Does not take advice easily. Values order, punctuality, cleanliness and obedience. Learns through experience and can be stubborn.

2 The peacemaker must work in co-operation with others. Gentle, warm, loving, tactful and considerate. Needs love peace and harmony. They will prefer to work in partnerships and associations. Marriage, home and family are important to them.

3 Self-expression, artistic, possesses a good imagination. These people are gifted with words, either spoken or written. Cheerful, optimistic, very enthusiastic, generous, friendly and good-natured. The natural leaders, sociable, their friends are important to them. They attract money and are usually lucky if they follow their hunches.

4 Loyal, patient, economical, a hard worker. These people are courageous and are prepared to put in what is required in the way of time and energy to build permanent and lasting things. Can be perfectionists and on occasions stubborn. Can always be relied upon and very dependable. They like routine work and exhibit good business sense.

5 Freedom, variety, expansive and active. These people do not like nine-five jobs. Very changeable, make quick decisions, enjoy travel and will try anything new. They communicate well with people; success comes through doing things with and for others. They have the ability to attract what they want to themselves. Marriage can be difficult.

6 Responsibility – These people like to be the centre of home, family and community. Understanding, sympathetic, reliable and stable. Like to work for the good of others. Excellent business ability. They will need to make adjustments throughout their life and are generally unselfish and generous with a keen sense of right and wrong.

7 Wise, secretive, the researchers, the thinkers are ruled by the number 7. They prefer to work alone. Intellectual, reserved, kind, a good companion when they feel they can trust you. Marriage will need to be built on mutual understanding of mind and soul. They dislike crowds prefer just a few close friends. Have interests in spirituality, religion or metaphysics.

8 Achievement usually within the business and commercial worlds if lived positively. They need to do good for others and to realise that money cannot buy everything. They prefer to lead, are the managers and are attracted to big business. Good organisers, efficient, courageous and should cultivate good ethical practices in business.

9 Humanitarian, compassionate. These people give love and charity, are intellectual, kind, tolerant and sympathetic. They like to travel have a magnetic personality and hate to be confined in small places. When problems strike they can be relied upon to help solve them.

The traits of the life path when read in relation to the personality, talents and motivations found in the name will, in the hands of an experienced numerologist, give detailed, constructive and helpful advice regarding the physical, emotional, mental and spiritual life of the individual.

Words of **Wisdom**

"It should be the function of medicine to help people die young as late in life as possible"

ERNST WYNDER

Nutrition

By Patrick Holford

A survey of patients at the Institute for Optimum Nutrition in London found that 86 per cent had a significant improvement in their health problem and 79 per cent of those following a personal nutrition programme designed by a nutritionist experienced a definite improvement in energy levels.

When you see a nutritional therapist she or he will work out your optimum nutrition needs, usually by using a questionnaire and by asking you questions in order to build up a picture of all the factors underlying your health status. The focus is on three main areas:

YOUR SYMPTOMS – which creates a picture of any imbalances you may have and which nutrients you may be lacking;

YOUR LIFESTYLE – which helps identify the factors that dictate your nutritional needs (such as your level of exercise, stress, pollution etc.);

YOUR DIET – examining what you should be eating to achieve optimum nutrition, taking into account the 'anti-nutrients' (substances that rob the body of nutrients) you may consume – such as alcohol, cigarettes, fried foods and refined foods.

Nutritional therapists also have access to biochemical tests that can accurately

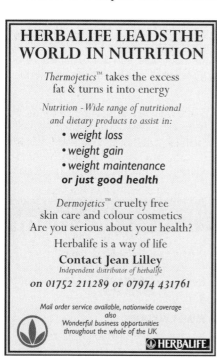

detect any imbalances and pinpoint your nutritional needs. Based on all this information and your main aims, your nutritionist will design a programme for you including dietary and supplement recommendations, clearly explaining the rationale behind these.

You only have to open a newspaper or magazine to grasp the massive increase in awareness of the link between diet and health. No longer is it cast to the minority world of a handful of so-called cranks.

It is a rare person in our society today who does not know that eating plenty of fried foods and animal fats is not good for your heart.

Yet nutritional therapy goes way beyond that – it provides an individual with a tailor-made programme, aimed not only at dealing with any current health complaint but also at setting the scene for minimising one's risk of illness and degenerative disease.

Taking vitamin C, for example, is not just for staving off the cold heralded by the sniffles that started this morning, but also for protecting your arteries and cells from damage that could lead to heart disease or cancer.

Nutritional therapy

We are literally made up of the food we eat, so good nutrition is the foundation of health. Nutritional therapy, the science of working out what nutrients are right for you, is not new. Many great visionaries have embraced it.

In 390AD Hippocrates said: "Let food be your medicine and medicine be your food". Edison, in the 20th century, said: "The doctor of the future will give no medicine but will interest his patients in the care of the human frame, diet, and the cause and prevention of disease."

In 1960 one of the geniuses of our time, twice Nobel Prize winner Dr Linus Pauling, coined the phrase 'ortho-molecular nutrition'.

By giving the body the right (ortho) molecules most disease would be eradicated – "Optimum nutrition," he said, "is the medicine of tomorrow."

Since then, modern science has uncovered the healing properties of dozens of nutrients, including vitamins, minerals, essential fats and amino acids.

Such concepts have now filtered down into mainstream consciousness to such an extent that the demand for information, products and nutritional therapists is booming.

Nutrition

By Dr. Liesbeth Ash M.B., Ch.B., Dip.Obst.(NZ)
& David Ash B.Sc. Nutrition (Lon)

Our health is at risk from the effects of stress, lack of exercise, pollution, soil depletion and eating processed and fatty food. Today, people are overfed but undernourished.

In a survey, conducted by the US Government (USDA 1982) of 21,500 people surveyed not a single person was receiving the minimum RDA of ten essential nutrients. Only three per cent were on a wholesome diet.

Dr. Walter Willet of Harvard University represents the winds of change in medicine: "Until quite recently, it was taught that everyone gets enough vitamins through their diet, and that taking vitamin supplements just creates expensive urine. I think we now have proof this isn't true." (*Newsweek,* June 7,1993)

According to the World Health Organisation, (WHO Report, May 1998 www.who.ch) every year more than 15 million adults aged 20-64 are dying premature and preventable deaths. In industrialised countries, heart disease, stroke and cancer are the leading causes of death.

- 7.2 million die of heart disease
- 4.6 million die of stroke,
- 6.2 million people died of cancer,
- 143 million suffer from diabetes
- 165 million suffer from arthritis

Research shows antioxidants and minerals can reduce the risk of chronic degenerative disease. Antioxidants scavenge free radicals generated by pollution and processed food. Minerals replace essential nutrients lost from depleted soil and processed food. Dr. Jeffery Blumberg, Director of Research of the USDA Human Nutrition Research Centre said: "We have the confidence that antioxidants really do work." (*Today*, March 4, 1994)

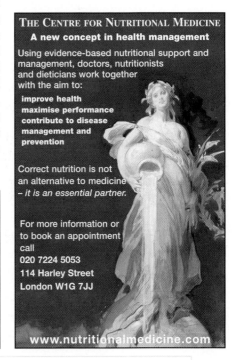

Our health is at risk – what nutrition supplements can we trust?

Dr. Jess Thoene of University of Michigan said: "In the marketplace today, the general public doesn't know what brand to trust." (*Newsweek* June 7, 1993)

Dr. Michael Colgan of the Institute of Optimum Nutrition said: "The majority of multi-vitamins are woefully inadequate. In a recent study at Yale… many were made with the wrong ratios of nutrients… or were missing some nutrients altogether." (*New Nutrition* p.100)

When buying supplements what should we look for?

Look for the words 'potency guaranteed' on the label. That tells you what is on the label is in the tablet. Without that the products are sub-standard. Look for tablets that are bioavailable e.g. their disintegration is guaranteed. They must disintegrate in your stomach within half an hour. Liquid minerals do not provide the levels required for optimum health. Clinical studies have proved that minerals are best absorbed if they are chelated – that is they are organic being linked to an amino acid. They are better absorbed than liquids in the inorganic, ionic, colloidal state. Look for a full spectrum of vitamins, minerals and antioxidants but avoid iron. Iron in supplements for general use can be a health hazard.

Look for synergy, balance and completeness in supplement formulations and go for optimum rather than RDA levels of vitamins and minerals. There is a lot to read on nutrition these days. Much is contradictory and confusing. We trust the research.

Clinical studies are proving the value of antioxidants and chelated minerals. Visit www.healthyfortune/products.com for well researched, easy-to-read articles – the latest in nutrition science.

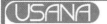

Nutritional Understanding

By M Willcocks PhD

The extremely complex processes that nutrients undergo in the body – how they affect one another, how they are broken down and released as energy, and how they are transported and used to rebuild countless specialised tissues and sustain the overall health of the individual – are understood only approximately.

Nevertheless, important nutrition decisions need to be made for the health of individuals, of groups such as the very young, the aged, and the malnourished.

Nutrients are classified into five major groups: proteins, carbohydrates, fats, vitamins and minerals. These groups comprise between 45 and 50 substances that scientists have established as essential for maintaining normal growth and health.

Besides water and oxygen, they include about eight amino acids from proteins, four fat-soluble and ten water-soluble vitamins, about ten minerals, and three electrolytes. Although carbohydrates are needed for the body's energy, they are not considered absolutely essential, because protein can be converted for this purpose.

The body uses energy to carry on vital activities and to maintain itself at a constant temperature. By using a calorimeter, scientists have been able to establish the energy amounts of the body's fuels – carbohydrates, fats, and protein. About 4 cal each are yielded by 1g (0.035 oz) of pure carbohydrate and 1g of pure protein; 1g of pure fat yields about 9 cal. A kilogram calorie, used in nutrition, is defined as the heat energy needed to raise the temperature of 1kg of water from 14.5° to 15.5°C.

Carbohydrates are the most abundant foods in the world, and fats are the most concentrated and easily stored fuel. If the body exhausts its available carbohydrates and fats, it can use proteins directly from the diet or break down its own protein tissue to make fuel. Alcohol is also a source of energy and yields 7cal. per g. Alcohol cannot be oxidised by the body cells but must be processed by the liver into fat, which is then stored by the liver or in the adipose tissue.

Functions of nutrients

PROTEINS: The primary function of protein is to build body tissue and to synthesise enzymes, some hormones such as insulin that regulate communication among organs and cells, and other complex substances that govern body processes.

Animal and plant proteins are not used in the form in which they are ingested but are broken down by digestive enzymes (proteases) into nitrogen-containing amino acids. Proteases disrupt the peptide bonds by which the ingested amino acids are linked, so that they can be absorbed through the intestine into the blood and recombined into the particular tissue needed.

Proteins are usually readily available from both animal and plant sources. Of the 20 amino acids that make up protein, eight are considered essential; that is, because the body cannot synthesise them, they must be supplied ready-made in foods.

If these essential amino acids are not all present at the same time and in specific proportions, the other amino acids, in whole or in part, cannot be used for metabolising human protein. Therefore, a diet containing these essential amino acids is very important for sustaining growth and health.

When any of the essential amino acids is lacking, the remaining ones are converted into energy-yielding compounds, and their nitrogen excreted. When an excess of protein is eaten, which is often the case with heavy meat diets, the extra protein is similarly broken down into energy-yielding compounds.

Because protein is far scarcer than carbohydrates and yields the same 4cal/g, the eating of meat beyond the tissue-building demands of the body becomes an inefficient way to procure energy. Foods from animal sources contain complete proteins because they include essential amino acids. In most diets, a combination of plant and animal protein is recommended: 0.8 g/kg of body weight is considered a safe daily allowance for normal adults.

Many illnesses and infections lead to an increased loss of nitrogen from the body. This needs to be replaced by a higher consumption of dietary protein. Infants and young children also require more protein per kilogram of body weight. A protein deficiency accompanied by energy deficits results in a form of malnutrition called kwashiorkor, which is characterised by loss of body fat and wasting of muscle.

MINERALS: Inorganic mineral nutrients are required in the structural composition of hard and soft body tissues; they also participate in such processes as the action of enzyme systems, the contraction of muscles, nerve reactions, and the clotting of blood. These mineral nutrients, all of which must be supplied in the diet, are of two classes: the so-called major elements such as calcium, phosphorus, magnesium, iron, iodine and potassium; and trace elements such as copper, cobalt, manganese, fluorine, and zinc.

Calcium is needed for developing the bones and maintaining their rigidity. It also contributes in forming intracellular cement and the cell membranes and in regulating nervous excitability and muscular contraction. About 90 per cent of calcium is stored in bone, where it can be reabsorbed by blood and tissue. Milk and milk products are the chief source of calcium.

Phosphorus, also present in many foods and especially in milk, combines with calcium in the bones and teeth. It plays an important role in energy metabolism of the cells, affecting carbohydrates, lipids, and proteins.

Magnesium, which is present in most foods, is essential for human metabolism and is important for maintaining the electrical potential in nerve and muscle cells. A deficiency in magnesium among malnourished persons, especially alcoholics, leads to tremors and convulsions.

Sodium, which is present in small and usually sufficient quantities in most natural foods, is found in liberal amounts in salted, prepared and cooked foods. It is present in extracellular fluid, which it plays a role in regulating. Too much sodium causes edema, an over-accumulation of extracellular fluid. Evidence now exists that excess dietary salt largely contributes to high blood pressure.

Iron is needed to form haemoglobin, which is the pigment in red blood cells responsible for transporting oxygen, but the mineral is not readily absorbed by the digestive system. It exists in sufficient amounts in men, but women of menstrual age, who need nearly twice as much iron because of blood loss, often have deficiencies and must take in absorbable iron.

Iodine is needed to synthesise hormones of the thyroid gland. A deficiency leads to goitre, a swelling of this gland in the lower neck. Low iodine intakes during pregnancy may result in the birth of cretinous or mentally retarded infants. Goitre remains prevalent in certain parts of Asia, Africa and South America. It is estimated that worldwide more than 150 million people suffer from iodine deficiency diseases.

Trace elements are other inorganic substances that appear in the body in minute amounts and are essential for good health. Little is known about how they function, and most knowledge about them comes from how their absence, especially in animals, affects health. Trace elements appear in sufficient amounts in most foods. Among the more important trace elements is copper, which is present in many enzymes and in copper-containing proteins found in the blood, brain, and liver. Copper deficiency is associated with the failure to use iron in the formation of lemoglobin. Zinc is also important in forming enzymes.

Deficiency in zinc is believed to impair growth and, in severe cases, to cause dwarfism. Fluorine, which is retained especially in the teeth and bones, has been found necessary for growth in animals. Fluorides, a category of fluorine compounds, are important for protecting against demineralisation of bone. The fluoridation of water supplies has proved an effective measure against tooth decay, reducing it by as much as 40 per cent. Other trace elements include chromium, molybdenum, and selenium.

VITAMINS: Vitamins are organic compounds that mainly function in enzyme systems to enhance the metabolism of proteins, carbohydrates, and fats. Without these substances, the breakdown and assimilation of foods could not occur. Certain vitamins also participate in the formation of blood cells, hormones, nervous system chemicals, and genetic materials.

Vitamins are classified into two groups, the fat-soluble and the water-soluble vitamins. Fat-soluble vitamins include vitamins A, D, E, and K. The water-soluble vitamins include vitamin C and the B-vitamin complex. Fat-soluble vitamins are usually absorbed with foods that contain fat. They are broken down by bile and the emulsified molecules pass through the lymphatics and veins to be distributed through the arteries. Excess amounts are stored in body fat and in the liver and kidneys. Because fat-soluble vitamins can be stored, they do not have to be consumed every day.

Vitamin A is essential for the health of epithelial cells and for normal growth. A deficiency leads to skin changes and to night blindness, or a failure of dark adaptation due to the effects of deficiency on the retina. Later, xerophthalmia, an eye condition characterised by dryness and thickening of the surface of the conjunctiva and cornea, may develop; untreated xerophthalmia may lead to blindness, especially in children.

Vitamin A can be obtained directly in the diet from foods of animal origin such as milk, eggs, and liver. In developing countries, most vitamin A is obtained from carotene, which is present in green and yellow fruits and vegetables. Carotene is converted to vitamin A in the body.

Vitamin D acts much like a hormone and regulates calcium and phosphorus absorption and metabolism. Some vitamin D is obtained from such foods as eggs, fish, liver, butter, margarine, and milk, some of which may have been fortified with vitamin D. But humans get most of their vitamin D from exposure of the skin to sunlight. A deficiency leads to rickets in children or osteomalacia in adults.

Vitamin E is an essential nutrient for many vertebrate animals, but its role in the human body has not been established. It has been popularly advocated for a great variety of afflictions, but no clear evidence exists that it alleviates any specific disease. Vitamin E is found in seed oils and wheat germ.

Vitamin K is necessary for the coagulation of blood. It assists in forming the enzyme prothrombin, which, in turn, is needed to produce fibrin for blood clots. Vitamin K is produced in sufficient quantities in the intestine by bacteria, but is also provided by leafy green vegetables such as spinach and kale, egg yolk and many other foods.

The water-soluble vitamins, C and B complex, cannot be stored and therefore need to be consumed daily to replenish the body's needs. Vitamin C, or ascorbic acid, is important in the synthesis and maintenance of connective tissue. It prevents scurvy, which attacks the gums, skin and mucous membranes, and its main source is citrus fruits.

The most important B-complex vitamins are thiamine (B1), riboflavin (B2), nicotinic acid or niacin (B3), pyraidoxine (B6), pantothenic acid, lecithin, choline, inositol, para-aminobenzoic acid (PABA), folic acid, and cyanocobalamin (B12). These vitamins serve a wide range of important metabolic functions and prevent such afflictions as beriberi and pellagra. They are found mostly in yeast and liver.

CARBOHYDRATES: Carbohydrates provide a great part of the energy in most human diets. Foods rich in carbohydrates are usually the most abundant and cheapest, when compared with foods high in their protein and fat content.

Carbohydrates are burned during metabolism to produce energy, liberating carbon dioxide and water. Humans also get energy less efficiently from fats and proteins in the diet, and also from alcohol. The two kinds of carbohydrates are starches, which are found mainly in grains, legumes, tubers and sugars, which are found in plants and fruits. Carbohydrates are used by the cells in the form of glucose, the body's main fuel.

After absorption from the small intestine, glucose is processed in the liver, which stores some as glycogen, a starchlike substance, and passes the rest into the bloodstream. In combination with fatty acids, glucose forms triglycerides, which are fat compounds that can be easily broken down into combustible ketones. Glucose and triglycerides are carried by the bloodstream to the muscles and organs to be oxidised, and excess quantities are stored as fat in the adipose and other tissues, to be retrieved and burned at times of low carbohydrate intake.

The carbohydrates containing the most nutrients are the complex carbohydrates, such as unrefined grains, tubers, vegetables and fruit, which also provide protein, vitamins, minerals, and fats. A less beneficial source is foods made from refined sugar, such as candy and soft drinks, which are high in calories but low in nutrients and fill the body with what nutritionists call empty calories.

FATS: Although scarcer than carbohydrates, fats produce more than twice as much energy. Being a compact fuel, fat is efficiently stored in the body for later use when carbohydrates are in short supply. Animals obviously need stored fat to tide them over dry or cold seasons, as do humans during times of scarce food supply. In industrial nations, however, with food always available and with machines replacing human labour, the accumulation of body fat has become a serious health concern.

In a way similar to that in which protein is broken down by digestive enzymes into amino acids to form the body's proteins, dietary fats are broken down into fatty acids that pass into the blood to form the body's own triglycerides. The fatty acids that contain as many hydrogen atoms as possible on the carbon chain are called saturated fatty acids and are derived mostly from animal sources.

Unsaturated fatty acids have some of the hydrogen atoms missing; this group includes mono-unsaturated fatty acids, which have a single pair of hydrogens missing, and polyunsaturated fatty acids, which have more than one pair missing. Polyunsaturated fats are found mostly in seed oils. Saturated fats in the bloodstream have been found to raise the level of cholesterol, while polyunsaturated fat tends to lower it. Saturated fats generally are solid at room temperature; polyunsaturated fats are liquid.

FOOD TYPES: Foods can be roughly classified into breads and cereals; pulses, or legumes; tubers, or starchy roots; vegetables and fruits; meat, fish, and eggs; milk and milk products; fats and oils; and sugars, preserves, and syrups. Breads and cereals include wheat, rice, maize, and millet. They are high in starches and are easily procured sources of calories.

Although protein is not abundant in whole cereals, the large quantity that is commonly consumed often supplies significant amounts, which, however, must be supplemented with other protein foods to supply all the essential amino acids. White wheat flour and polished rice are low in nutrients, but whole grain wheat and rice supply the body with needed fibre; the B vitamins thiamine, niacin, and riboflavin; and the minerals zinc, copper, manganese, and molybdenum.

Pulses, or legumes, include a wide variety of beans, peas, lentils and grains, and even peanuts. All are rich in starch but may provide considerably more protein than do cereals or tubers. Their amino acid patterns often compliment those of rice, maize, and wheat, which are staples in many poor countries.

Tubers and starch roots such as potatoes are rich in starch and relatively low in protein content, but provide a variety of minerals and vitamins.

Vegetables and fruits are a direct source of many minerals and vitamins lacking in cereal diets, especially vitamin C from citrus fruits and vitamin A from the carotene of leafy vegetables and carrots. Sodium, cobalt, chloride, copper, magnesium, manganese, phosphorus, and potassium are present in vegetables, which supply the roughage needed to pass food through the digestive tract. Many of the more fragile, water-soluble vitamins exist in vegetables and fruit and can be easily destroyed by overcooking.

Meat, fish, and eggs supply all the essential amino acids that the body needs to assemble its own proteins. Meats usually contain about 20 per cent protein, 20 per cent fat, and 60 per cent water. Organ meats are rich sources of vitamins and minerals. All fish are high in protein, and the oils of some are rich in vitamins D and A. Egg white is the most concentrated form of protein.

Milk and milk products include whole milk, cheese, yogurt, and ice cream, all of which are well known for their abundant protein, phosphorus, and especially calcium. Milk is also rich in vitamins but contains no iron and, if pasteurised, no vitamin C. Although milk is essential for children, for adults too much can cause unsaturated fatty acids to build in the blood system.

Fats and oils include butter, lard, suet, and vegetable oils. They are all high in calories, but, apart from butter and certain vegetable oils, contain few nutrients.

Sugars, preserves, and syrups are heavily consumed in more affluent countries, where they make up a large portion of the carbohydrate intake. Honey is composed of over 75 per cent sugar and contain few nutrients. Sugar causes tooth decay.

The science of nutrition is still far from explaining how foods affect certain individuals. Why some people stop eating at a certain point and why others eat obsessively, for example, is still a mystery. Researchers recently found that shortly after ingestion, foods influence the release of important brain chemicals and that carbohydrate foods in particular trigger the release of serotonin, which, in turn, suppresses the desire for carbohydrates. This mechanism may have evolved to prevent people from gorging themselves on carbohydrates and failing to procure harder-to-find protein.

Until recently, carbohydrate foods were far more accessible than protein. Serotonin is believed to work in complex relationships with insulin and several amino acids, especially tryptophan, all of which participate in monitoring the appetite for various food types.

Why Organic

By M. Willcocks PhD

Organic living, natural medicine and an awareness of damage to our natural environment are intrinsically linked. Are you doing your bit to protect nature? Do you want gigantic synthetic vegetables and fruits; is there an argument for organically produced foods, cosmetics, clothes and other consumables?

What is the difference? The simple answer is that organic producers don't use synthetic fertilisers or pesticides on their plants.

But producing organically is much more than what you don't do. When you farm/garden organically, you think of your plants as part of a whole system within nature that starts in the soil and includes the water supply, people, wildlife and even insects.

An organic producer strives to work in harmony with natural systems and to minimise and continually replenish any resources the soil consumes. Organic farming, then, begins with attention to the soil by regularly adding organic matter to the soil, using locally available resources wherever possible.

There are surprisingly raw ingredients of organic matter available in our everyday lives, from corn stubble, weed control, animal slurry, hedge and lawn clippings, autumn leaves etc, even some of the kitchen waste is suitable.

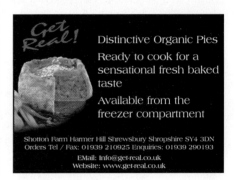

We understand
that you care about what you eat

⬡rganic

With over 700 products in some of our largest stores, you can trust Tesco to provide you with a fantastic range of quality Organic food at low prices.

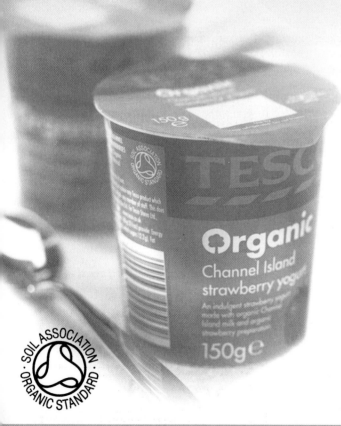

If you've ever thought that choo organics meant limiting your ch think again. We've re-launched organic range to ensure we offe an organic alternative for all yo everyday products. But that's no we also offer a selection of mor exotic organic lines so you can organic products to suit every occasion.

You can trust us to provide you the highest quality organic food low prices. All our organic prod are grown and produced to regulations laid down by the Un Kingdom Register of Organic Fo Standards. And all our products certified by approval bodies suc the Soil Association who ensure these strict standards are adher

TESCO **'The UK's favourite Organic Retaile**

These products of natures natural evolution, are the building blocks of compost, the ideal organic matter for the soil. If you add compost to your soil, you're already well on your way to raising beautiful, healthy crops organically. The other key to producing organically is to choose plants suited to the site. Plants adapted to climate and conditions are better able to grow without a lot of attention or input; on the other hand, plants that are not right for a particular site will probably require a boost to their natural defences to maintain health and productivity.

The alternative

Most crops, organic or otherwise, are produced with identical procedures, the difference is that organically grown crops are not treated with chemicals or genetically altered to enhance productivity. It is therefore much safer to consume/use products that do not contain synthetics or have been scientifically generated.

An example would be a province in the hinterland of China which has not been contaminated by modern living, there are no machines, electricity, cars or other trappings we in the Western world consider to be essential, here only produce from the land sustains life. The average age is 150 with a funeral every 50 years.

The gardener and his flower

The gardener started his flower garden with the smallest of seeds. With complete love, gentleness and the greatest of care, he placed each of his seeds in the fertile ground.

Over an expanse of immeasurable time, he tended to his seeds and nurtured them. His heart swelled with love for his seeds and the hope he had for their growth. Each seed grew at its own rate and appeared as a different flower. His garden was becoming

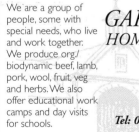

Eden with the beauty each flower brought to the collective garden.

He loved each of his seeds equally and completely, and patiently waited for each seed to flower. On this particular day a seed germinated and began to grow, pushing up through the ground to meet its father gardener and the sun. The flower's petals were rays of love extending from its centre, growing towards the other flowers, the sun, and the gardener. The beauty of this flower was radiant and shone over the whole garden.

The other flowers were attracted to this flower and grew from their association. The sun shone more brightly on all the flowers, it was so filled with the joy that this flower brought. The gardener fully experienced the beauty and love of his entire garden, which was his utmost desire.

He knelt over this radiant flower and cupped his hands around it. He gently touches his lips to its petals, letting the flower know of his unconditional love and joy, at what it is bringing and becoming.

An unconditional love and joy that is shared by all the flowers, the sun and the

ORGANIC FOOD & DRINK

MRS J COLLIER, Orchard Wholefoods, 16 High Street, Budleigh Salterton, Devon. EX9 6LQ. Tel: 01395-442508. We sell a wide range of gluten free/diabetic products & fresh organic bread. Herbal & Homeopathic remedies are also available

MOUNT PLEASANT WINDMILL – Kirton-in-Lindsey – Lincolnshire. Traditional four-sailed brick tower mill built in 1875, renovated in 1991 and producing today pure organic stoneground flour by windpower. Tearooms with home-made cakes, wholefood shop and organic bakery. Tel 01652 640177

GREEN ACRES ORGANIC FARM Shop, Dinmore, Herefordshire HR4 8ED. Tel: 01568 797045. Established 1982 and producing over 80 veg. Also stocking organic meat, fish, cider, dried and tinned goods, bread, ice cream etc. Open: Tues – Sat. 9.00am – 5.30pm.

NEW FARM ORGANICS – growers and suppliers of quality organic produce. For further information please contact J Edwards, Lincs. Tel 01205 087 0500 Fax 01205 087 1001 Email newfarmorganics@zoom.co.uk www.newfarmorganics.co.uk

FRESH & WILD, London's leading organic food and natural remedy retailer with supplements, herbs, homeopathy, books, bodycare. Stores in Camden Town, City, Lavender Hill, Notting Hill, Soho, Stoke Newington (April 01) Tel 0800 9175 175 www.freshandwild.com

HEALTH WISE, 27 North Walk, Yate, Bristol, BS37 4AP. 01454 322168

ORGANIC FOOD & DRINK

RUSSELL SMITH FARMS, College Farm, Grange Road, Duxford, Cambridgeshire, CB2 4QF. 01223 839002

WHITEHOLM FARM, Whiteholm, Roweltown, Carlisle, Cumbria, CA6 6LJ. 01697 748058

NATURAL CHOICE, 24 St John Street, Ashbourne, Derbyshire, DE6 1GH. 01335 346096

CHORLTON WHOLEFOODS, 64 Beech Road, Chorlton-Cum-Hardy, Greater Manchester, M21 9EG. 0161 881 6399

SUNNYBANK VINE NURSERY, The Old Trout Inn, Dulas, Herefordshire, HR2 0HL. 01981 240256

FIELDFARE ORGANICS LTD, Oakcroft, Dudswell Lane, Berkhamstead, Hertfordshire. 01442 877363

FRUGAL FOOD, 17 West St Helen Street, Abingdon, Oxfordshire, OX14 5BL. 01235 522239

MYRIAD ORGANICS, 22 Corve Street, Ludlow, Shropshire, SY8 1DA. 01584 872665

D J PRODUCE, Unit 1 Griffiths Yard, Gazely Rd, Moulton, Newmarket, Suffolk, CB8 8SR. 01638 552709

HARVEST SUPPLIES, Harvest Home, Chuck Hatch, Hartfield, Sussex, TN7 4EN. 01342 823392

holiest of spirits that behold the garden. The beauty of this one flower makes all the difference in their world. The love, joy, and light that radiates from this flower is felt so strongly. What is the flower?

The effect of human consumption

What we eat and the foods we buy dramatically influence the health of the environment. It is not just individual acts that can be harmful; it's our collective actions over time that threatens the Earth's incredible diversity of life – its biodiversity.

As consumers, we play a vital role in shaping how our food is produced and what foods are available. Making small changes in our food choices is one of the simplest ways we can protect the Earth. From fruits and vegetables to fish and poultry, the Earth's biodiversity is the source of our food supply.

We rely on the variety of life for our basic nutritional needs. But biodiversity is also important in several, less obvious ways: One of the Earth's most vital processes, pollination is necessary for fruit and vegetable production. Bees and other insects, birds, bats, and other small mammals pollinate 75 per cent of the world's staple crops.

The productivity of our agricultural lands depends upon the fertility of the Earth's topsoil. This thin layer – only 15 centimetres deep – contains organic matter, nutrients, minerals, insects, microbes, worms and other elements needed for plants to survive. The health of the soil depends on this diversity of organisms. They break down and recycle organic matter, providing nutrients that enable crops, pastures, and forests to grow.

Over thousands of years, people have domesticated some 12,000 wild plant species and 20 to 30 animal species, primarily for agricultural uses. But agriculture still depends upon wild relatives of domesticated species for genetic material that provides resistance to disease, enhances productivity, and improves adaptability to ever-changing environmental conditions.

Farmers around the world spend nearly £25 billion annually on pesticides; however, natural parasites and predators, like some wasps and birds, provide an estimated five to ten times this amount of free 'pest control'. Without these wild species, pest damage would be catastrophic.

Many of the Earth's most important species – pollinators and soil organisms – are threatened by toxic chemical sprays used on crops for pest control. Chemical pesticides and fertilisers also release harmful chemicals into the air, water, and soil.

In fact, fertiliser that has washed into lakes and rivers is a major cause of water pollution.

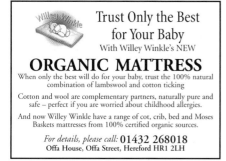
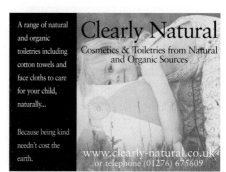

Living with Nature

There is no randomness or coincidences in Nature. When one lives with awareness of and in harmony with the laws of Nature, life is less hardship and more of a flow. The effort to achieve or create circumstances is lessened. The opportunities to create the circumstances you desire are increased. The plan or purpose of your life can become clearer and easier to follow.

Your health, whether it is physical, emotional, mental, or spiritual, is directly dependent on and reflects the harmony in which you live with Nature. The greater the harmony and unification with Nature, the greater your health. The less harmony and more separation from Nature, the less your health.

The correlates of harmony and disharmony are love and fear, respectively. The laws of nature are immutable. It is your feelings, thoughts, words, and deeds that must change to create harmony and health.

All in nature, whether it is animal, mineral, vegetable, or human, share the same life force. There is a shared and unified consciousness among all of nature. The evolution of nature is the ultimate truth from which countless philosophies, religions, and interpretations have been derived.

Are you doing your bit?

Choose organic products; Buy produce that is grown locally; Buy produce that is in season; Avoid eating over-exploited species; Draw on the Earth's biodiversity; Eat foods that are lower on the food chain; Buy products with minimal packaging; Minimise your food waste.

For every pound of shrimp caught, an average of 7lbs of other sea life is killed. Over two-thirds of the world's fisheries are presently over exploited, fully exploited or depleted.

Food makes up about ten per cent of the rubbish we send to waste tips. Packaging of food alone accounts for six per cent of the energy consumption in the EEC.

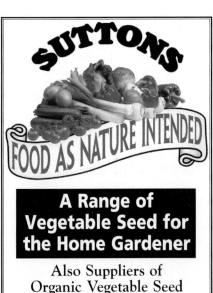

ORGANIC PRODUCTS & SERVICES

LAMBS SKIN BABY RUGS. Organically reared and tanned. Machine washable. £50.00 + £4.50 p.& p. Also a family camp, 1st two weeks August, on our organic farm. Information from, Golden Fleeces, Coachgard Cottage, Sharpham, Ashprington, Totnes, Devon. TQ9 7UT. Tel: 01803 732324.

SUNNYBANK VINE NURSERY, The Old Trout Inn, Dulas, Herefordshire, HR2 0HL. 01981 240256

NATURAL INSTINCTS, Killar, Co Donegal. 00353 7338256

Osteopathy

By the Osteopathic Information Service

Osteopathy is an established, recognised system of diagnosis and treatment that lays its main emphasis on the structural integrity of the body. It is distinctive in the fact that it recognises much of the pain and disability we suffer stems from abnormalities in the function of the body structure as well as damage caused to it by disease.

Osteopathy uses many of the diagnostic procedures used in conventional medical assessment and diagnosis. Its main strength' however, lies in the unique way the patient is assessed from a mechanical, functional and postural standpoint and the manual methods of treatment applied to suit the needs of the patient.

Osteopaths use their hands both to investigate the underlying causes of pain and to carry out treatment using a variety of manipulative techniques. These may include muscle and connective tissue stretching, rhythmic joint movements or high velocity thrust techniques to improve the range of movement.

When you visit an osteopath for the first time a full case history will be taken and you will be given an examination.

The osteopath will then use a highly developed sense of touch, called palpation, to identify any points of weakness or excessive strain.

The osteopath may also refer you for additional investigations such as x-rays or blood tests. Then full diagnosis and a suitable treatment plan will be developed for you as an individual.

Osteopathy is the first of the professions previously outside conventional medical services to achieve statutory recognition. The Osteopaths Act 1993 set up a single body, the General Osteopathic Council, to regulate the profession in the UK.

The legislation came into force in May 2000 and now all practising osteopaths must be registered and the title 'osteopath' is protected. In this way patients have the same protection as they have when currently visiting a doctor or dentist.

Words of **Wisdom**

"The beneficent effects of the regular quarter-hour's exercise before breakfast is more than offset by the mental wear and tear involved in getting out of bed fifteen minutes earlier than one otherwise would"

SIMEON STRUNSKY

Past Life Regression

By the College of Past Life Regression

Past life regression therapy is a way of exploring the past in order to make sense of the present. Many of our problems in relationships, business or health are rooted in old patterns, traumas or decisions made in past lives.

Awareness and processing of the past life causes that have led up to present circumstances can often be life changing and enables us to move forward in our present lifetime.

This therapy developed from hypnotherapy in the 1960s. Hypnotherapists such as Edith Fiore found that clients would spontaneously regress into what appeared to be past lives when directed to go to the first time they felt a particular emotion or to find the source of an issue.

This occurred even if the client didn't believe in reincarnation! It is a powerful tool that can be used to gain insight into and bring relief from phobias, fears, relationship problems, physical symptoms and sexual dysfunction.

It can help people to gain a sense of direction and purpose in life. Most people an be regressed successfully, however, it is not suitable for children, pregnant women or anyone suffering a severe mental disorder. If you are considering having regression therapy it is important to find a trained therapist. It is not advisable to attempt a DIY regression using tapes as it is possible to bring far memories into the conscious mind that may be disturbing; it is the role of the therapist to help you to resolve the issues to enable the healing to take place.

One typical example of a past life regression case is that of James, a man in his 30s who worked in advertising. He came for regression therapy to try to find the cause of his fear of water. He also spoke of recurring disturbing dreams in which he lost his wife and sons. Under regression, he accessed memories of drowning after falling from a bridge. His dying thoughts were of his wife and family in that lifetime and his overwhelming sadness at being parted from them.

After remembering this event his fear of water subsided and he has now learnt to swim and enjoys taking his children to the swimming baths. He also sleeps better and has not had any more nightmares about losing his family.

An example of how relationship issues can be clarified with the help of past life regression is the case of Elizabeth, a secretary in her 30s. Involved with an unhappy and destructive relationship with a married man, Elizabeth wanted to know why she felt so powerless to break free. It transpired that in a previous lifetime she had been married to the man who was now her 'lover' and their relationship had been good. On his deathbed he had declared his undying love for her and promised that they would be reunited. He said he would always love her.

Meeting up again in this lifetime they felt an irresistible pull towards each other. Unfortunately the promises made in the previous lifetime were no longer appropriate as he was married to another. During the regression Elizabeth released him from the promise and was able to see her present situation in a new light. She was finally able to distance herself from him and went on to form a new and happy relationship.

Regress into your past lives
By M Willcocks PhD

Is it necessary to see a therapist in order to discover one's past lives ? It is not always necessary to see a therapist in order to discover one's past lives. Meditation on your own or by using audiotapes can help you to have your own experiences.

Learn and practice meditation regularly. This will help a great deal. After a while, the answers to your questions will come to you, but you must be persistent and patient and not get discouraged. This is a practice for a lifetime.

Are all problems helped by past life therapy ?

It is not always necessary to discover our past lives in order to live better lives in the present. Not all of our problems have their source in the past. Many people have enough understanding about themselves without delving in the past so that they can live this life in a healthy fulfilling way.

Perhaps everybody reincarnates because we have many lessons to learn; lessons about love, compassion, charity, non-violence, inner peace, patience, etc. It would be hard to learn them all in only one life. Also, some people come back voluntarily to help others.

Do all souls reincarnate ?

Perhaps that sometimes you have to come back. If your learning is not finished, you find yourself being born into another lifetime. There may be some choices involved, however, but apparently there are limits to the choices. Highly evolved souls do not have to come back but often choose to reincarnate to help as teachers.

What is the role of physical health ?

We have tasks to do and much to learn. The healthier the body, the easier it is and the more time and energy there are to do what we came here to do. Your actions regarding your body can shorten your life and can thus limit your spiritual growth. Also, it's one of our lessons to respect our bodies.

PAST LIFE REGRESSION

PHEONIX HEALING CENTRE. Tel: 01332 702018. Experience the 'Inner Healing Journey' for Self Discovery, which gently releases blockages from the Past that have hindered fulfilment, whilst revealing your direction and purpose in Life. Cathie Shepherd H.dip.C.th. N.F.S.H. P.M.I.A.C.

Personal Care

By Sheila Gill

How safe is your bathroom? Have your ever considered whether or not you are harming yourself when you take your morning shower and wash your hair? Is the anti-perspirant you use safe? Is your moisturiser potentially harmful?

According to several sources, including Professor Samuel Epstein, founder of the Cancer Prevention Coalition, and author of the Safe Shoppers' Bible, we could be harming ourselves when using many of the everyday products in our home. Philip Day, author of 'Cancer – Why we are still dying to know the truth', agrees with Professor Epstein.

Is Fluoride safe? Check it out before buying Fluoride toothpaste, so that you are making an informed choice. Does your toothpaste carry a child health warning? Is this because of Sodium Lauryl Sulphate? Is it true that Sodium Lauryl Sulphate and Sodium Laureth Sulphate are potentially harmful? Check these out before buying bath and hair cleaners that contain them. Be sure you know the origins of these chemicals. Some are used as engine degreasers and their use in other areas carries a health warning and says to avoid contact with skin.

Is there any Propylene Glycol in the moisturiser you buy? Check out what this may do to the body. Would you knowingly buy a product that contained potentially harmful ingredients? Would you bath your child in these products?

The following ingredients are all claimed by some experts to be potentially harmful.

Potentially harmful ingredients

There are many potentially harmful ingredients including: alcohol, alpha hydroxy acid, aluminium, animal fat (tallow), bentonite, collagen, dioxins, elastin of high molecular weight, fluorocarbons, formaldehyde, glycerin, kaolin, lanolin, lye, mineral oil, petrolatum, and talcum powder.

The three most commonly used are –

PROPYLENE GLYCOL present in many moisturisers and nappy wipes. A cosmetic form of mineral oil found in automatic brake and hydraulic fluid and industrial antifreeze. In skin and hair products, propylene glycol works as a humecent, which is a substance that retains the moisture content of skin or cosmetic products by preventing the escape of moisture or water.

Material Safety Data Sheets (MSDS) warn users to avoid skin contact with propylene glycol as this strong skin irritant can cause liver abnormalities and kidney damage.

SODIUM LAURYL SULPHATE (SLS) present in many shampoos and toothpastes. Harsh detergents and wetting agents used in garage floor cleaners, engine degreasers and auto cleaning products. SLS is well known in the scientific community as a common skin irritant. It is rapidly absorbed and retained in the eyes, brain, heart and liver, which may result in harmful long-term effects.

SLS could retard healing, cause cataracts in adults and prevent children's eyes from developing properly.

SODIUM LAURETH SULPHATE (SLES) present in many shampoos. SLES is the alcohol form (ethoxylated) of SLS. It is slightly less irritating than SLS, but may cause more drying.

Both SLS and SLES may cause potentially carcinogenic formations of nitrates and dioxins to form in the shampoos and cleansers by reacting with other ingredients. Large amounts of nitrates may enter the blood system from just one shampooing.

While the debate goes on about their safety perhaps you may want to find out as much as possible from unbiased sources and make your own decisions from informed choice rather than from ignorance.

There are one or two companies who are now committed to leaving out the potentially harmful ingredients, you may wish to shop with them.

Care about what you wear

Some 8,000 chemicals are used in the modern textile industry. Most of the waste from these chemicals ends up in our rivers, many are highly toxic and harmful to the environment. Organic wool minimises the use of chemicals.

At present there are no UK Organic Standards for organic wool. However, the Soil Association, the regulatory body governing organic produce, is currently working to produce a set of rules covering all aspects of organic textiles.

Not only must the wool be from organic sheep, but the system used for processing the wool, from fleece to finished garment, must also be carried out along organic lines. Organic processing aims to minimise the impact of chemicals on both human health and the environment.

Many shops now offer clothing made from organically produced materials, from nappies to designer outfits.

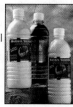

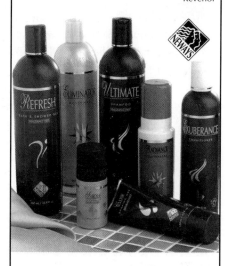

Personal Development

By Richard Morgan

Society in the 21st century is passionate about its health, and staying healthy. Yet with today's pace of life, and the need to combine our family and personal lives with our professional commitments, its vital that we adopt an individual, contemporary approach to caring for ourselves, caring for our health.

The dawning of a new century has brought with it a consensus about how we can best nurture our well-being. There have emerged two clear approaches – one based on modern scientific methodology, and the other on knowledge and wisdom rooted in ancient times.

The truth is, that for all of us, staying healthy is about making the right lifestyle choices. With medical healthiness as its bedrock, Lifestyle Management is a process, which recognises and celebrates the ingredients that make up our lifestyle, restoring or discovering as appropriate.

It embraces a Whole Health approach – connecting our emotional and spiritual side, whilst satisfying our physical and medical needs. In short, a personal and professional health check.

What's involved

The process begins with a refreshing analysis of your health and well-being. We harness energy and fun in developing new ways of thinking about our circumstances. You will work with a Lifestyle Management Practitioner, on a one-to-one basis. The initial consultation is focused on talking about individual needs, and what you want to achieve in becoming involved in the process.

Embracing the Whole Health approach the process will then, where appropriate, incorporate medical treatment. This can either be as part of the consultative process, or embarked upon separately. For example, combined with Reflexology we treat the whole body. The mind benefits with a lessening of tension and the body's digestive system is boosted. It is also ideal treatment to tackle feelings of stress and fatigue.

How long do I stay involved with the process?

There are no rules here! Some people seek a consultation for dealing with a particular issue or situation. Still others value the opportunity of having someone not directly involved with their lives providing an input, integrating the process into their schedules on a weekly, or monthly basis. Consultations can be in person, or once the key topics have been outlined, many people conduct some sessions telephonically or electronically. On major matters though, there is no substitute for human interaction and discussion.

MARIE HERBERT
AUTHOR, SOUND HEALER,
PSYCHOSYNTHESIS GUIDE, OFFERS SACRED
QUESTS, RITES OF PASSAGE & SOUND
WORKSHOPS FOR ALL AGES

Address:
**Rowan Cottage, Catlodge, Laggan,
Inverness-shire PH20 1AH**
Telephone:
01528 544396
e-mail:
healingqst@aol.com

The benefits

The energy of the process is particularly suited to dealing with prevention as opposed to cure. You'll further develop a positive and pro-active view in respect of people and situations. You will think less about coping with life, and more about excelling in life's aspects and opportunities. You will feel an enhanced sense of wellbeing, together with greater clarity and direction in life.

Who is it for?

The process is best suited to those individuals who want to achieve more, but would value the assistance of an 'external touchstone'. For busy people who will however commit the necessary time to integrate the process into the lifestyle, and who will act on, and implement the results of the consultations and treatments in their daily lives.

Common Sense Personal Care Ideas
By M Willcocks PhD

STRESS: Sit down with a friend if you can, and talk about a problem. Find out what things in your work or life are causing stress. Even just talking to someone can bring relief from stress. You can you work out better ways of handling stressful things in your life? Perhaps they are not as important as they seem? These things seem bigger than they really are, but it may be possible to work out ways of keeping them to their real size. Learn to find ways of relaxing and thinking of other things

WORK TIPS: Learn to make priorities (i.e. to put the most important things first) How? At the beginning of the day, write down everything you plan to do that day, on a piece of paper, a 'To Do' list. List jobs according to importance – A must be done today; B can be left until tomorrow; C can be left for some days; D is it really necessary? Then carry out the tasks according to your list of importance, with A tasks being done immediately. At the end of the day, don't worry about things that have not been done. Write them down on the list for the next day, perhaps giving them a different priority. Then forget them till the next day! This little idea is so effective that many businesses pay big money to consultants who suggest exactly this approach to improving efficiency!

Remember you are not perfect – you will always make mistakes. Learn to say 'no' politely to extra work. Always take time for a proper meal break. Maybe it will help to take a quiet meal break away from everyone else. Don't leave things till the last minute. Allow spare time for travel, for appointments, for the unexpected.

Don't drive yourself hard all the time. Everyone has a breaking point. Recognise where yours is. If it is less than for other people in your place of work, don't worry. You can only do your own best.

Learn to relax at home – do things you enjoy. Take time out to do other relaxing things or hobbies. Take days off, and go somewhere completely different.

Get plenty of exercise – our bodies are made to be used. If your job keeps you always sitting in one place you must get your blood circulating another way! And eat a good balanced mixture of healthy food, with plenty of fruit, fibre, and green vegetables.

Get involved in helping other people – this always brings our own problems down to their proper size. You cannot change some things! Learning to live with, and get on top of, struggles, is what helps us to grow and mature.

Physiotherapy

By Darren Higgins, the Vanburgh Physiotherapy Clinic

Physiotherapy has been around for over 100 years yet there are many people today that are still unsure as to what physiotherapists do and why we need them.

Physiotherapy is the science of rehabilitation and treatment that aims to return people to their optimum health and fitness after illness or injury. Physiotherapists treat many people suffering with painful backs and necks as well as those that suffer from arthritis and other joint problems.

Physiotherapists also work with sporting athletes both amateur and professional providing treatment and rehabilitation programs after injury.

Most professional and semi-professional sporting teams will have their own physiotherapist. The British Olympic Team took a team of physiotherapists with them to the Sydney games to look after the athletes.

But you don't have to be an athlete or even participate in sport to need a physiotherapist. Many people today suffer from work related injuries and muscular pain and these problems are expertly managed by Chartered Physiotherapists.

Back and neck pain is the largest single problem facing society today. It causes severe disability for thousands of people, and prevents many from working and living active healthy lives.

Physiotherapy is at the forefront of management for back pain. Much research is being done by physiotherapists looking at better ways of treating sufferers as well as looking at ways of preventing back pain from recurring.

The name given to physiotherapists specialising in the treatment and management of problems with the body's joints and muscles is musculo-skeletal physiotherapist. These physiotherapist work both in the NHS and in private practice.

If you have been in hospital for an operation, then you may have been treated by a physiotherapist. Following surgery, especially orthopaedic surgery (where joints and fractures are fixed by a surgeon), then physiotherapy is vital to assist you in strengthening the muscles affected by the surgery.

Often with leg and hip surgery, it is the physiotherapist who will rehabilitate you so that you can walk, run and fully function as soon as possible. Physiotherapy also involves the rehabilitation of other medical and neurological problems including strokes, open heart and lung surgery, as well as looking after people with chronic lung diseases, teaching them how to manage their problem, exercise safely and how to breathe effectively.

Physiotherapists also work with children of all ages: we forget that children can have the same problems that adults do. Some physiotherapist train specially to look after children who have physical disabilities from birth or who develop problems as a result of a disease or accident.

When do we need physiotherapy?

For the most part the human body has an innate power of healing itself, but sometimes there are muscle and joint problems – back pain, neck pain, arthritic pain or sporting injury – which doesn't respond or the pain is so severe that we cannot function.

That is the time to seek assessment and treatment from a physiotherapist. Very often the physiotherapist is better able to diagnose a musculo-skeletal injury or problem far better than your local GP – that is because the physiotherapist has had four years intensive training specifically in this field.

That is not to say that your GP is not important. Physiotherapists and GPs work together to provide the optimum management for your problem. If necessary, a referral can be made for you to see a consultant, but for the far majority of people, a visit to their physiotherapist is the best solution.

To see a physiotherapist privately, you don't need a doctor's referral. The most important thing when looking for a physiotherapist, is that you seek out a Chartered Physiotherapist – they will have the initials MCSP SRP after their name.

This is the public's guarantee that the physiotherapist has been properly trained and is fully qualified to look after you. If these initials are not displayed after the name, then they are NOT a qualified physiotherapist.

Some therapists claim to be physiotherapists but in fact do not hold the correct qualifications.

If you are unsure, then you should contact the Chartered Society of Physiotherapy, Bedford Row, London. They will be able to assist you.

Remember that the early diagnosis and treatment of any problem, whether it be medical, or to do with the muscles and joints in your body, is the best way of ensuring that the correct management occurs. Physiotherapists are best placed to help with any musculo-skeletal problem you may have.

Physiotherapy – getting into shape

By M Willcocks PhD

Physiotherapists can help you achieve your highest level of physical functioning (at any stage in life) by providing you with a personalised treatment plan based on your specific needs.

Listed below are some general tips to keep you fit and physically healthy. Remember, though, if you are experiencing severe mobility and functioning problems, you should see a physiotherapist for a personalised assessment and treatment plan.

Remember, after extensive immobility or just simply limited activity, you aren't what you used to be. A physiotherapist can give you guidelines for a graduated exercise program to have you climbing those mountains again.

Be fit to sit! There is no one chair which suits everyone. You should try to adjust your sitting position to the one that suits you best. For safe digging in your garden, don't stoop. When lifting or shovelling, take the strain with your legs rather than you back.

Desk-bound jobs and increasingly sedentary lifestyles put a strain on our health in general - but especially on our backs and necks. In fact, back and neck pain is thought to be one of the most common causes of illness in all types of work.

The following simple adjustments to the way you sit at your computer could help take at least some of the pain out of working and will help you to stay fresh and focussed.

Use a chair with a proper backrest as this reduces pressure on the lower back. A portable lumbar support can be used on chairs with poor back support, and chairs with armrests help by supporting the weight of your arms.

Make sure your computer is at the right height - you shouldn't need to lean towards or away from your screen. A correct desk/seat height allows your arms to rest lightly on the desks surface, with the keyboard a comfortable distance away, and about 60cm between your screen (which should ideally be at eye level) and your eyes.

Adjust your position to make the most of lighting arrangements, especially if you find that you hunch over and peer at papers. Move the items you need most frequently within easy reach. Input materials should be at eye level so that you don't have to bend your neck over your work.

Rest your feet flat on the floor or use a foot support to prevent the weight of the lower legs being supported by the front of the thighs. Don't cross your legs or have your thighs pressing against your chair seat too firmly, as this puts pressure on the veins situated on the underside of your thighs.

Get up and walk round as often as possible - try setting an alarm or reminder function to help you remember. Anyone who enjoys sport will at some time suffer from aches and pains. Sometimes these small injuries recover naturally, but often we just learn to live with them...which can lead to more serious problems.

Physiotherapy can be extremely beneficial in many cases of back, neck pain and sport injuries, but as always see your Doctor for advice if your pain is new, unusual or relentless, and to find out its cause and discuss possible treatment.

Pilates

By the Pilates Association

The primary goal of the Pilates Method is to enhance functional stability and functional movement throughout the body. The body itself is always treated as an integrated, whole system, instead of a series of independent muscle groups and parts.

Key emphasis is placed on identifying faulty postural and movement patterns, and then correcting these by working with both the skeletal and muscular systems. So often when we exercise we concentrate almost exclusively on the muscular system. What Pilates helps us remember is that muscles only work efficiently and properly when our skeletons and all our joints move freely and smoothly.

All Pilates exercises focus on building functional strength and endurance in 'core' postural muscles to create what Joseph Pilates called a 'girdle of support' for the spine and pelvis. Attention to correct positioning and diaphragmatic breathing are integral components of each exercise. Above all though, clients are encouraged to sharpen their mental focus, and keep their minds on what their bodies are doing. After all, Joe liked to remind people: "It is the mind itself which builds the body."

As clients work on core postural muscles and joints, their bodies begin to change shape and move differently. Their abdominals strengthen and flatten, their lower backs become better supported, and their overall posture improves. Time and again clients tell us they have never felt their abdominals work as hard as they do in a Pilates session. In addition, they begin to integrate what they learn about posture and alignment into other exercise routines, sports activities, and even daily activities like driving and sitting at a computer. People often comment that they look and feel longer, leaner, and more graceful. Many even say they feel taller!

When I see Pilates Advertised, I always see expensive machines. Can I learn to do Pilates without machines?

The short answer is yes. Originally Joseph Pilates developed some elaborate machines for special needs situations. Today, most people associate Pilates with one of those machines, The Universal Reformer. There is also an extensive repertoire of Pilates exercises designed to be done on a mat on the floor. It is the mat-work above all that has proved the most versatile for large numbers of people. It requires only a mat, a small towel, and a stretchy rubber band. This way, Pilates is always portable, practical, and affordable for everyone.

Because the Pilates Method emphasises functional stability and functional movement, virtually everyone can benefit from it. It is ideal for three specific types of conditioning needs:

Postural correction and rehabilitation

Freedom of movement helps to reduce pain, tension and strain. The key here is emphasis on simple and safe techniques. People with chronic back pain, neck and shoulder tension, repetitive strain injuries, fibromyalgia, MVAs, Multiple Sclerosis, osteoarthritis and rheumatoid arthritis, scoliosis, and osteoporosis to name a few, have all found our Pilates-based programs beneficial.

The main reason for this is that there is no impact, so there is little or no stain on your joints. A lot of time is spent increasing joint mobility, breathing capacity, and body awareness. In addition, exercises are executed in a variety of positions including sitting, standing, and lying on a mat, which all simulate typical positions of daily life, that can often be problematic and painful. Clients learn exercises in all of these positions that help them increase movement and support in their spine and pelvis so they can reduce pain, and prevent future flare-ups and recurring injuries.

Core conditioning

Pilates helps build strong, lean muscles from the inside out. For the general public the Pilates Method offers a refreshing change to more traditional types of exercise.

In a nutshell, Pilates teaches you to access muscles and move bones in new ways so that you get the maximal benefits out of an exercise session. Emphasis on the trunk, and creating functional strength throughout the torso keep people flocking to Pilates. One of the benefits people notice first is newfound strength and definition in those hard to target abdominal muscles. What keeps people hooked is the continuous learning they do as they gain awareness about their bodies and how they move. People find they feel 'different' after a single Pilates session – some even say they feel taller.

Performance enhancement

Tight muscles cannot feel. Athletes and dancers use Pilates consistently to help them stay in peak performance condition. The attention to muscle balance and effective range of motion training makes Pilates an obvious choice for all serious athletes because it helps the muscular and skeletal systems function at optimal levels.

An integral component of performance enhancement is fine-tuning of our kinesthetic awareness, or in lay terms – our body awareness both internally and externally in relation to the environment around us.

The quality of a movement is emphasised rather than the quantity, as well as attention to what and how you are executing a particular movement. Pilates for performance enhancement encourages us to use our muscular and skeletal systems more effectively so that we move freely and powerfully, without strain or risk of injury.

Is Pilates good for cardiovascular conditioning?

Pilates conditions your muscular and skeletal systems. It does not condition your heart directly so it is not cardiovascular by definition. What Pilates really helps you do is prepare your body so that you are better able to meet the demands of cardiovascular activities. Pilates is an excellent way to strengthen and stretch muscles throughout your body. It also teaches you to move your bones efficiently so that you can reduce your chances of joint pain and strain while you do your favourite activities.

Before starting any conditioning programme it is important to check with your health care professional. Luckily though, Pilates can be modified for almost any level of ability. There's no impact so it is easy on joints. The priority at all times is to ensure the integrity of the spine.

Emphasis on functional movement and functional stability means that individuals work at their own pace and always within a comfortable range.

PILATES

LEIGHTON BUZZARD centre for Osteopathy, Physiotherapy and Clinical Pilates. Tel: 01525 211444 for information and appointments. We aim to provide the most affordable and effective treatment possible

Body Control Pilates

With Lynne Robinson

Body Control Pilates is a body conditioning system that works in a different way to other fitness techniques. Targeting the deep postural muscles, Pilates works by building strength from the inside out, rebalancing the body and bringing it into correct alignment.

The Body Control Pilates movements figurehead, Lynne Robinson, explains: "Essentially, Body Control Pilates is a body conditioning method which offers both mental, and physical training. By improving focus and body awareness you learn how to release unnecessary tension and how to align your body correctly, with the pelvis, spine and joints all in their natural 'neutral' settings.

"The next step is to learn how to breathe more efficiently, breathing into your sides and back, expanding the lower ribcage; we call this lateral thoracic breathing. You are then taught how to engage the postural muscles which stabilise the lumbar spine in particular, the pelvic floor muscles, tranversus abdominis, and a deep back muscle called multifidus.

"Once you have mastered stabilising the lumbar spine, you need to learn how to stabilise the shoulder blades, ensuring good upper body use. Relaxed, aligned, breathing correctly and with the stabilising muscles working to create a 'girdle of strength' around the trunk, you can then add movement, simple movements at first but becoming increasingly challenging as co-ordination skills develop. Lightweights may then be used or resistance added with the use of specially designed studio equipment," says Lynne.

The beginning of 2001 will see Body Control Pilates on packets of a well-known breakfast cereal. This is wonderful as it will bring Pilates to the attention of yet more new people.

Meanwhile Pilates is being integrated into all sorts of areas, with the support of leading physiotherapists, chiropractors and osteopaths. Top athletes from many sports have taken notice. Pat Cash (tennis) and Michael Atherton (cricket) helped to show what could be done in terms of recovery from long term injury, and there are approaches from the authorities from various sports asking for advice. This has included the England and Wales Cricket Board and the Football Association.

Lynne has recommended that Body Control is used with young athletes. In this way correct postural and exercise patterns can be established before any persistent injury problems occur. Prevention has to be the better long term solution. With this in mind the Body Control Pilates Group been working regularly with the England cricket teams for the last year, right down to the under 16 age group. Other sports, such as tennis and soccer are showing interest in a similar approach for use in the future."

Meanwhile interest in Pilates continues to spread dramatically, both here, in the United States, and in other parts of the world.

The first Body Control Pilates book is available in six languages worldwide. You may well have noticed Pilates classes appearing at your local gym or leisure centre. Body Control Pilates is bridging a gap between natural health care and the maintenance of fitness, as well as prevention of injury.

Lynne believes that we all need a mix of activities to provide the ideal balance between strength and flexibility, stamina and cardiovascular strength. Before you start it is advisable to seek advice from a Pilates practitioner to be sure that you are doing the right things?

Balanced workouts can re-educate, realign and reshape you. The basic principles of Pilates are applied to a range of activities including mat exercises and popular gym machines.

Some of the alterations you will be encouraged to make to your technique and fitness programme are subtle and may seem minor, but they can help to provide profound and lasting results. This is the whole point of Pilates, to provide a long-lasting state of balanced health. It is applicable to many areas of our lives.

Body Control Pilates exercises are suitable for everyone – irrespective of age and levels of fitness. What I am finding now is that interest is coming from so many different areas. I can see that Pilates will be linked to other areas, such as nutrition and beauty, in the near future.

The correct alignment restored by Body Control Pilates allows natural, normal movement. The body can then function more efficiently resulting in general benefits for overall health and appearance.

So it seems that the future for Body Control Pilates is bright. As holistic approaches to health care and natural living become more and more popular, so the principles of Pilates are being seen as an integral part of the way we can choose to live.

An ideal case study of the difference Pilates can make is that of Lynne Robinson herself: She says: "I attended my first Pilates class whilst I was living in Australia, and, quite simply, it turned my world upside down!

"I had been suffering from chronic back and neck problems for five years, the result of lack of exercise, two large babies, stress and terrible posture. I had given up hope of resuming normal life. In my heart I knew exercise held the key to restoring my health and yet aerobics and gym work were far too strenuous; even gentle yoga aggravated my problems. And then I discovered Pilates… Within ten minutes of my first class I thought to myself, 'Where has this been all my life?' My second thought was 'Why have I never heard of Pilates before, everyone should know about it?'

"What I loved about it most was that not only could I do the exercises without pain but that I instantly felt differently about my body.

"Joseph Pilates had promised that 'in ten sessions you'll feel the difference, in 20 you'll see the difference and in 30 you'll have a new body.' Almost instantly, I found that I was so much more aware of my posture, my breathing and also the deep abdominal muscles which I needed to support my spine.

"The regular tension headaches I had suffered with for years disappeared, as did the chronic pain in my back. I felt a new woman at 35! It wasn't long before friends started to notice the difference.

"Delighted with the newfound strength in my abdominals and back, the cosmetic benefits a flatter stomach; trimmer thighs and toned buttocks were side effects I certainly welcomed. Now, at 45, I've a better figure than I had at 25!

"I first worked in the Body Control system because I found the classical Pilates movements difficult. My background was in teaching (History and Religious Education) and I wanted to be able to teach and help others to access the amazing benefits of Pilates.

"This was where the Body Control emphasis started for me. I suppose I have carried on my original career path, but in a different direction!

"By bringing together body and mind and by heightening body awareness, Body Control Pilates literally teaches you to be in control of your body, allowing you to handle stress more effectively and achieve relaxation more easily. I certainly wish I had known how to do this when I was a secondary school teacher.

"Now I find myself working with a fantastic team of leading physiotherapists to run weekend Pilates workshops in hospitals across the country and to give presentations at medical and specialist conferences, such as those run by the Society of Orthopaedic Medicine and the British Institute of Musculoskeletal Medicine.

"I often have reminded myself that I was once one of their typical 'case' patients."

PILATES

LOUISE STEARN North Glasgow, Scotland. Body Control Pilates Tutor. Matwork. Classes and Private Tuition available. Tel: 01360 860050.

MRS K BOYLE, 72 Dells Lane, Biggleswade, Bedfordshire, SG18 8HN. 01767 312582

MS C EALES, The Willow House, 25 New Road, Little Kingshill, Buckinghamshire, HP16 0EZ. 01494 890111

THE PURE PILATES Studio, 25 New Street, Torrington, Devon, EX38 8BN. 01805 625025

MS L HATCH, Heron Stone Barn, Cockshutt, Ellesmere, Shropshire, SY12 0JL. 01939 270804

PILATES

MISS K LOCHER, 56 Vicarage Lane, Kings Langley, Hertfordshire, WD4 9HR. 01923 400454

MRS P BURNETT, Nottinghamshire. philippa@pilates.fsbusiness.co.uk 01636 673931

BRIGID MCCARTHY Pilates Studio, 16 Canning Street, Edingburgh, West Lothian, EH3 8EG. 0131 221 1131

EDINGBURGH PILATES CENTRE, 45a George Street, Edingburgh, West Lothian, EH2 2HT. 0131 226 1815

Polarity Therapy
By Liz Welch

There is much talk of energy these days, but how can we say what energy is? When we are tired or stressed we say that we are 'low in energy', and if we are enjoying ourselves or relaxing we frequently feel energised.

We know that it is electrical energy that we depend upon for heat and light as well as running all our modern appliances, and the energy from burning petrol drives our cars. In our bodies we also obtain energy by slowly 'burning' the food we eat. It is true to say that energy is always needed for movement and activity. If we go a little deeper, we learn that Albert Einstein discovered that everything in the universe, including our own bodies, is actually made of tiny bundles of energy, known as elementary particles, which are in continuous vibration and motion.

It could also be said that thoughts, creative ideas and emotions are expressed as movement of energy in the physical body, as seen for example in the flow of electrical impulses in the brain, and the movement of hormones or chemical messengers throughout the body. So we can think of all these layers in a living human being as connected and working together as one thing. Dr. Randolph Stone, 1890-1973, the founder of Polarity Therapy, spent 50 years researching how the energy in our bodies flows and how a blockage in that flow can result in physical, emotional or mental problems. He said: "Disease is not an entity, nor a fixed thing. It is nothing but a blockage of the currents of life in their flow and pattern circuits. All pain is but an obstruction to this energy flow. A cure constitutes reaching the life currents within and re-establishing a free flow... Anything short of this is but a relief measure."

Why 'Polarity' Therapy?

Dr. Stone realised that the energy flow in the human body works in a similar way to what happens in a magnet. A magnet has a North Pole and South Pole and an energy field, which extends around it. On every level of organisation the idea of opposite poles is found in the body. This works for example as a simple structural balance between the left and right sides of the body, or the sensory and motor aspects of the nervous system, or the flow of blood away from and towards the heart.

There are also subtler flows of energy of which we are generally less aware. Dr. Stone has described these patterns in some detail, in terms of positive, negative and neutral poles. Energy flows between these poles until a neutral balance is found. Ideally everything would be in balance, but of course this is seldom the case.

How does Polarity Therapy work?

A Polarity Therapist uses a number of different ways of helping a person to balance their energy. Firstly there is a system of hands on bodywork where the therapist uses a variety of different kinds of touch. This could involve applying a gentle pressure to points on the body in a similar manner to reflexology or acupressure, working gently to release tension in muscles or joints, the more subtle touch of cranio-sacral work, or even working off the body with the person's energy field. Contact is always made with respect and regard for what the person needs at that moment. The therapist may teach the person some of Dr. Stone's special energy postures and movements, which are known as

Polarity Yoga. These can be used at home to continue the work begun in the session. If appropriate, the therapist may suggest ways of modifying the diet to aid energy flow. This could include the use of special cleansing diets to help detoxify the body. The therapist may also help the person to look at patterns of thinking and lifestyle which may be affecting their health and well being. In this respect it is helpful if the person receiving treatment is prepared to work for positive change in themselves and in their life generally. If a person comes with a particular complaint the therapist will tend to work with their whole system and not simply the affected part. They may work to correct imbalances in the different qualities of energy known as the five elements.

These are earth, water, fire, air and ether. For instance, if you have a problem in your colon this is likely to relate mainly to the earth and air elements, whereas if you are suffering from depression it may be helpful to encourage your fire energy to flow better. There are no rules to this as we are all unique, and the skill of the therapist is in tuning in to each client and following what needs to happen for them.

Why Polarity Therapy?

By M Willcocks PhD

You appear well but feel in yourself that something is not quite right; perhaps a feeling of being out of balance. Alternatively, you may have physical symptoms that need attention. If you decide on Polarity Therapy, a case history will be taken at the first session, followed by appropriate treatment. Where appropriate, the therapist will liaise with your doctor. A trained Polarity Therapist can incorporate any of the following aspects:

BODYWORK: The therapist uses a series of subtle and/or deep qualities of touch which allows the client's energy system to seek balance through facilitating previously unconscious tissue memory to surface. This process can be relaxing and restorative; it can also allow emotional and personal issues to surface and become clearer.

AWARENESS/PROCESS SKILLS: A Polarity Therapist will allow the client's own inherent 'knowing' to emerge in its own time, by building a secure therapeutic relationship. This increased awareness, together with the release of unconscious tissue memory, enables us to realise our own potential.

HEALTH BUILDING AND/OR CLEANSING DIETS AND PROCEDURES: These can be used to help detoxify the system. This in turn will free up the held life giving energy. Each person is assessed individually, as no one procedure is correct for everyone.

POLARITY STRETCHING EXERCISES: these not only release stagnation, but also allow the client to continue and maintain their own healing process.

Case history

'I found Polarity to be a gentle, relaxing therapy. An initial in-depth questionnaire provided information on all aspects of my life, birth, diet, mental and physical.

"One positive response for me was the eradication of lower back aching which I've experienced for some time. Most memorable was stretching out of my little toes, neck and head. I really did feel longer! During the treatment I had some memories raised from the past on which I reflected and then let them pass. This could mean some unfinished business to deal with, in my own time, when I want to. You may experience various reactions during and following your session. It is reassuring to have a treatment that deals with both mental, physical, diet and lifestyle in a practical way."

Pranic Healing

By Sally Humby & Caroline Nelson

Pranic healing is a revolutionary and comprehensive system of natural healing techniques, which utilises prana to treat various illnesses. Prana is a Sanskrit word literally meaning 'life-force', the invisible bio-energy or vital energy that keeps the body alive and maintains a good sense of health.

The Japanese call this subtle energy 'ki' and the Chinese 'Chi'. As an art and science, Pranic Healing was widely practiced in the ancient civilisations of China, Egypt and India. Pranic Healing enables you to:

• Improve your physical, emotional, mental and spiritual well-being

• Learn about subtle energies and their connection to health

• Feel and see energy fields, auras and chakras – and analyse their condition

• Brighten your aura, strengthen your energy, immune system and healing power

• Awaken your intuition, clarity and clairvoyance

No previous experience is necessary, although if you are a medical practitioner, therapist or nursing professional you can systematically improve your analytical skills, reduce side effects of many allopathic therapies and drugs, and improve almost any other form of therapy you practice. Using a scientific non touch methodology, Pranic Healing utilises prana to initiate specific biochemical changes to accelerate the body's innate ability to prevent, alleviate and heal a whole spectrum of physical, emotional and mental ailments.

Physical touch is not necessary because the practitioner applies Pranic Healing on the energy body rather than the physical body. Scientific experiments conducted by the eminent Russian scientist Semyon Kirlian using ultra sensitive photographic process, showed a colourful radiant energy field surrounding the physical bodies of humans, animals and plants.

This energy field (or aura) interpenetrates the visible physical body, extending about four to five inches from the surface of the skin. These experiments have also revealed that diseased energies appear first in the energy body before manifesting as a physical ailment. In Pranic Healing wellness is effected by the trained practitioner by removing the congested or diseased energy from the patient's invisible energy body and then by transmitting fresh vital prana to the effected areas.

What ailments can be treated?

Simple disorders such as headaches, coughs, fevers, stomach aches, menstrual pain, muscle pain, sprains and minor burns; emotional and mental disorders like stress, tension, anxiety and depression, phobias, schizophrenia and other related ailments; severe conditions like tuberculosis, hypertension, heart problems, arthritis, cancer, epilepsy and ME. Pranic healing is not intended to replace modern medicine. However this ancient healing methodology can complement conventional medical practices as well as alternative healing methods.

Its founder, Master Choa Kok Sui, is a Chinese Filipino scientist, educator and philanthropist. His teachings are the distillation of over 25 years of study and research. His work is published in five books and in more than 20 languages. He founded the Institute of Inner Studies and the World Pranic Healing Foundation to spread his profound teachings across the globe. Pranic Healing is taught in hundreds of schools and centres, to health professionals and laymen alike. The Trainer, Rainer Krell, is a research scientist and direct student of Master Choa Kok Sui. As a biologist he has been experimenting for many years with the use of subtle energies in agriculture, bee keeping, ecology and human health.

Case histories

Eight years ago I was diagnosed with a platelet disorder, hypercoagulable state, which left me legally blind in my left eye from a central retinal vein occlusion. I was placed on many different medications ranging from blood thinners, steroids and blood pressure sedatives and had nine laser and cryonics surgeries on my eye.

Two and a half months ago, after receiving Pranic Healing, not only could I see clearly out of my left eye but there was no indication of a blood clotting disorder and my bleeding was normal. I have been off all medication for almost three months. I am still seeing clearly out of my left eye and I feel normal for the first time in years. Now I, too, can have a future free of pain and confusion and hardship.

Barbara, Northumbria

After a fall in a car park the pain in my knees for over a year was constant. I was unable to bend, squat or kneel without intense pain. I was unable to walk up or down stairs without pain as well. After my Pranic Healing, all of these symptoms disappeared. Miraculously, in less than 30 minutes, I was released from my pain. I had been under a doctor's care before with the usual treatment of motrin and cortisone. The doctor said it was permanent and was as cured as was possible by Western medicine. Now I am pain free, and I walked up and down a flight of stairs without any negative effect!.

Burt, Nottingham

I have had MS since my early 20s. I am now 53. I have been seeing a Pranic Healer for 3½ years and in this time Pranic Healing has enabled me to control my bladder without the use of drugs. My headaches have virtually disappeared and the numbness and tingling leaves after a session. When I have had a relapse, with the full blown symptoms, Pranic Healing has cleared it immediately and I have been able to return to remission. A recent MRI was clear of any new lesions. I believe with all my heart that Pranic Healing has kept the MS in remission."

John, Plymouth

Preconceptual Care

By Belinda Barnes

People have been having children for a very long time – it is a truism that has been pointed out to me! Surely, they imply, we don't need all this fuss? Indeed, Foresight, the Association for the Promotion of Preconceptual Care, might be thought to be making a meal of the whole thing.

But, in preparing people for pregnancy, we try to eliminate factors known to inhibit conception or cause damage to the baby in the womb. We feel, as do parents who come to us, that this is fairer to the baby.

Pollution, impoverished food grown in exhausted soil, lead and copper in the water, smoking, alcohol, street drugs, hazardous food additives, mercury from dental repairs, – the list could go on. You name it, it's out there, and it has foeto-toxic potential. It is no coincidence that, as the level of dubious substances in the environment has risen, so the level of infertility, miscarriage, malformations, premature birth and chronic child ill health has risen commensurately.

It is said that asthma afflicts one child in seven, eczema one child in five, and the ubiquitous 'AHDD' – the all-embracing term for hyperactivity/dyslexia/retardation is now being attributed to one child in four. It is harder to have a baby, harder to have a fit baby, and harder to keep him/her fit when you do. So is there something we can do? Yes there is! The Foresight programme comprises nine main facets, although advice and help may not always be confined to these areas.

OPTIMISING DIET: We advise fresh, whole, organically grown foods (no refined carbohydrate) and no artificial additives known to have delatorious side-effects. We have a booklet on these. We produce a wholefood cookbook, with menus and nutritional advice. We advise filtering water, or, if your area is fluoridated, drinking bottled water.

Farming with artificial fertilisers and pesticides can denature and contaminate food, as can some processing methods. The best foods are those grown organically and interfered with as little as possible.

We help partners to stop all smoking, alcohol and street drugs, OTC drugs and to minimise the intake of tea and coffee. This eliminates many of the toxins proven to be harmful to foetal development. We encourage couples to learn Natural Family Planning (NFP) as this eliminates the need for the contraceptive pill, or the copper coil, as both of these

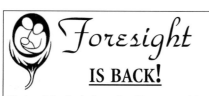

methods tend to raise the body levels of copper. Three minerals particularly crucial for normal foetal development are selenium, manganese and zinc.

We help people to be checked for genito-urinary infection and have found that around 50 per cent of couples with reproductive problems test positive for one or more infections. Few have symptoms but with estrogens released into the blood, infections tend to manifest and sadly terminate the pregnancy. If the baby survives chlamydia, and there is a live birth, the baby may suffer from damage to the eyes or lungs, or may later suffer recurring middle ear infection or gastro-enteritis that is chlamydial in origin. Where prospective parents are on medication for asthma, eczema or migraine, we help them to find a practitioner who understands allergy to see if the condition can be controlled by means other than drugs. Homeopathy may also be useful.

Where irritable bowel syndrome is a problem, we can arrange stool tests to identify any condition such as coeliac disease or intestinal parasites. It is important this is eliminated prior to conception, as the bugs will be competing for nutrients with the baby.

We arrange hair analysis to look for heavy metals – lead, calcium, mercury and/or aluminium, which are dangerous to the foetus – and trace mineral deficiencies. Numerous studies show that deficiencies of vitamins and minerals can cause deformity – spina bifida, cleft palate, talipes, genital anomalies, heart defects, eye defects and so on. Heavy metals can also cause skeletal anomaly and mental retardation.

Hypoglycaemia, or 'swinging' blood sugar is another condition we commonly see, where the pancreas is responding to an overload of sugar, coffee, alcohol, chocolate and white flour. The blood sugar handling mechanism is disrupted by exhaustion and energy levels rise and fall rapidly. This will respond to dietary change, and supplements of chromium and B complex vitamins.

We are studying the role of electro-magnetic pollution in the origins of chromosomal defects. We are also studying strategies for avoidance. Obvious first steps are avoiding eating microwaved food within four minutes of cooking (preferably avoiding it altogether, as so many nutrients are destroyed); turning luminous clocks away from your head at night; turning off electric blankets when you go to bed; avoiding too many hours in front of the VDU etc. For more sophisticated work; pylons, leylines, radar dishes, mobile telephone masts etc. it is worth seeking help from the National Society of Dowsers (01233 750750 x253) at www.dowsers.demon.co.uk.

This is the bare bones of the Foresight programme. We are constantly updating and improving our methods, and recruiting new practitioners to help the ever-growing army of dedicated prospective parents.

At the last count, conducted with the help of Surrey University, of the 367 couples who came to us, 327 conceived within the timescale of the study, and 327 healthy babies were born. The earliest birth was 36 weeks, and this was the lightest baby, born at 5lb 3oz. There were no malformations, and no baby went into a Special Care Baby Unit. Of the 204 couples that came to us with a fertility problem, 175 (86 per cent) gave birth within the timescale of the study.

Practical Psychology

By M Willcocks PhD

The opening stance in any negotiation is meant to build bridges between yourself and your prospect. There are many ways to establish that rapport; you can open the discussion on a neutral subject, allay suspicion, assure that you want to gain mutual agreement.

To negotiate successfully requires that both parties are prepared to give and take, and that both parties have some understanding of the other person.

Communication is never easy. Communicating so that someone else will do what you want – can be very difficult, and often seem impossible. Several events can take place when someone hears your request; the other person thinks to themselves, 'I am important and want to be respected'. Next they silently say 'You must consider MY needs'. Next they ask themselves, as you blurb away, 'How will the ideas of this person help ME?' Getting more rational, and beginning to accept your case, they then ask, ' What are the facts'

It is imperative that you listen at these formative stages.

People

Get to know people involved – have a preliminary chat, perhaps about another subject. Find out something about them, if a lasting relationship is to work it is good to know as much as you can about the other party – their personal life, the progress of their business/ambitions.

Objectives

What are the objectives, what are the priorities, what variables exist and what is your attitude to each of them. Can you afford to lose out on some points, in order to gain advantage elsewhere. It will be a give-and-take process.

Conduct

The tactics of negotiation and the interpersonal behaviour that will take place during the discussions that lead up to closing the 'deal'. Never accept promises, only congratulate performance i.e. when you have got what you want irrevocably signed and sealed.

Negotiating power

Promise a reward – you have something the other side actually needs.

Legitimacy – you know the facts, and your statements are true.

Other variables – knowing a personal friend, using a sympathy vote, insisting on a small detail as being of vital importance.

Confidence

You know what you want, and exude that knowledge.

Steps in Planning Negotiations

Aim High – it is easier to come down from the mountain. Separate out the elements that; You must have to make the 'deal' worthwhile. The ideals, what you would really like to achieve. Once you understand your needs – look carefully at what your prospect will require, they may want to increase their profit, remember profit is not a dirty word, without such incentives business becomes an unworkable sham. Or they may want to emulate your success, there are a million variables. Planning will have identified the concessions you are prepared to make. Concessions must be traded, very reluctantly, never given. Be seen to be driving a hard bargain (albeit sweetly), there will only be a limited number of concessions you can make – make each one count, draw as much out of each point as possible.

When making a concession

Stress the cost/effort to you. Exaggerate – but truthfully. Do not overstate, and provide evidence. Refer to major problems that you will suffer as a result of conceding. Imply that the concession is exceptional – I would never normally do that but ....

When the other party makes a concession

Do not overdo any expression of thanks, a curt acceptance is sufficient. Underplay the concession when it is made – say 'that is a small point, I suppose.' Treat them as expected, not concessions at all. Accept, but imply that it was not really necessary. Deny that the concession has any value. Underplay any offer they make, inflate any concession you are forced into.

Tips to use when negotiating

Keep thinking all the time. Each word is important and keeps looking for the unstated implications. Take time – there is no need to keep talking, silence can be very effective, especially when you have asked a difficult question. Wait and make them answer. Take notes, make any calculations necessary – involve the other party in that process, use it as a time to restate the case. Go through each step, and confirm the progress made. Make sure the prospect is happy to proceed, and feels good about the negotiation.

Build an agreement, do not have a fight. Try and remain neutral – imagine that this 'deal' is not for you, often talking in the third person can help,. contain yourself until everything has been revealed before making that final offer on the 'deal.' Time is rarely important – be flexible – and accommodating, eventually, time is a negotiating variable – and rarely will you find it so important that a final time/deadline cannot be extended. Remember nothing is ever fixed; everything can be changed with negotiation. Your personal behaviour is important – be aware of body language and or of verbal signs. Phrases like 'I do not have the authority' – Your response can be 'Well who does, let me talk to them'.

Make sure your motives are clear – hidden motives will state that you have something to hide. Understand and be sure that you have had a clear answer to any question asked. If it is avoided, sidestepped or ignored you will damage your presentation of fact. Keep calm, summarise the discussion at frequent intervals. This is not the place to consider the complications of negotiation in which you set out to deliberately unbalance the opposition, but that can really be fun.

Closing the negotiation.

Then move on to that crucial closing stage in the game, ' What shall I do?' Finally, you get, 'I approve', and they agree the 'deal', or 'I do not approve' and you have a hill to climb, and you will have to go back over the who scenario, identify the points of disagreement and obtain a 'yes' before moving on to the close once more. You may have to do this several times before you achieve your objective.

Psychoneuroimmunology
By Andina Seers

T he idea that the mind could influence the immune system would have been considered far-fetched even as recently as 20 years ago. The notion that stress exerts its adverse effects upon our health has entered popular culture in an all-pervasive way. Terms like 'stressed out', 'freaked out', 'burned out', 'adrenaline buzz', 'flight-or-fight', testify to the widespread general knowledge that the direct or indirect effects of stress can cause heart attacks, exacerbate pre-existing health complaints, lead to depression or even be a factor in the onset and/or outcome of cancer.

The word Psychoneuroimmunology was coined in the 1980s when different branches of specialist sciences joined each other for the first time.

Three of the main disciplines that came together were:

• **PSYCHO**: of the mind & thinking.

• **NEURO**: of the nerve system.

• **IMMUNOLOGY**: of the body's defence/immune system.

During the final decades of the 20th Century scientists and health practitioners were beginning to come to a greater understanding of the workings of the physical body and so ways of treating health problems and diseases also began to themselves evolve:

1st Stage medical model standard up to the 1950s

Initially it was believed that in order to deal with a disease the best treatment was usually to either remove, radiate or else poison with it chemicals. At this time there simply wasn't the knowledge that who we were as a person effected our body and so disease was seen as an isolated dysfunction.

The phrase 'Magic Bullet' stems from this time, when it was believed that it was possible to simply deal with a physical problem as separate from the person. If only the right bullet was found which would target just the disease, that was all that was needed.

2nd Stage mind & body 1960s-1970s

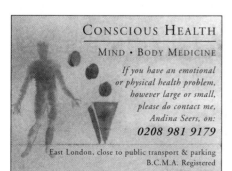

CONSCIOUS HEALTH

MIND • BODY MEDICINE

If you have an emotional or physical health problem, however large or small, please do contact me, Andina Seers, on:

0208 981 9179

East London, close to public transport & parking
B.C.M.A. Registered

However as knowledge about the body increased, there started to develop the realisation that our minds and thinking processes could also be very powerful tools for promoting recovery from disease. So began a greater exploration and utilisation of such methods as guided imagery and bio-feedback Both techniques used the power of the mind to create measurable changes in the body.

At this time there also began to

develop a growing interest in stress management, meditation and 'positive thinking' as ways of both supporting the body to heal and also to prevent disease. The realisation was beginning to dawn that who we were as a person and also our lifestyle had significant implications for our health or lack of it.

3rd Stage mind/body/emotions up to the present day

However 1972 heralded the discovery of the body's own cellular communication system by Professor Candace Pert, USA. This provided the scientific proof that thoughts and emotions were transported round the body by messenger molecules. These messenger molecules were shown to be constantly effecting and altering all our cells, including the immune system's, and so our very thoughts and emotions were implicated in disease.

It was also now beginning to be realised that a health problem was more than just a physical or pattern of thinking issue, our bodies were being actively and continuously changed by not only or thoughts, but by feelings and emotions as well.

At this same time a large amount of information was also coming out of long-term studies on the effects of trauma on Vietnam War Veterans and survivors of the Holocaust. These studies were showing that past emotional trauma became stored as changes in body cells.

The studies also explored and refined ways to release and finally heal this stored up trauma. In terms of health and recovery from disease, it was becoming clearer that it was now at last possible to significantly effect immune system functioning using emotional therapy and that patients could actually actively and effectively participate in their own healing processes.

Whole new ways of working with disease began to be explored, building on from and complementing those that had already been developed in mainstream medicine, and leading to the birth of the Science of Psychoneuroimmunology.

Freaking out!

By M Willcocks PhD

Tables have been compiled scoring stress factors including divorce, moving house, changing jobs – the higher your tally, the more likely it is that you may suffer a major illness. There is now an expanding body of published evidence which documents the biochemical and even molecular level, how and to what extent states of mind such as anxiety, depression and anger affect the functioning of immune cells – T-cells, B-cells, natural killer cells, and macrophages. Hence it would appear that a level of cure may be possible in the not too far distant future.

Support and counselling

It cannot be emphasised enough how important support groups are to cancer patients and their carers and families. Despite the concern of loved ones, and the professional involvement of health care professionals, there is almost a metaphysically therapeutic process in getting together with other cancer patients who are in the same boat to share feelings of anger, despair, grief, depression, hope, love. There is so much fear and unspoken terror surrounding cancer. Patients who participate and share with other their honest feelings as part of such support groups actually live longer.

Qigong and Hua Gong

By Dario Gerchi

Everybody wants mental peace, physical relaxation, balanced and harmonious energy, and good health in their life. It can be frustrating, however, to find that we do not always know how to achieve these qualities. Even when we do know the way, we may still find that we cannot follow it properly.

Qigong/Hua Gong provides an invaluable way for us to realise these desirable qualities. The art of Qigong originated in China several thousand years ago. Throughout its history it has been practised by Taoist and Buddhist monks, Confucian scholars, indigenous doctors and Martial Arts practitioners as a source of power, knowledge and wisdom. It embodies the essence of the Chinese civilisation.

Qi is the vital subtle energy that gives us life and connects us to the universe. Gong means the practice of cultivating the Qi. The way of Qigong is to awaken and cultivate the Qi to prevent or conquer illness, to improve physical and mental health, and to realise our inner potential, creativity and inner intelligence.

Hua Gong is the style of Qigong developed by Zhixing and Zhendi Wang and taught by them and their senior students. Hua means transformation, integration and simple body movements. Relaxation, visualisation, breathing techniques, sounds and mantras are the various techniques used in Hua Gong. To integrate Qigong principles into daily life is also an important part of the practice.

It is simple enough for beginners to learn, and profound and sophisticated enough as a lifelong practice.

Benefits of Hua Gong practice

GOOD HEALTH – Prevention is always better than cure. Those who are considered healthy can prevent future illness and improve their health greatly

HEALING EFFECTS – Its healing power is probably the most important reason for the popularity of Qigong. Many people have experienced profound transformation in their lives through their Qigong practice. For example people coming into a class on crutches (because of M.S. or accidents) have been able to walk without them after attending one morning or one weekend with Zhixing Wang.

LONGEVITY – Qigong has been practised for longevity and immortality for centuries. With Hua Gong practice, instead of feeling the aches and pains and weakness as years go by, we can become more supple and energetic. Many students in their 50s and 60s have experienced this rejuvenating effect.

MORE FREEDOM IN LIFE – Our health is more in our own hands with Hua Gong practice. We Learn how to take care of our own health. It becomes possible to recover from illness and to improve our health through our own efforts. We are better able to restore the balance when we occasionally feel unwell. This frees us greatly from the suffering due to illness and old age.

MENTAL CLARITY AND SPIRITUAL REALISATION – By deepening our perception to the subtle level and widening our awareness into the spiritual aspect, our view of life can change fundamentally. Mental clarity and spiritual realisation will become the fruit of our practice.

UNUSUAL ABILITIES – It is possible to develop unusual abilities in healing, arts and spiritual aspects.

Confucius, he say...

By M Willcocks PhD

To many people, Confucius is no more than the set-up to a one-line joke. Few have heard or read any of his teachings. Yet the truth and importance of his words resonate today because Confucius's teachings, although developed in response to the times in China in which he lived, are just as applicable today.

Confucius lived through a time of moral chaos. Common values were being widely rejected or simply disregarded. Crime was on the rise, with robbery and theft increasing in the countryside and murders a serious problem in the cities. There was a general lack of interest in trying to reintegrate criminals into society. The gulf between rich and poor was broad and growing, with the rich living extravagantly in enormous mansions, while the abundance of food somehow failed to reach the hungry who needed it.

Government was routinely corrupt and distrusted by the people, who didn't fail to observe the lack of productivity among the rich and powerful: as the chronicler Shu Xiang noted: "The ministers never go out to work in the field."

The economy was changing as well. The productive class, mostly farmers, was shrinking, while the mercantile sector was growing. The market places were flooded with goods described as being costly and of 'no real utility'. Part of the growing middle class was a sector of scholars, who had great difficulty finding employment.

While reformers such as Confucius existed, they were a minority; society was dominated by pessimists and conservatives. Pessimists, perhaps predecessors of today's millennial survivalists, militiamen and 'patriots', withdrew from society in disillusionment, convinced that the social order was irreparably corrupt and resistant to reform and that the best thing to do was to look after one's own.

Conservatives were either ordinary people wrapped up in their own lives and indifferent to social and political problems, or men of society with good reputations and a vested interest in maintaining the status quo, determined to block social reform and new ideas wherever they popped up. Their private conduct may have been unimpeachable, but in the public sphere they were fierce defenders of an unpleasant system. Sound familiar? That's why Confucianism is still significant.

Radionics

By Linda Fellows

The fundamental proposition of Radionics is that a living body has a subtle, invisible energy field which vitalises it, and that if this energy field is weakened for any reason physical problems may arise.

Exposure to toxic substances and stress are two common causes of malfunction. The aim of Radionic treatment is to keep the subtle energy field in good shape – whether it be that of a human, animal or even a plant.

Practitioners ask for some information about your health problem, a small sample of hair (just to represent the real 'you' – a 'witness') and a signed request for treatment. Equipped with these, they claim to be able to assess what is impeding the flow of your subtle energies. This they do by means of pendulum dowsing, after 'tuning in' to this invisible 'you'. They then aim to restore a healthy distribution of energy in the subtle field by means of an instrument which makes little sense to a conventional physicist – it may just look like a box with dials on the front, and with puzzling circuitry inside.

During treatment, the dials are set to coded numbers which represent states of imbalance in the subtle energies, and also the concepts needed to restore them. Treatment seems to be equally fast and effective wherever the patient is in the world – distance is quite irrelevant. For those of us brought up on the 'common sense' view of the world, Radionics sounds absurd, but dip into its history and you will find, not a long line of gullible amateurs, but hard-headed scientists who were convinced that Radionics was both real and medically useful.

One of the early pioneers was American neurologist Albert Abrams. After his death in 1921 many of his methods were enthusiastically taken up by doctors on both sides of the Atlantic. Originally, the patient was always present, but in the USA, chiropractor Ruth Drown (who is believed to have invented the word Radionics) discovered that she could both analyse and treat at a distance, using a drop of the patient's blood as a 'witness'.

In post-war Britain, engineer George De La Warr and others developed new instruments for analysis and treatment, even inventing a camera for capturing images of diseased tissue at a distance. But the processes involved in Radionics, particularly distant analysis and healing defied 'common sense', and it was ignored by mainstream science despite a growing band of satisfied customers.

By the 1980s the Radionic community was divided between those who strove for a physical explanation of Radionics, and those who had concluded that it was essentially a 'psychic' phenomenon.

One leading figure of the day, David Tansley, said that it was 'magic' and that a scientific explanation would never be found. What Tansley could not have

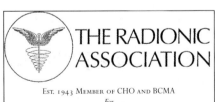

THE RADIONIC ASSOCIATION

Est. 1943 Member of CHO and BCMA
For
Practitioner Register
and
Training Course Details
T/F +44 (0) 1869 338852
radionics@association.freeserve.co.uk
Web: www.radionic.co.uk

foreseen was that the scientific view of the world was about to experience a massive shake-up. The common-sense view of world which we hold dear today is of matter in three dimensional space moving through time: to get to one part of it from another you have to move through space, and the greater the distance the greater the time it takes. The idea of instant communication between different parts of it is impossible, and so the claims of Radionic practitioners to analyse and treat people equally quickly wherever they were in the world was quite unacceptable. But in the last 20 years evidence has accumulated that the familiar time/space world and everything in it emerges from a different level of reality where time and space do not exist.

The revised world view proposes that all matter is born from, and guided from, this subtle, primary reality which neither our physical senses, nor our electronic gadgets which are only an extension of them, can reach.

Radionics practitioners suspect that the disciplined dowsing sense which they employ enables them to reach into this hidden area of nature to get to the programming behind the body and to restore it.

Abrams offered a reward, still available, to anyone who could come up with a machine which would replace a human operator in his system, but so far there have been no takers. It seems that so far only man himself can get behind man. It doesn't matter where in the world patient and practitioner are situated because the connection between them is outside of the space/time framework.

But what does all this mean in practical terms for those with health concerns? It means that in Radionics we seem to have a powerful additional strategy for managing illness.

Satisfied customers contend that radionic techniques, as a supplement to conventional care, are helpful in a wide range of physical and emotional problems, and can often help when conventional strategies have little to offer. They also believe that disturbances in the subtle energies can be detected and dealt with before illness takes hold in the physical body, and have regular checks as a health 'M.O.T'.

One advantage is that those unable to travel can be treated as readily as those who can. Animals respond well to radionic techniques, and 'putting him on the box' is commonplace in equestrian circles. Many people use it to promote the health of garden plants and crops.

There are signs that the mainstream scientific community may at last be ready to look at what Radionics has to offer. In the latest edition of his book, Richard Gerber M.D.* writes: "Radionics is a unique healing modality in that it is a system of diagnosis and treatment geared to more than just the physical body. It may ultimately teach us the most about the nature of healing and human consciousness itself."

We are all unique individuals and need to find the complementary healing strategies which suit us best. With Radionics there is no risk of adverse side effects, and a long history of satisfied customers. Talk to a qualified practitioner about your health concerns – maybe it will help you.

RADIONICS

JOHN TEMPLE BSC, MSc, MRadA, Radionic Practitioner. PO Box 75, Ripon, HG4 1AP. Tel/Fax +44 (0) 176 560 2705 email john@balancingenergies.co.uk

MRS C A STEWART, Charles Cottage, 6 New Road, Brockhampton, Cheltenham, Gloucestershire, GL54 5XQ. 01242 820250

Rebirthing

By Chris Retzler

The core technique of Rebirthing is conscious connected breathing, a continual in-breath and out-breath with no gaps in between. Usually done lying down, it has the effect of energising and activating you emotionally, allowing images and sensations to surface. These may be connected to past events and often feel quite birth-like.

An example would be that of Alan, who in a breathing session felt pressure on his head and face, twisting and turning in response. At the end of the session he recalled how at his birth he had stuck halfway, and a forceps delivery had been performed.

Alan explored how this related to his adult experiences of starting projects, then undergoing a crisis of confidence halfway through and either leaving the project unfinished or relying on others to rescue him. In later sessions, when he considered it further, it also related to his childhood experiences of never getting things right for his mother. The breathing stimulated a birth-like experience that was a graphic symbol of his frustration and 'stuckness't. Such symbols are clues from the unconscious, and because they arise from within, are safe clues to follow – we seem to have an instinct for suggesting to ourselves what we are ready to encounter and to change.

The breathing is the chance to experience feelings in a physical, non-intellectual way. The experience may have been dramatic and revelatory, or just relaxing and constructive in a quieter way. Rebirthing is integrative – that is to say it allows emotional material to arise, be resolved and made part of a new, healthier you. It is the remedy for the human tendency to evade uncomfortable experiences by postponement or suppression.

Alan used Rebirthing to recover feelings about his mother: pain and anger at her for the coldness and disapproval he had experienced from her, and grief for the love he had yearned to receive. Also, he took responsibility for the love he had not expressed. By the end of his sessions he had forgiven both his mother and himself, and had completed a loving letter of reconciliation to her. Perhaps forgiveness is both a component of and a metaphor for therapy – when we forgive someone, essentially we are signalling our willingness to re-establish a relationship with them. Likewise, in therapy we re-encounter the parts of ourselves we have cut off and disowned; and with compassion and a new understanding we welcome them back, making ourselves whole again, allowing ourselves to move forward.

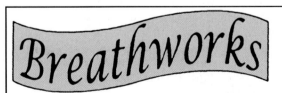

Conscious Connected Breathing

By Gerd Lange of the British Rebirth Society

Rebirthing or Integrated Breathwork is a wonderful tool for self-exploration. It is a simple, gentle yet powerful technique which allows you to access, release and integrate memories, emotions and patterns stored in your body, mind and soul that hinder you to live your full potential, physically, emotionally and mentally.

After discussing your particular needs with your rebirther, the session itself is done sitting up or lying down. Having been guided through a relaxation sequence, you consciously connect your breathing so that there are no pauses between the inhale and the exhale. The breathing is relaxed, yet full. Slowly you will be guided to find your own rhythm, probably slightly faster and fuller than you are used to. Every breathing session has its own cycle which includes an activation phase – 20 to 40 minutes depending on the individual – an expression phase where we work with the material that surfaces and an integration phase. The length of a 'breathe' is generally one to one and a half hours, a full session usually lasts for two hours.

The breath is the bridge between the conscious and the subconscious. You can control your breathing consciously (e.g. pranayama breathing exercises) but if you don't think about your breathing even for the whole day, you still are breathing. Rebirthing works on the principle that there is a direct connection between mental and physical well being and the openness of the breathing. Relaxing and releasing the breath dissolves tension in the body and mind.

Through breathing continuously without break, your body becomes mom oxygenated than usual, which changes the CO_2 level in your brain. You enter a self-induced trance state where memories, pictures or emotions can come up to the surface to be reviewed, released and integrated. The power of rebirthing is that in this state you are the experienced and the observer of a past incident at the same time, and therefore able to release or re-interpret what happened then from a new and conscious angle.

Through conscious connected breathing you accumulate life force, prana, chi, ki, which starts to move freely through your body – experienced as tingling, energy rushes or waves. This loosens up stored blockages held in your four-body energy system, physical, emotional, mental and spiritual, thus working on all four levels at the same time. Therefore possible experiences can be manifold and may vary every time. The spectrum ranges from physical sensations of pain or pleasure to release of emotions (sadness, anger etc.), realisations of dysfunctional thought patterns or new thought connections and insights, and deeply spiritual or energetic experiences.

Rebirthing has an innate self-control mechanism. Your subconscious and your higher self decide what is most appropriate for you to experience right now and how much to release. Whatever will surface might be challenging for you, but is never more than can safely be integrated.

You don't necessarily have to understand or review certain incidents as pictures or thoughts to be able to release the charge around them as the whole process has its own innate intelligence. All you have to do is to trust the breath. It will take you where you need to go, and it will bring up what is most important for you in this moment, to be able to take your next step towards becoming whole and happy.

The rebirther is your guide on the journey. He or she will manoeuvre you through the surfacing material, witness and validate your experiences, help you to stay present and to maintain your mental clarity. To integrate what has come up a skilled rebirther will use various psychotherapeutic integration tools ranging from counselling, family dynamics, the inner child, psychic surgery, past life etc.

The rebirther's most needed qualities, besides being professionally highly trained and experienced, are unconditional personal regard and to be non-judgmental and compassionate.

Together you form a morphogenetic energy field consisting of the rebirther's self-experience and integration plus yourself and your willingness and trust. Therefore it is very important that you feel comfortable with your rebirther. Check out a few till you find the person who feels right for you. Rebirthing with a man will be different from Rebirthing with a woman and will bring up different issues.

Most rebirthers offer a free initial consultation to discuss your particular needs and to find out if you are suited to each other. Cost and length of session may vary widely.

Reflexology

By Simon Duncan, the Association of Reflexologists

Reflexology is an approach to health that emphasises the health care of the whole person, not only on the physical, but also on the emotional, psychological and spiritual levels. It recognises every individual's capacity for self-healing and accepts that disease is often the result of stress, faulty habits, destructive thought patterns and unfavourable social conditions.

Patients are expected to take a responsible, active part in any treatment programme, which may include orthodox medical care using drugs and surgery, a variety of complementary methods and remedies, and instruction in self-help skills.

Reflexology, besides being a therapy in its own right, is ideally suited for use in collaboration with orthodox medicine or other complementary therapies. It is a safe, non-invasive treatment, co-operating with the body's own healing processes to induce a state of balance and well-being. It may also help the body to counteract the side effects of drugs and is very valuable in aiding recovery after illness, operations or fractures.

The history of Reflexology

Treatment of the body by using pressure points on the feet is not new. It was used in China and India over 5,000 years ago, and a wall painting in an ancient Egyptian

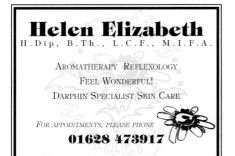
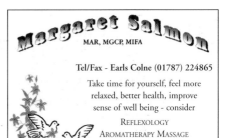

tomb illustrates its usage there in 2350BC. A number of American Indian tribes also used similar methods for treating disease and relieving pain for many centuries.

Whether 'folk medicine' in the West ever used such methods is not recorded though in the 16th Century a number of European doctors published papers describing ways of treating internal organs through the use of pressure points.

The Italian sculptor, Benvenuto Cellini is said to have used pressure on his hands and feet to relieve pain. However, it wasn't until the end of the 19th Century that reflexology was rediscovered and introduced to the western world by an American ear, nose, and throat specialist, Dr. William Fitzgerald.

His main interest was in the use of pressure points on the hands, and to a lesser extent on the feet, to relieve pain and induce anaesthesia in specific areas enabling him to perform minor surgery on his patients without anaesthetics. He used a variety of mechanical devices for stimulating the points including rubber bands and metal combs; and on a number of occasions he publicly demonstrated the effects on his colleagues by pressing points and then sticking pins into the anaesthetised parts!

In 1917 Dr. Fitzgerald and Dr. Bowers jointly published a book called: 'Zone Therapy or Relieving Pain at Home', describing their methods, and presenting a rough map of the internal organs on the soles of the feet. He also coined the term 'reflexology' for the study of the reflexes.

Since then a great deal of research has been carried out and a number of people have made important contributions to the development and acceptability of reflexology.

The study of reflexology was developed by the work of Eunice Ingham Stopfel, an

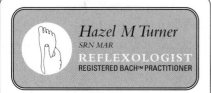
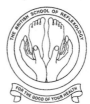

American physiotherapist and follower of Dr. Fitzgerald, who spent many years painstakingly locating the reflexes on the feet, compiling and evolving her own method of 'compression massage'. Doreen Bayley, a student of Eunice Ingham, first brought reflexology to England in 1966 where she established the Bayley School of Reflexology. Reflexology is now available in every town in the UK.

Research into reflexology in many parts of the world is accumulating an impressive tome of evidence of successful treatment in a great variety of circumstances, and is also widening our understanding of its application.

What is Reflexology?

Reflexology is a method of bringing about relaxation, balance and healing through the stimulation of particular points on the feet, or sometimes on the hands. Reflex points on the feet and hands are linked to other areas and organs of the body. Tension or congestion in any part of the foot mirrors tension or congestion in a corresponding part, and treating the whole foot can have a deeply relaxing and healing effect on the whole body.

How does Reflexology work?

The body has the ability to heal itself. Correct stimulation of the reflex points on the feet can have a beneficial effect on the whole body. Following illness, stress, injury or disease, it is in a state of 'imbalance', and vital energy pathways are blocked, preventing the body from functioning properly. Reflexology can be used to restore and maintain the body's natural equilibrium and encourage healing.

Reflexologists use their thumbs and fingers to apply a particular type of pressure to the feet. For each person the application and effect of the therapy is unique. Sensitive,

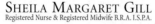
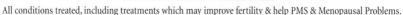

trained hands can detect tiny deposits and imbalances in the feet and by working on these points, the reflexologist can release blockages and restore the free flow of energy to the whole body.

Tensions are eased and circulation and elimination are improved. This gentle therapy encourages the body to heal itself at its own pace, often counteracting a lifetime of misuse. This can be an opportunity for you to give time to yourself, time to relax and to replenish your energies.

How or why an image of the body is projected onto the feet has not, as yet, been fully explained. Perhaps it can be understood as working in a similar way to the hologram, which is a three-dimensional picture produced by laser beams, which fix a coded image onto a two-dimensional photographic plate.

One unusual attribute of a hologram is that, if the plate is broken, any fragment can be used to reconstruct the whole image, which means that all the information about the whole picture is contained in every part.

It could be that systems which use reflections or pictures of the whole body projected onto a part are based on the concept that every part of the body, indeed every cell, contains a complete image and understanding of the whole; and that therapies such as reflexology are utilising the body's ability for self-perception and self-knowledge.

What happens when you go for Reflexology?

When you go for a treatment, there will be a preliminary talk with the practitioner during which time they will take a case history to establish medical history, lifestyle, diet etc. Then you will remove your shoes and socks and relax on a treatment couch while the reflexologist begins to work on your feet, (or hands if necessary), noting the problem areas. For the most part the treatment is pleasant and soothing.

There may be discomfort in some places but this is fleeting, and is an indication of tension or imbalance in a corresponding part of the body.

Treatment usually lasts for up to an hour. A number of sessions will normally be necessary as the benefits of reflexology build up gently and gradually. Weekly treatments are often recommended to begin with, and the total number of sessions will depend on your own body's requirements.

The reflexologist will discuss this at the first session. After the first treatment or two, the body may respond in a very definite way. There may be a feeling of well-being and relaxation.

Occasionally the client may be lethargic, nauseous or tearful for a short time. This is transitory and is simply part of the healing process. Once the body is back in tune, it is wise to have regular maintenance treatments.

Our modern lifestyle creates all kinds of physical, emotional and mental stresses. Often we are unable to release these in a natural way and they become 'locked up' in our body, producing a wide range of different symptoms. It has been estimated that more than 75 per cent of all illness is stress-related.

Stress can lead to a weakening of our body's defence system so we become more vulnerable to illness and disease. When we are stressed we are tense. Tense muscles restrict the blood flow, reduce the transportation of oxygen and nutrients to all the cells of the body and prevent the proper disposal of waste products.

The whole system becomes sluggish and is unable to function efficiently. We may get muscle aches and pains, or we may develop problems in underlying organs. By helping to relax the muscles, by encouraging the process of circulation and the elimination of toxins, and by stimulating the production of natural chemicals in the brain, reflexology can ease pain and discomfort.

As tension and irritation are soothed away, and as the client becomes calmer, they will find improvements occurring in many different areas of their life: relationships become more rewarding; they are able to handle work or study more effectively; they sleep better, throw off fatigue more easily, gain mental alertness and generally enjoy life more.

The actual thumb and finger technique used in reflexology is unlike any other massage movement. Work is done mostly by the thumb which, by moving only the distal joint, crawls like a caterpillar in a forward direction over the reflex areas in a specific sequence.

Needless to say, the nails must be kept very short to avoid digging in to the feet. Treatment usually starts on the toes, or head area, then proceeds over the sole, round the ankles, and finally, using fingers in the same 'caterpillar walk', the dorsal aspect of the foot is covered. Thumb and finger movements will be slow and rhythmic and the pressure even.

Reflex points to the glands and organs are pressed by a 'hook-in and back-up' technique, which accurately pinpoints the reflex. Points can be tender and people's sensitivity varies, but usually any pain felt is quickly dispersed with treatment and the reflexologist will adapt pressure to suit. Any very tender places may need a little extra attention as this can mean a blockage or depletion of energy in that area. The aim is to provide the body with the opportunity to heal itself and bring relief, not to inflict pain, so pressure should always be adjusted to the feet being 'worked'.

During treatment the foot will be held in such a way as to give a sense of comfort and security. Both hands remain in contact with the foot throughout, providing leverage and support. Most schools advocate starting on the right and working over that foot before moving to the left, although this in not always the case.

There is a great proliferation of schools, particularly in the United States and they all have their own individual variations. However, it is universally accepted that as reflexology is aimed at helping to restore health and balance to the whole person on all levels and not just relieving symptoms, the whole of both feet are usually worked in every treatment although emphasis can be given to symptomatic or causal areas.

The hands-on reflexology part of a treatment usually lasts for between half and three-quarters of an hour and, if possible, the patient should rest for a while after the session.

Occasionally there is a temporary reaction as the body rids itself of released toxins. This will not last long and should be seen as part of the healing process. If there is a reaction the patient should be advised to eat lightly and drink plenty of water.

Rebalancing through Reflexology.

Working on the feet with reflexology helps to re-establish the close contact between the feet and the whole body, and between the body and the environment by stimulating nerve endings and providing a deep sensory experience.

As we get older the body's functioning is influenced by the accumulated experiences of a lifetime. Both the mind and the body store memories of past illnesses, physical hurts, emotional pain, and psychological and social stresses. We shift weight to relieve pain in joints or organs, tense some muscle fibres to ease others, droop or hunch our shoulders when unhappy, tighten our stomachs, clench our jaws, find excuses, become anxious, or otherwise modify the way we use our minds and bodies.

These modifications become habitual and effect our posture, functioning and thinking. Much of the body's 'wear and tear', often attributed to ageing, is due to the way we misuse ourselves.

Reflexology can help in reprogramming the mind and body by sending signals through the feet to encourage the body to reassess and rebalance its internal environment allowing the body to heal at every level, physically, mentally, and emotionally.

Conditions helped by Reflexology.

The main benefits of reflexology are relaxation and the normalisation of the body's functions. A great many of today's diseases and disorders are the result of stress which causes disruptions to the normal functioning of the body.

By inducing a state of relaxation, muscular and emotional tension is released, circulation is improved, blood supply to vital organs increased and the elimination of toxins and waste matter is encouraged.

Treatment helps the body's internal communication systems to work more efficiently which is particularly important if there is any hormonal imbalance, especially during menopause or in cases of dysmenorrhoea.

LEONIE H. DACK
BSc(Hons) MAR

Traditional & Universal
Reflexology. Reiki Healing

Home visits & Gift Vouchers
available Kent/East Sussex Area
01797 362794 / 07979 244669

Linda J. McIntyre
MRQA, MAR

REMEDIAL MASSAGE THERAPY
AROMATHERAPY, REIKI, REFLEXOLOGY

Tel: 01904 623833
7 TERRY STREET BISHOPTHORPE ROAD YORK YO23 1LR

Reflexologist

Mary Higgins
M.I.I.R, Reg

For appointment telephone
Kilkeel (016937) 64136 after 5.00 p.m.

Lorna Goudie, MAR, MBSR, CIMI
Reflexologist and Infant Massage Instructor

Armorel, 1 Staneypark, Gulberwick, Shetland Isles. ZE2 9JX
Tel/Fax: 01595 695389 (answerphone)
e.mail: lorna_goudie@yahoo.co.uk

Reflexology is a totally natural holistic therapy which can help with a variety of common complaints including: asthma, arthritis, back pain, circulation, migrain, PMT, sciatic pain, sinusitis and stress, to name a few. Try a painfree solution that really works.

Infant Massage relaxes and soothes your baby, deepens bonding, improves development, aids sleep and help relieve wind/colic.

There is, indeed, a wide range of conditions which may be helped by reflexology: stress related problems such as allergies, asthma, insomnia, depression, anxiety, migraine and so on; disorders due to muscular tension, back pain, fibrositis, neck and shoulder problems, and it is of great benefit in restoring balance to the endocrine and autonomic nervous systems.

In fact there are few conditions that do not derive some benefit from reflexology. However, it is not an alternative to, nor a replacement for, other forms of treatment and a therapist will always refer patients to doctors or other therapists for treatment or examination when necessary. Reflexology works well in conjunction with other medical remedies and is a great aid to recovery.

Contra-indications in Reflexology

Although reflexology is a safe and effective way of aiding the body to restore health and balance, there are some occasions or conditions when it is not appropriate. When visiting a Reflexologist they will assess the suitability of the client for reflexology at that time.

This will mean that the Reflexologist can adapt the approach to the treatment session to suit their needs. Occasionally they may advise that any form of reflexology would not be appropriate for them on that visit.

Children can be treated with reflexology and usually love it, but pressure must be light and the session short. Elderly or frail patients may also need light, gentle handling and babies' feet should only be held, caressed and lightly stroked.

If the foot itself has corns, calluses, bruises, sores or fungal infections those areas may be avoided. If it is not possible to work on the foot at all because of injury,

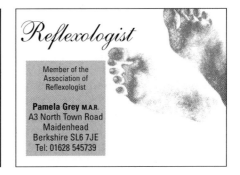

verrucas, infectious skin diseases, oedema, etc., then reflexology may be given on the hands.

Hand Reflexology

The structure of the hand is similar to that of the foot and the location of the reflexes correspond closely, although most are closer together on the hand. There are some situations when it is easier to work on the hands than on the feet and the technique and procedure is the same.

Even though it may feel slightly different to foot reflexology, it is nevertheless a very beneficial and pleasurable experience.

Holding and working on the hand is a natural way to bring comfort to another person and any hand massage, given with compassion, will help the patient to relax and release tension.

Self-treatment

It is fairly easy to give oneself a hand or foot reflexology treatment. The main disadvantage in treating oneself is that it is not possible to obtain the deep relaxation that comes when receiving a treatment from a qualified reflexologist.

However, there are nevertheless great benefits to be obtained from self-treatment.

Sensory signals are transmitted from the reflexes to the corresponding body areas increasing self-perception and evaluation, and mobilising the healing process; circulation is improved with all the advantages that it entails; nerve pathways are cleared, and the foot or hand is made more flexible and receptive.

Also, of course, hands and feet are always with us so it is possible to fit in short treatments while watching television, for instance, travelling or taking a bath. It is recommended in every case to consult a qualified Reflexologist before carrying out any self-treatment.

Professional status

Unlike any other country in the Western World, common law in England permits the practice of any therapy or treatment which has not been specifically prescribed, provided, of course, that the practitioner does not contravene any other civil or criminal laws. This is an important freedom and, is less open to abuse than is sometimes claimed.

A practitioner who is poorly trained is not likely to get many clients, and the public is protected from misrepresentations or negligence under existing legislation. However therapists who work with patients and who wish to be responsible co-workers with the medical profession should be properly trained, maintain a high standard of ethical conduct and work consciously on their own health and development on all levels.

There is a growing impetus from within the complementary health movement towards regulation and quality assurance for all practitioners. Reflexology as a profession is very much at the forefront of this development.

Associations are working together to bring about national training standards and common codes of practice and ethics.

They are also talking with the government and licensed bodies to develop an appropriate system of regulation which government, Reflexologists and the public alike can rely on.

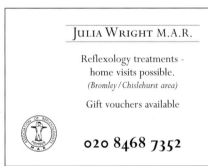
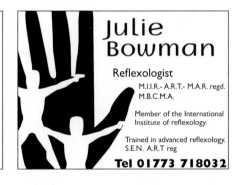
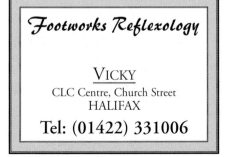
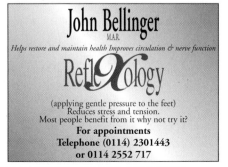

Training as a Reflexologist

The majority of the main reflexology organisations are in agreement that a reflexology course should last a minimum of 100 hours contact teaching. Indeed it is recognised by these organisations that there will need to be a significant increase in the length of reflexology training in order to accommodate the push for higher standards and regulation.

As well as the 100 hours contact teaching, there will be a considerable amount of home study required – a minimum of 300 hours is usual. This home study will include the presentation of at least 6 case studies amounting to 60 treatment sessions.

This level of practical must be considered as an absolute minimum. There is no substitute for hands on experience. This in turn must be backed up by supervised treatments on other students and non-students.

There will be a required minimum level of Anatomy and Physiology (A&P), and Integrated Biology. A minimum level is currently regarded as GCSE or Level 3, though there is a strong push to upgrade this to A level or Level 4.

In addition to practical work and A&P a good reflexology course will have units covering many areas, and allow the time to investigate each of these to the appropriate level. These must be backed up by the direction and delivery of a qualified teacher.

The provision of training

The Association of Reflexologists is the largest reflexology organisation in the UK, and holds a reputation for high quality and integrity. Other reflexology organisations with a reputable standing based on similar standards to those mentioned include the

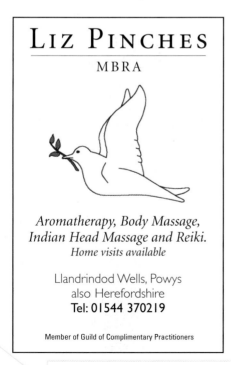
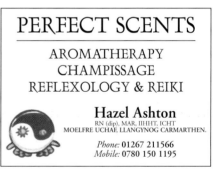
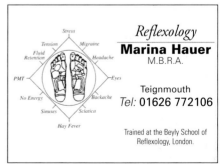

British Reflexology Association, the Holistic Association of Reflexologists, the Reflexologists Society, the International Institute of Reflexology and the International Federation of Reflexologists to name a few.

Each organisation can provide information on training courses, curriculum, tutors and certificates.

Many reflexology schools are private and provide a prospectus laying out all the details involved in training. This information is very helpful in establishing how one course compares with others in each area and around the country.

The tutors delivering the courses are an integral part of the training and it is important to be able to interact well with them. Each organisation will have a code of conduct for their schools and tutors are required to operate within that code.

The organisation may also have an accreditation procedure for the school laying out the requirements for the content, delivery and assessment of the course. Tutors may be required to hold teaching qualifications and have a certain amount of experience – five years in practice, as a Reflexologist is not unusual or unreasonable. Like so much else in life, there is no substitute for experience in reflexology.

The reflexology school will provide information on the cost of training as a Reflexologist, and will include all additional costs such as books, charts, treatment couches and exams. All these should be clearly stated in the pre-course information.

They will also provide you with a contract prior to the beginning of the course. This will lay out exactly what is expected from the student and what is expected from the tutor, school or college. It also makes the financial position clear.

Many people who go for reflexology have chronic conditions which orthodox medicine has been unable to help. Their doctors have told them that, apart from drugs to relieve the symptoms, there is no cure for their arthritis, or hardened arteries, multiple sclerosis, or persistent back ache, and so on.

Reflexology is not a miracle cure and not everyone is helped, but treatment is based on the premise that, given the right circumstances, every cell in the body will work together to promote total health and balance.

Some patients make remarkable progress for, by refusing to accept a hopeless prognosis and assuming the responsibility for their own sickness, they are taking the first big step towards creating the right conditions for self-healing.

Disorders, which are the result of years of bad habits, poor posture and wrong diet, for instance, will not be remedied by a few reflexology treatments, although often much relief is obtained.

However, reflexology may help the body to reassess its own internal environment. Cells are constantly being replaced within the body and by enlisting the body's innate healing powers, sickly cells can be replaced by healthy ones and a process of regeneration and rejuvenation can take place.

Seeking and co-operating with treatment is another step towards health; however it is also helpful for the patient to examine those attitudes, habits and conditions which contributed to the disorder in the first place, and to correct them with proper diet, exercise, posture and positive thinking. The future of healthcare in the UK is for doctors, nurses, complementary therapists, healers, social workers, dieticians and psychotherapists all work together in the Health Centres of the future to provide a comprehensive holistic health care service for everyone.

In 1984 the Association of Reflexologists was founded with the aim of maintaining a high standard of practice among reflexologists, encouraging research, furthering the work of practitioners, accrediting high quality training courses and providing information to the public. Membership is limited to those with approved qualifications but it is not affiliated to any particular school.

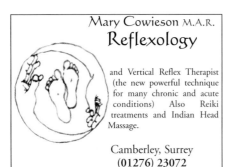
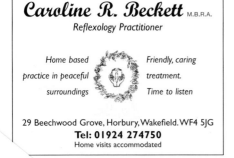
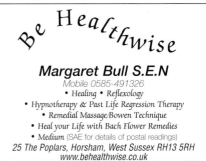

The unique pressure points of the hand and foot

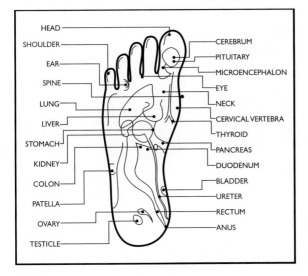

These diagrams show the unique pressure points of the foot and hands

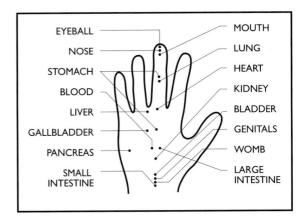

The pressure points

Whatever problem there is in the body, the relative part of the foot will be very sensitive when the reflexes are stimulated. The hands and feet tell a story; a sensitive reaction reveals that all is not well in that part of the body.

Maybe there is congestion or inflammation as the result of a recent illness or injury. Maybe the body, mind and spirit are in a state of turmoil due to a particularly stressful period of time. Whatever the cause, reflexology can offer great relaxation to the body, mind and spirit.

REFLEXOLOGY

RAINBOW FEET Enjoy holistic reflexology in your own home, using advanced techniques for a healing, relaxing and revitalising experience by Jane, M.A.R. qualified reflexologist. Gift vouchers available. Herts/South Beds Area. Ring Jane 01727 760609

SALLY LOGAN M.A.R., ART (Regd.) Wren House 14b Over Norton Road, Chipping Norton, Oxfordshire, OX7 5NR Tel: 01608 645319. "Reflexology is a unique therapy that works on the body through the fleet, flushing out toxins renewing energy."

ENJOY LIFE WITH REFLEXOLOGY. Help to relieve stress, aches and pains, improve circulation, and enabling you to experience a feeling of well being. Linda Rumbles MIIR ART(Regd) appointments : Yeovil/Somerton. Home visits by arrangement. Tel: 01935 840132

HELEN G BROWN MAR. The Cardiff Health Practice, 9 Tydfil Place, Roath Park, Cardiff CF23 5HP. Tel: 029 2048 4555. Experienced reflexologist and lifeskills coach, with a background in nursing, having lived in Iran, Zimbabwe and Switzerland.

ANN EDMONDS M.A.R. Thatcham, Berkshire. RG18 4BZ. Tel. 01635 865612. Gentle technique used, making the treatment particularly relaxing and suitable for all ages and conditions. Lifestyle counselling included.

JUDITH WRIGHT RGN MAR Reflexologist. 40 Victoria Ave, Cheadle Hulme. Home Visits available on request. Take a step in the right direction and telephone. 0161 485 3518 or 0771 2211760

CORINNE EVERT MSSCH MBCHA MIIR MAR ART Hons Reflexology and Meridian EFT Therapist. Fosse Road, South Leicester. Tel/fax 0116 2857833

LONDON NORTH-WEST. Relax with Reflexology – tension released, aches and pains soothed away; many medical conditions helped. Feel good with Reflexology. Fully insured. Phone Sharon Carr (associate member of AOR) on 020 8933 8491; e-mail: Sharon.carr@cwcom.net.

HELEN PEARSE BA, MAR Reflexologist. 41 Marksbury Avenue, Kew, Richmond, Surrey, TW9 4JE.Appointments: Tel/Fax: 0208 876 8970. Special interest in woman and children's reflexology. Articles published on the use of reflexology in pregnancy and unexplained infertility.

REFLEXOLOGY

REFLEXOLOGY helps the body to heal itself naturally. For information and appointment. Eveline Brooks. Member of The British Reflexology Association. 54 , Greencourt Drive, Bognor Regis, West Sussex. PO21 5EU. Tel: 01243 824973. Home visits available.

REFLEXOLOGIST. Mavis Lowther, A member of The British Reflexology Association. 1 Boswell Road, Bessacarr, Doncaster, DN4 7BJ. Tel: 01302 539681. Mobile: 07714 037001.

FEEING STRESSED, tired and irritable? Get life back on track by giving me a call. Angela Byrne, AoR Registered Mobile therapist. Giving treatments in Reflexology/Reiki and Indian Head Massage. Tel: 020 8949 4787. Mobile: 07719 588 410.

REFLEXOLOGY. Wendy Mackintosh BSc MBRA. Fedaland, Aultvaich, By Beauly, Inverness-shire, IV4 7AN. Tel: 01463 870634. Appointment by telephone only. Member of the British Reflexology Association. Trained in Vertical Reflex Therapy and Synergistic Reflexology (the Booth Method).

PRECISION REFLEXOLOGIST and Integrated Therapist can assist with stress related disorders and teach relaxation techniques. Back problems, migraine, minor ailments and general health all benefit from treatments. Margaret Moger. Tel: 01395 265603, East Devon/Exeter.

REFLEXOLOGY, Health Kinesiology. Cynthia Prior, M.B.S.R., M.A.R., Assoc. Member, B.C.M.A., Reg. Bach Flower Consultant. Brock's Hollow, Vann Road, Fernhurst, Haslemere, Surrey GU27 3NL. Tel: 01428 658780, Fax: 01428 645093. e-mail: cynthiaprior@hotmail.com

CAROL FERGUSON MAR MBRA. 28 Patricia Road, Norwich NR1 2PE Tel: 01603 663153 and at Focus Organic, 76 High Street, Southworld, Suffolk Tel: 01502 725299. Reflexology And Metamorphosis. For relaxation and to support your good health and wellbeing.

MS J EVANS, 418 Milton Road, Cambridge, Cambridgeshire, CB4 1ST. 01223 510047

MS T MCGLOIN, 71 Mora Road, London, NW2 6TB. 020 8208 0401

MR B MAZURKE, 101 Woodkirk Gardens, Dewsbury, Yorkshire, WF12 7JA. 01924 47665

Reiki

By the Reiki College

Reiki answers who am I, what am I doing, where did I come from and where am I going, the happenings in life. Today there are many different aspects of Reiki being taught. You deserve the best, as with all things you buy, ensure its quality.

You know yourself better than anyone else in the universe so trust in your ability to discern what's simply the best for you. What happens for you after learning Reiki? It opens up whole new worlds/perspectives. Reiki is different for every one and expresses itself differently in each of our lives, almost as though it's a completely different wisdom. That's the beauty and the fun of it.

No matter where you are at in your life, if you want to enhance or improve any bit of it (and who doesn't?) or to simply redesign your life the way you want it, Reiki is for you. I promise you 'if you never, ever go, you will never ever know'.

Reiki is incited by our imaginations. No matter what it is, if we can perceive it there is a way to relieve it with Reiki. This incredibly simple and beautiful energy is free of limitation (apart from the ones we place upon it ourselves).

Reiki is a completely safe, natural, simple, easy-to-learn system (either by self-study or Clarence style) and requires no special knowledge or equipment. Anyone can learn Reiki from children to the elderly, from those who are healthy to those who are participating in various degrees of disease. Reiki balances, harmonises and restores your energy systems and you experience peace, love, happiness, joy in all aspects of your lives. It puts the fun, the joy, the happiness and magic beck into your life and a sparkle in your eyes.

Through Reiki you get back in touch with yourself, who you really are, not who you think you are and your lives have meaning, purpose and direction. You feel good about yourself and happy with who you are and your self esteem escalates.

"To be what we are, and to become what we are capable of becoming is the only end of life' – Robert Louis Stevenson.

He would have loved Reiki because this is what it does. Reiki restores balance and harmony in our lives including health, wealth and love (the three main items that keep us awake at night) and takes the loneliness out of life.

Health is often thought to be merely the absence of disease/sickness, however it's much more than this. Reiki enables us to function in a more balanced way and totally embraces our being – body, mind, emotions, spirit.

Until recently, there's been a focus on the application of Reiki to treat root causes of disease for both ourselves and others. This has resulted in Reiki being labelled as an alternative therapy, however it's also much more than this.

We've ignored to a large extent, Reiki's power for our personal growth and the quality of our life.

It can also be used as a guide for the way we live our life and to open up the 'mysterious' parts of ourselves (our inner secrets and surprises).

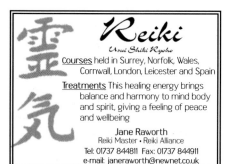
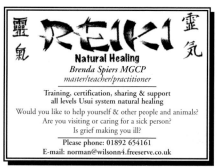
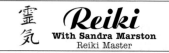

Reiki can be easily integrated into our lives (no matter what religion we are) from day one. When we are healthy our body energy systems flow finely and they meet in harmony (good relationships) with each other. When we feel healthy, good about ourselves and generally happy we treat those around us (our world) similarly. How can we succeed and be happy in life if we aren't healthy?

Perhaps it's time to smooth some of the bumps, life isn't a random chaotic assembly of parts – it's a unified whole governed by a pattern of world of energy. Reiki connects and interfaces us with this web and gives us back control of our lives.

The last millennium was not a wonderful success in terms of human behaviour and the way we treated each other and ourselves. Epstein commented that 'everything has changed except our thinking'.

In spite of fantastic discoveries in science and technological fields, our thinking has become firmly implanted in what has been (we learn from history, however it is also possible to get stuck in it and then history repeats itself.

Another way of looking at this is, where the eyes go, the body will follow; so if we continually look backwards – remember Lot's wife who looked back and was turned into a pillar of salt?).

People who learn Reiki comment on the 'coincidences' or sequence of events that triggered them to learn Reiki and offer a myriad of reasons for being at a class.

Ultimately it comes down to the simple reason that, the time is right. Reiki is unconditional, i.e. it asks nothing of you, the giver, or your receiver, and requires no specific belief in a supreme being, creed/dogma or even in Reiki itself.

Reiki

By Christine Green

Reiki is an ancient healing form, originally used by Tibetan monks. For a long time, it was lost to the world but it was rediscovered at the end of the 19th century by a Japanese Christian Minister and teacher, Dr Mikao Usui.

The story goes that his students asked him why we couldn't heal as Jesus was able to, even through Jesus had said, "go and do likewise". Over many years, and after travelling to America and Tibet to study both modern Christian and ancient Sanskrit writings, Dr. Usui felt he had found all the intellectual answers, but he still could not activate the healing energy.

Eventually, after fasting and meditating for twenty one days on Mount Kuriyama, a sacred mountain near Kyoto, he achieved enlightenment and found he could heal.

He became the first modern Reiki Master, and it is from him that all current Reiki practitioners descend.

How does Reiki work?

Reiki healers channel concentrated 'ki' ('chi') or Universal Life Force Energy. Reiki energy boosts, enhances and kick-starts their own natural abilities, healing abilities, self-healing abilities, creativity, wisdom and physical energy – the very essence of themselves at the deepest, most profound spiritual level.

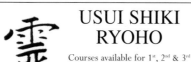

This enhancement enables the recipient of the energy to use it in accordance with their soul's and for their whole situation's highest good. It enables them to galvanise all their resources – physical, mental, emotional and spiritual – towards a positive and beneficial outcome.

Since this galvanisation is not miraculous but natural, it may not register as something different. It isn't different – it is more. It is more of what is good and positive, healthy and constructive.Working with Reiki energy sets you on a course of profound inner development.

The beauty of Reiki is that it will enhance, boost and kick-start the goodness in everyone. This goodness manifests in different ways in different people. It will bring out the gifts and talents you have. It will create a way forward through stuckness. It will enhance all that is good, lovely and true in all whom it encounters.It will work at many and various levels which is why, when you send energy to situations, they just seem to resolve.

The Reiki is enhancing, activating, kick-starting and unblocking everything in its path. When a Reiki healer does a hands-on session they are sending energy to all the chakras in the recipient's body. They are sending energy to every cell in that body, and to all the spaces in between.

This energy will work at all levels, bringing the body back into balance in the most appropriate way. Once the body is back in balance, the need for the physical manifestation of imbalance dissolves and the body heals.

The body, mind and spirit are our soul's vehicle for experiencing itself, for connecting with others, and for connecting with God.

Every imbalance on every level is a communication to us from our soul about something we need to heal or bring into our conscious awareness.

This healing process requires energy. Reiki will provide more of that energy, faster. Reiki will speed up the natural processes, which occur at every level.

Bringing the body, mind and spirit back into balance is a complex and intricate process.

There are so many factors and mechanisms, all interlocking and interacting at so many different levels.

The Reiki will work at all of these

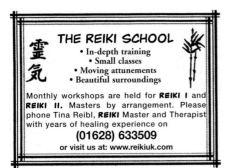

levels, bringing about all the many changes required. Many of the changes will be subtle, and one obvious change may be achieved through a myriad of tiny changes.

What happens during a Reiki session?

The recipient will normally be asked to lie down on a massage couch, fully clothed. The Reiki energy is channelled through the practitioner's hands to find its own course to and within the recipient. It can work at a physical, emotional or mental level.

The Reiki flows to the areas in need, soothing pain and supporting the recipient's natural ability to heal themselves physically, emotionally and mentally.

What does it feel like?

Most people have a feeling of deep relaxation and inner calm whilst receiving Reiki. The energy can be perceived in many different ways, such as warmth or chill, tingling or slight pulsing – both by the practitioner (through his/her hands) and by the recipient.

Becoming a Reiki healer

When you make a commitment to use Reiki energy in your life, you are making a commitment to value, train, develop, enhance, bring out and boost all that is good, kind, honest, beautiful and true in you.

When you use Reiki in your life you will find that you attract everything you need to encounter to help you shift whatever is blocking you from being the best you you can be.

Whether this comes in the form of experiences which make things clearer for you, situations which demand that you grow, people who can teach you skills you need, or challenges which call forth more and more strength, faith, skill or dedication, it will come.

The best thing you can do for yourself is to channel more Reiki energy into more areas of your life. The more you do this, the faster, the easier and the smoother your transformation into the fully actualised you will be.

As a Reiki healer, you are a channel for Reiki – the Universal Life Force.Energy does not come from you, it comes through you. Thus, whenever you give a Reiki treatment, you too will feel the peaceful and healing Reiki energy.

You receive Reiki when you give it. One of the most wonderful things about Reiki is that it assists you to take responsibility for your own health and healing, as you can treat yourself.

You can use Reiki when you are feeling good to assist you to maintain that balance, and you can use Reiki when you are not feeling well. Use Reiki to calm your emotions, relieve the pain of a headache or stomach ache, hasten the healing of burns, or to treat more serious illnesses such as cancer and the many opportunistic viruses.

Reiki practitioners are not medical specialists. They are channels for healing energy. Reiki is not a substitute for conventional medicine. However, it will enhance any other form of treatment: therapy, medicine or natural remedies.

Sekhem

By Helen Belot

Sekhem is more than just channelled energy. It is a complete healing system that can be used in any situation or crisis. Even more importantly it can be used to prevent the illness, disease or crisis happening.

It brings balance, clarity and understanding in these times of rapid global and personal change which force us to choose our own personal spiritual path and the direction of our self-development. This is the energy that will take mankind safely into the 21st century and a different dimension. It will guide and assist you to make the right decisions and to be in the right place at the right time. Sekhem works at the soul level and will always go to the deep underlying cause that needs to be resolved rather than just addressing the symptoms. It bonds together your conscious mind with your higher self or higher mind.

Sekhem is a relatively new channelled energy with a very high vibrational frequency. It was developed by Helen Belot and came into being in Australia in 1992. Its origins are from the ancient temples of very early Egyptian times and is gentle, compassionate and loving energy but awesome in its power. This is the energy used by the great masters of the past to heal the sick and to perform their miracles.

Because of its gentleness, compassion and feeling of great love it is considered to be Goddess energy but it also has a beautiful angelic quality. It can take you to a place beyond pain and suffering, to where you have always been whole and at peace, and so enable you to heal. You feel nurtured, cared for, and above all loved. It is the most natural

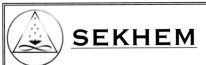

thing in the world to love and honour yourself and others. This is not selfishness, rather the complete opposite, for it is honouring the immortal spark within yourself that gives such a sense of self-worth. Of being worthy. You know that in the greater scheme of things you do matter and you as an individual can make a difference in this lifetime.

This loving energy helps to cut through blocks and restrictions with ease. There are no long drawn out traumas and dramas, the changes happen easily and gently as understanding flows in. You open up to love and life becomes easier. No more doing things the hard way unless that is your choice. For Sekhem will never take away your right of choice. There are no prerequisites to learning to use this energy, which has the highest vibration of any channelled energy at this time. All will benefit from experiencing the closest thing to unconditional love that can be imagined. Whether learning to channel or receiving a treatment, your life will be enriched beyond measure.

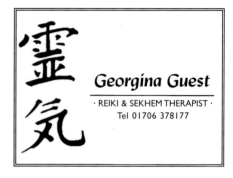

Shamanism
By Nick Redcloud

The Shaman of all the continents of the world, throughout time have been sought by their local people to perform the role of teacher, healer and counsellor.

The bedrock foundation of love and respect for the earth and connection to all things are fundamental to Shamans the world over and yet each tradition has developed its own gloriously unique ways of working when called upon to give guidance for the benefit of the people.

If one studies the shamans on many of the continents of the earth one comes to certain understandings about the customs, the philosophy, the spirituality of the shamanic traditions. It becomes clear then, that there are certain core beliefs and fundamental knowings that are common to all, which are at the very heart of shamanism. One example of this is that the shamans know that although the things on this earth might be put together and look differently to us, in essence, man and everything around us is made of the same stuff – energy.

If everything is energy then we are connected to everything else. We are not separate. We are part of everyone and everything. On the shamanic level there is no difference between a man, a tree, a rock, a dog, a cloud or a fish. We are all connected and are all part of the same system – planet Earth.

It was only the emergence of modern religions that tried to tell man that he was superior, in charge, and therefore had all other things to use for his benefit, as he thought fit. As a result to achieve certain things we poison the air, the rivers, the sea and the earth. The Shamans of the world including the Hawaiian Kahuna Shamans and the Native American spiritual leaders, have no idea, no comprehension at all about how we in the modern world can do this.

It is so clear to them that because we are all connected, if we poison even one tiny stream, we poison ourselves. I use this as but one example of the many many teachings and learnings that are common to all the shamanic traditions of the world.

With a clear understanding of these fundamental truths, it is possible to take a glimpse at how specific traditions built on their understandings in order to develop their unique customs and rituals for life. Now we can learn about the

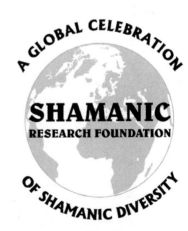

Nick RedCloud
Director of Studies
The Shamanic Research Foundation
The Grove Hotel, The Grove, Ilkley
West Yorkshire, England LS29 9PA
Tel: 01943 817471 - Fax: 0870 706 5587
e-mail:nickredcloud@shamanics.co.uk
www.shamanics.co.uk

powerful techniques they use for spiritual harmony, community development, emotional health and personal growth. We can study and take immense benefit from the wonderful practices from this fascinating world of shamanic diversity.

The origins of Shamanism

Shamans and shamanistic religion were first identified among the peoples of Siberia and continue to be associated mainly with Siberian and American Indian peoples, although closely related phenomena exist in other parts of Asia and in Oceania. The word shaman is derived from a Tungus word meaning 'he who knows'. The term medicine man is frequently used as a synonym for shaman in American Indian cultures. Eskimo shamans are called angakoks.

Russian accounts of Siberian shamanism date back to the 17th and 18th centuries, but German-Russian scholar Wilhelm Radloff, one of the pioneers of Siberian ethnology, was first to treat shamanism seriously as a subject for scholarly research.

The shaman may be grouped with the healer or diviner but is distinguished from that general class by the specific nature of his or her religious experience and practices.

Shamanic power is said to come from a supernatural force; a spirit (sometimes associated with a particular animal) takes possession of the shaman during an ecstasy or trance and gives the shaman powers of healing and knowing, often after transporting him or her to a spirit world. Sometimes the ecstatic state may be induced by hallucinogens. It is the shaman's function to regulate relations between the spirits and the community. Shamans concern themselves with such matters as locating and attracting game or fish, controlling the weather, detecting broken taboos that bring misfortune, expelling harmful spirits, and especially with curing the sick and guiding the souls of the dead to the spirit world. Because of their special powers, shamans may gain considerable political influence in their communities, as, for example, among the Colorado people of Ecuador.

A shaman is said to be chosen by the spirits, selected from among persons of an excitable temperament who are given to daydreaming and visionary experience. Sometimes a shaman is marked for the vocation by repeated illnesses or mental disturbance.

Shamanism as practised among the Ona, Yaghan, and Alacaluf peoples of Tierra del Fuego, at the southern tip of South America, exhibits the same features as exist among the Buryat, Yakut, Khant-Mansi, Samoyed, and other peoples of Siberia.

This evidence links even these remote peoples of the Western Hemisphere to what scholars believe was their prehistoric origin in northern Asia. Shamanism crossed the Bering Straits in prehistoric times and is found among the Eskimos, Aleuts, and American Indian tribes throughout North and South America.

Closely allied systems occur in the Malay Peninsula, in Indonesia, and among Australian Aborigines; until recent times, remote tribal groups in India and Korea maintained shamanistic systems as well.

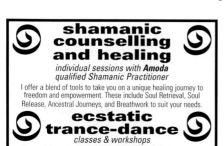

SHEN® Physio Emotional Release Therapy

By The SHEN Therapy Institute

SHEN® Physio-Emotional Release Therapy is a non-traditional, alternative approach to emotional health and wellness, one that can bring profound change for those whose lives or bodies are upset by painful emotions.

SHEN's methods, a remarkably effective process of healing old emotional wounds and accelerating positive emotional change, are not based on the current medical concept that emotions are neurological – mental processes that take place in a special portion of the brain.

SHEN's basic principle states that emotions are not in the cells of the brain or in the cells of the body either, but are disturbances and conditions that occur within the biofield (sometimes called the 'energy field') that permeates both the physical body and brain and therefore affects them both.

The reason why our emotions and emotional states are so difficult to change or control by mental effort is that they are not neurological and are not under control of the brain. It is the reason why unpleasant emotions can, in spite of our best intentions, upset the body in the many ways they often do. The biofield is the 'link' in the term 'mind-body link'.

SHEN's singular techniques are unusually effective because they are all based on conventional physics rather than on the metaphysical principles that others have used to try to explain them.

Through a series of careful experiments, it has been shown that the biofield is regulated by the same patterns of nature that guide all other moving fields in nature such as electricity, magnetism, oceanic currents and weather currents.

SHEN Practitioners are taught to apply the field between their hands to the recipient according to these patterns in ways that will produce the greatest effect. SHEN's unique concepts have been thoroughly validated by its clinical results and its methods and techniques are firmly established.

SHEN's unique hands-on procedures do not include physical pressure or manipulation; the practitioners work entirely by properly applying the biofield between the practitioner's hands to and through the client's body. The biofield can be applied by direct contact with the skin but is usually applied through normal clothing.

During the SHEN session the recipient reclines fully clothed on a table that is fitted with a special 'cradle' which allows the practitioner access to both the front and back of the body. The client is encouraged to relax while the Practitioner places his or her hands in a carefully organised sequence of several different positions around the regions in the body where we experience or feel the individual emotions.

These are: the heart, the upper abdomen, the lower abdomen, and the junction of the legs and torso. The client often feels tingles or warmth as the field between the practitioner's hands flows through their body.

Often they drift into a light sleep or trance state, similar to what one experiences just before falling fully asleep or just before becoming fully awake.

While in this state, the contractions surrounding and trapping deeply held emotions can be loosened and emotions or emotionally charged, dream-like images are able to emerge.

Sometimes memories of forgotten, emotionally painful events from earlier times in one's life come to the surface and are relived and the emotions in them brought to completion.

The rising of the emotions in this process is not frightening. Whenever emotions come to the surface in a SHEN session they are experienced differently from the way we usually experience them.

Instead of being driven to physically respond to, or act out, the effects of the emotion – or to be overpowered by them, the person feels the emotion strongly in one of the body's regions of emotion but in a non-threatening way.

This occurs in a way they can more easily handle and absorb than when they occur in day-to-day living. Recall of previous emotional states and the resolution of troubling emotions through their experience are the hallmarks of the SHEN session; emotional empowerment is its intent.

An American scientist, Richard R. Pavek, developed SHEN's alternative approach to understanding and treating emotional complaints and physio-emotional conditions after he left a career in chemistry and electronics to devote his efforts to the alternative medical field.

He began formulating his original concepts about emotions and their effects on the body and mind in 1977 from observations he made as he was studying the effects of physics in the biofield. He noticed that when he placed his hands on others in certain patterns some of those patterns of hand placements produced the release of emotions in surprising ways – ways that left the person free of their debilitating effects. He also noticed that very frequently long-standing physio-emotional disorders cleared up and disappeared after these applications.

At that point he diverted his attention from studying the physics of the biofield into developing the process that is now

ELIZABETH WARD CSP:
0131 447 6513
Edinburgh/Lothians
MARGARET MCCATHIE CSP:
01786 832 030
Central/Fife
FIONA MORTON CSP:
0141 334 7145
Glasgow/West
CAROLYN BARLOW:
01556 640 353
South West/Borders

Develop your Emotional Intelligence with

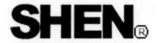

'Emotional Health is the basis of physical and psychological health...

..SHEN Therapy is the missing link which can provide this.'

See the article on SHEN Physio Emotional Release Therapy in this issue.

For further information contact: SHEN THERAPY CENTRE

LONDON : 020 8658 6505
EDINBURGH : 0131 478 4780

know as SHEN Therapy. By combining his emerging theory of emotions with his observations of the physics of the biofield, he was able to develop several essential hands-on applications of the biofield that successfully clear painful emotional blockages from the physical body and restore the proper and normal experience of the emotions.

As he began to establish the effects emotions had on the body, Richard noticed a consistent relationship between the locations of painful emotions and the physical disorders with which they were associated.

He realised that anger and fear, emotions that are prominently associated with eating disorders, are experienced in the same regions of the body that contain the digestive organs. This same relationship of the emotions being felt in the body where related disorders occur is also true for long-term grief and heart disorders, as it is for shame, guilt and the dysfunctions they produce.

This was the key for which he had been looking; he realised that the organs in that region of our bodies must be adversely affected by those emotions because they are experienced there. Somehow, the emotions were controlling the body.

The puzzle of how emotions controlled the body fell into place when he observed that, when our bodies feel painful emotions, such as fear, grief and shame, our bodies always clench tightly around the locations where these emotions are felt. He reasoned that the clenching traps the painful emotions inside the body and prevents their completion and escape.

He further reasoned that the physical tension trapping the emotion would have to interfere with normal flow of blood and other nutrients; this alone would prevent the physical organs in the region from functioning normally.

Obviously, breaking the tensions would release the emotions and the body would no longer react by clenching and the bodily functions would return to normal.

With these principles firmly established, Richard began developing the specific SHEN techniques that are now being used to release trapped emotional trauma within the recipient's body.

Using these new techniques, he was able to demonstrate that release and resolution of these emotions does restore normal functioning of the organs, just as it produces positive behavioural change.

SHEN THERAPY

SHEN THERAPY – Extremely effective for stress, bereavement, separation, migraine, irritable bowel, PMT, anxiety, panic attacks, loss of confidence, eating disorders, phobias, chronic pain, recovery from abuse, childhood terrors. Rhona & Duncan Campbell, Dunblane. Tel: 01786 821311. Email: rhonac@onet.co.uk

IRENE MCLANE. Certified Shen Practitioner, Newcastle upon Tyne, Tel: 0191 2667075. I work from home as a stand alone Shen Therapy Practitioner. Shen is a very powerful tool, creating personal unfolding and emotional growth.

SHEN THERAPY

GLASGOW AREA. Jeni McLennan, C. S. P., Tel: 0141 6476424, (Rutherglen), e-mail : jeni@shen.fsnet.co.uk Irene M. Phillips, C. S . P., Tel: 0141 6324098, (Shawlands). Both Jeni and Irene have been practising Shen for over 5 years, and have experienced how effective, empowering and life-changing this therapy can be.

MR T BAILEY, Heart Of England Centre, 11 Severn Side South, Bewdley, Worcestershire, DY12 2DX. 01299 401407

Shiatsu

By the Shiatsu Society

Shiatsu is a traditional Japanese healing art. It can help a wide range of conditions – from specific injuries to more general symptoms of poor health.

Shiatsu is a deeply relaxing experience and regular Shiatsu sessions help to prevent build up of stress in our daily lives. Conditions which have been helped by Shiatsu:

- Back pain
- Whiplash injuries and neck stiffness
- Menstrual problems
- Asthmatic symptoms
- Depression
- Headaches / Migraines
- Joint pain and reduced motability
- Digestive problems
- Sports injuries

Each Shiatsu session lasts approximately an hour. The first session may be slightly longer since your practitioner will take a detailed case history in order to develop a complete picture of your health according to the principles of oriental medicine. The session usually takes place on a padded mat or futon at floor level, although it is possible to receive Shiatsu sitting on a chair if you are unable to lie down. The client stays fully clothed. Following a treatment, there can be a feeling of increased vitality and you may feel invigorated yet relaxed. The benefits of Shiatsu include:

- It relaxes mind and body
- It eases tension and stiffness
- It improves posture
- It enhances well being
- It restores and balances energy
- It improves breathing
- It improves circulation
- It heals

Tao Shiatsu includes an abbreviated basic form for children. It is technically very simple and can be performed easily, even by non-professionals. With children, the palm and heel of the hand and the thumbs and fingers are used, all of which give soft pressure. The knees and elbows are not used. Shiatsu may be practised on sick children by professional healers, but it can be more usefully practised by a child's mother or father. This is because nothing is more beneficial for children than a parent's loving hands. In fact, diseases such as asthma can actually be cured by the parent's hands.

Skenar Therapy

By Roger S. Meacock

Quantum Physics tells us that all matter at the sub-atomic level is based in Energy. This is encompassed by Einstein's equation $e=mc^2$. All bonds between atoms vibrate with a frequency determined by the energy of the bond. Bonds between different atoms have different characteristic bond energies measured at a standard temperature.

The combination of the bond energies within a molecule give an overall vibrational energy to the molecule itself with its own characteristic frequency of vibration. These energies and vibrations themselves combine together to give different tissues, organs and ultimately the body as a whole, their own vibrational resonances.

It is plain therefore that all matter is fundamentally energy, and thus the health of all living organisms is based in energy. This has led to the re-emergence of Energy Medicine in all its various forms, through any of the senses with colour, sound, magnetic and electrical energy being the most obvious forms of energy influence. More subtle Energy Medicines include Homeopathy, Aromatherapy, Bach Flower remedies, gem therapy etc where 'signatures' of the different remedies are chosen according their known effects.

Everybody has the ability to varying degrees to channel energy to promote healing of themselves and others, e.g. Reiki. However, the vast majority of people have lost the belief in their own ability and consequently cannot heal in this way.

The development of technology with the ability to detect and measure these life energies is making this paradigm shift impossible to refute. The vast number of people who have experienced healing from Energy Medicine and who now are no longer afraid to question conventional medical practices, are moving medical practitioners to look into other forms of treating, the most popular at present probably being Homeopathy and Acupuncture. The use of many of these therapies for the successful treatment of animals provides greater credibility to the arguments for Energy Medicine and negates the commonly expressed cry of 'placebo' from non-believers. Technology is also developing on the treatment side with electro-acupuncture breaking the ice for devices such as the Skenar, which combines advanced skin electro-stimulation with a sophisticated biofeedback mechanism such that the patient effectively controls his or her own treatment.

Sound Therapy

By Pauline Allen

For those with perfect hearing, it may be hard to imagine what it must be like for people who have problems with their auditory system. Yet, research has shown that hearing dysfunction is linked to a wide variety of problems.

Hearing dysfunction is not the same as being deaf. In fact, far from being deaf many people suffer from really painful hearing, due to abnormal sensitivity to specific frequencies. This can have enormous repercussions in many areas of life. People, and especially children, who have problems processing auditory information frequently experience many learning and behavioural difficulties as a result.

For example, they may find it extremely difficult to follow conversations and become irritable, frustrated, tired, aggressive, unsociable, withdrawn, introverted or depressed.

Children who have such problems are the worst affected, because it interferes with their basic development. It hinders learning on all levels – they may not learn to read properly, because they simply cannot perceive the meaning of speech sounds correctly in order to comprehend what's going on.

This means they fall behind in all subjects. Sometimes, where auditory problems are undiagnosed, poor academic or social performance is often interpreted as uncooperative behaviour and an unwillingness to comply. Some children are even diagnosed as dyslexic.

Hearing dysfunction is also frequently accompanied by related problems with balance, co-ordination, tinnitus, sleep disorders, and overriding fatigue and stress.

Research carried out by Eric Courhesne at the University of California at San Diego has also shown that autistic individuals typically often have hearing problems. This only exacerbates the condition. Research has also shown that auditory processing problems may also be linked to several autistic characteristics such as inattentiveness, unresponsiveness and general socio-interactive problems. It can also make some children hyperactive.

One way of helping individuals with hearing dysfunction is through Auditory Integration Training (AIT). This is a

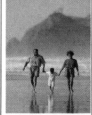

process whereby the ears are re-trained to hear sounds in a more balanced manner, and this helps to improve any related problems.

The system, which is based on 30 years of research, was developed by Dr. Guy Bérard, a French ENT specialist, who identified a link between hearing dysfunction and many behavioural and learning difficulties.

AIT has been shown to be extremely beneficial for adults and children who suffer from dyslexia, hypersensitive or painful hearing, tinnitus, poor sound recognition, stammering, general learning difficulties such as poor memory, organisation and concentration, hyperactivity, motor problems (e.g. clumsiness, dyspraxia), autism, asperger's syndrome, depression and even suicidal tendencies. Some people have even reported benefits related to eating disorders and allergies.

To begin with, individuals (apart from the very young, autistic or other non-verbal clients) have an initial hearing assessment. This is done by conducting a pure tone audiogram, together with laterality and selectivity tests. The results of these tests show the extent of the problem and they also show whether there is a left and right ear imbalance, which can cause difficulties in making sense of speech and processing language.

Together with other presenting and historical indicators the auditory patterns indicate whether AIT may be helpful. Further audiograms are taken at the mid point and at the end of treatment to monitor progress. During the actual treatment, the individual sits in a chair listening to music through headphones. The music is specially modulated and filtered through an electronic device, the Audiokinetron. This helps to retrain the ears so that hearing becomes more balanced. It also helps to improve phonological awareness (e.g.: sound awareness) and listening skills.

AIT helps to reduce or eliminate hyperacute peaks, in order to alleviate painful hearing. As a result, the hearing threshold of different frequencies tends to flatten out, and finally an individual is able to start processing sounds better. Once, normal hearing is restored, many behavioural and learning difficulties can now be resolved.

The treatment involves two 30-minute sessions a day (at four hour intervals) for ten days. These are normally consecutive, but breaks may be allowed for the weekend. Both adults and children show improvements in academic and social performance.

Also, in some cases of non-verbal autism, AIT, has triggered the development of speech. Many people suffering from suicidal depression have also reported that AIT has transformed their lives. The initial benefits of AIT are often seen within days and progress continues to develop over several months.

Space Clearing
By Ali Northcott

Space clearing is a way of energising your living space or any area in which you spend time, creating a positive atmosphere that feels good and supports your personal energy.

It can be used to clear away any negative or stagnant energy left by past events and replace them with a positive charge to the atmosphere which feels good. Or simply to enhance and improve the energy so that we feel uplifted.

Most people would recognise the need for an energetic clear out when they move into a new home, as it is a great way of clearing out the old and inviting in the new.

Once a place has been Space Cleared, you can see and feel the difference, everything feels lighter, and gains a clarity and vibrance. The atmosphere becomes charged with positive energy, which is conducive to positive experiences, good health, and new opportunity, which benefits everyone.

Space clearing can be used in our every day lives to maintain the energy in our homes and keep it flowing. It is also very effective when used after illnesses or any traumatic event to clear the air and restore balance.

Negative atmospheres

We are all aware of the impact of a negative atmosphere. We are able to feel and describe changes in the atmosphere after a negative event, even from a minor incident. For example after an argument we say that 'you could cut the atmosphere with a knife'. Negative experiences and behaviour patterns, such as unhappiness, misfortune and ill health, leave a negative imprint on the energy and presence of a place.

This can be unsettling to our energy, and feel unwelcoming. These negatively charged atmospheres have the ability to attract negative events and feelings, which effect the way that we behave and function.

Past events

Space Clearing techniques are excellent for transforming spaces where a negative energy or presence has been building up in the atmosphere over a period of time. Some times we can find ourselves repeating the same pattern in the same place, such as arguments which always seem to start off in a certain area of the home.

The same old issues get triggered, it is as though we are replaying the same event. We can even find that we seem to pick up on the way that person felt that used to live in our home. It is helpful to free the atmosphere of these old patterns and create new ones for our selves.

Clearing clutter

Clutter is the physical aspect of blocked and stagnant atmospheres. Our physical space or external landscape

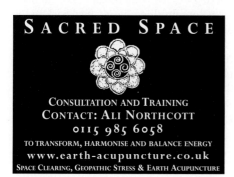

reflects of our internal landscape. When we store clutter, this reflects unresolved area in our lives. Letting go of clutter can be hard but extremely fruitful as it shows a readiness for new experiences and creates space for new opportunities.

Practitioners

The techniques used in Space Clearing come from a rich heritage of traditions that have been kept alive in the East and are now undergoing a revival in the West. A practitioner will bring techniques that have been past down from ancient cultures, such as Bali and the American Indian traditions.

They will have a wide range of tools including singing bowls, rattles, bell, candles, incense, smudge sticks, crystals, tinctures and essences. Also working with rituals, sometimes including movement and voice in order to perform ceremonies to bless and purify the space.

The space is cleared and a new pattern of energy is initiated into the atmosphere, by focusing energy and intention along with the appropriate ritual and elemental tool.

This can differ according to the spirit of the place and the needs of the people living there. If it is appropriate then some practitioners will invite you to get involved in the process of Space Clearing, and teach you some basic ways of maintaining the energy.

The benefits

Space Clearing is a very creative process, it is a great way of inviting positive change and transforming the way a place feels. Places that feel good uplift us; we immediately connect with those places. People who have had their space cleared experience a wide range of benefits, from improvements in their personal energy, health and wellbeing.

They often find it easier to let go of old and negative patterns in their lives, which assist in their relationships to themselves and other people. People find a renewed energy and commitment to the place that they live in.

Case history

Clearing out my rooms had been on my mind for some time, but it was always 'a job to do tomorrow' and then a Feng Shui practitioner told me that cluttered space was characteristic of a disorganised person. This made me think of how cluttered my mind was – not concentrating on or finishing any one particular task, thus doing, but not finishing, a dozen things all at the same time. This made me determined to take the advice of my Feng Shiu friend.

So there I was enjoying great success clearing out 14 years of collected 'rubbish', things I though that I needed at the time, but before finishing I was called back to the office to deal with an insurmountable problem, and I was frantic with anxiety. On reaching home in the evening my partner asked me why I was so edgy and why the lounge was full of junk. By this time I was distraught. Then I remembered why I had put the junk in the lounge in the first place. I had intended sorting it out, as I explained to my partner. He fell about with laughter and I got so angry that I threw everything in the bin. Strangely enough I enjoyed doing it and realised that clearing my home had definitely had a therapeutic effect and that the problem in the office would take nothing to solve!

Melissa, Plymouth

Spinal Touch Therapy

By Major Hugh M Jones, School of Spinal Touch Therapy

Spinal Touch is a century-old therapy for people of all ages which is drug-free, non-invasive and painless – it is so gentle it can tickle! The sufferer stands in front of a hanging plumb line which shows where the spine should be and where it is and the therapist makes some simple assessments showing how the therapy should be applied.

Next, the client is placed face down on a therapy table where the spine is supported by carefully-placed cushions; in many cases the pain will ease even before therapy starts. The body relies for its control and reporting function upon the nerves, which mainly emerge from the spine.

Our life-style – bad car seats, loads carried on one shoulder or in front, fashion shoes, poor diet, slouching and so on – can distort the spine so the muscles around it have to work overtime to hold it up and can't relax.

Two things happen: the muscles don't release used go-juice so it converts to poison, making the muscles ache, and the bunched muscles press on the nerve roots at the spine, which causes pain and makes organs malfunction.

Back pain is by far the biggest single reason for time off work and the cause is almost entirely bad posture; distorted spines 'lock in' today's work effort so it's still there when you start tomorrow, and the cumulative load can take the back beyond its ability to recover.

The therapy itself is given by a thumb being placed under a selected buttock and the other hand being used to gently rub a host of places over the buttocks, spine, shoulders, neck, head and abdomen.

This instructs the muscles holding the spine to relax – and in almost every case the muscles obey! Once the muscles are relaxed the spine straightens so pressure is taken off the nerve roots. Pain and sickness go, but the therapist will usually give advice about life-style changes to keep them away. On average people need about four or five treatments to ensure complete relief and should thereafter have treatment every few months as a 'top-up'.

So what sort of cases can Spinal Touch handle? The answer is just about everything. Success has been achieved treating piles, prostate trouble, St Vitus's Dance, impotence, bed-wetting, allergies, breathing difficulty, headaches, constipation, nerves, poor eyesight, hay fever, lack of energy – you name it!

For back pain it is the absolute tops; while other treatments can relieve the pain, it will return unless in addition the spine is put back where it should be and Spinal Touch does exactly that.

Spiritual and Psychic Development

By Kamini Alena Hola

Times are a-changing in the new Millennium... and fast! Over the last few hundred years society has undergone a tremendous development in the technological and material sense; this century in particular has witnessed change at an ever-accelerating rate.

But what about us humble human beings? How are we coping? A look at the levels of stress, violence and breakdown in traditional values in society today reveals that an equally major adjustment is needed in other areas of our lives.

Indeed, the rapid growth in recent years in the areas of healing, holistic learning, personal and spiritual development has been phenomenal and shows that society is evolving.

The growing number of therapists who offer a variety of physical and emotional healing methods is spreading to the traditionally allopathic sector. Who would have thought, just a few years ago, that some NHS physiotherapists would be able to offer acupuncture as part of their daily work? Or that kinesiology, massage and aromatherapy practitioners would be found affiliated to doctor's surgeries?

The need for change is particularly acute in the area of education. While the school curriculum aims to teach subjects necessary for the individual to earn a living, what about teaching the skills that we really need in order to live life?

Life skills such as compassion communication, patience, listening, awareness, service, sharing, storytelling and a willingness to see life as a wonderful adventure to experience rather than a problem to resolve. Skills that nurture the creative being in each of us.

Workshops, courses, lectures and group experiences offering an alternative teaching to parents and children have changed the lives of millions.

This sea of change has been supported and nurtured in Personal Development Centres throughout the UK.

Such centres, whether situated in a quiet former stately home, or in a busy city centre, all have one general purpose in common: to provide an environment, facilities and support for creative expression, healing and reaming with a spiritual basis.

It is here that workshops and courses take place and that healing therapies can be learnt and experienced. Retreats allow people to find a supportive refuge from the pressures and conflicts of their daily lives.

Many centres do not subscribe to a single spiritual path, but promote a general involvement in the profound meaning and value of life. Often elements of what was traditionally ascribed to eastern culture are found on the daily programme, such as meditation, yoga and tai chi.

These centres of personal and spiritual development provide a vital reaming space, one which encourages self-enquiry, care for each other and the environment, and a deep search for peace and oneness, in a non-dogmatic and non-heretical way.

Some call this profound reaming – learning the essence of life within and in all things, as well as bringing our connection into everyday reality.

Perhaps one of the greatest challenges for many, and the greatest opportunity for the future, is remaining to live and communicate with others in peace and harmony. For this reason, several centres offer an experience of community life, short or long term, residential or more temporary.

Some offer a free, long-term programme for young adults as well, which involves participating in the day to day activities of the centre, in return for free board and lodgings and lots of free time to spend in nature and in which to reflect upon the meaning of life.

As society is undergoing tremendous technological change, it is naturally creating alternative places of holistic healing and learning, personal growth and spiritual development to help humans adapt while maintaining their integrity. Long may theses centres serve as beacons of light, and guide society through this era of extraordinary change.

Spirit Release Therapy

By Alan Sanderson MB, BS, DPM,MRCP, MRCPsych

Spirit release is not a complete treatment. It will only have lasting success if it is used as part of a comprehensive approach to the spiritual health of the individual. It may be necessary also to treat the effects of trauma, both in this life and in previous lives. Soul integration and inner child healing may be called for.

The client is instructed in spiritual protection. More important than the use of protective techniques, is a life in which fear and anger are replaced by love and forgiveness and where there is an acceptance of the spiritual basis of existence.

Spirit release, as now practised, is a new therapy. True, its roots reach back to ancient times, but the beliefs and practices of contemporary spirit release therapists are based not on faith, but upon experience with many thousands of cases.

Spirit release therapy differs fundamentally from the religious rite of exorcism, for it is non-confrontational and shows concern for the attached spirit as well as for the host. It is a love-based, secular therapy, developed in the consulting room and still developing.

SRT, as practised in the US over the last 15 years, comes largely from the work of two outstanding pioneers, Edith Fiore and Bill Baldwin.

Fiore, a clinical psychologist specialising in past-life regression, came across discarnate spirits in many of her clients. 'The Unquiet Dead' (1987) gives a riveting account of this work.

Baldwin, a one-time dentist, took the subject further. In addition to earthbound spirits of deceased humans, he described thought forms and non-human entities, principally the dark force entities, which are to be found particularly in cases of depression and addiction.

Soul fragments of living humans are also described. Baldwin (1992) gives detailed protocols for diagnosing and releasing the different types of entity.

Another method, practised on the Continent, and recently introduced into the UK, is that of Karl Nowotny, a leading Austrian psychiatrist whose death, in the 1964 was followed by six channelled volumes, first published in German in 1972.

Nowotny states that emotional disturbance comes from an incorrect attitude, basically a lack of love for humanity, and is often exacerbated by spirit interference.

The focus of treatment is upon the patient taking responsibility for his/her own condition and progress. Once this happens, Nowotny and his team in spirit, rehabilitate the attached entities.

Spirit attachment is a common occurrence, which is usually unsuspected by the host. It can present in many ways. Unexplained fatigue, depression, anxiety, sudden changes in mood, addictions of all sorts, hearing voices, uncharacteristic changes in personality or behaviour, problems of sexual orientation, unexplained somatic symptoms – these have all been described in association with attached spirits. Diagnosis is achieved by having the subject focus inward, in an altered state of consciousness, then by dialogue, through the subject, with the attached entity. After identification, including the reason for attaching and the ways in which the entity has affected the subject, it is helped to leave.

This can involve negotiation and treatment for the entity, which will have its own problems. Angelic help is often necessary, always so in dealing with dark force entities. Spirits from the light are asked to assist in recovering any of the client's missing soul fragments and in healing the soul. Treatment may require one (occasionally) or many sessions, depending on individual need.

What conditions are most likely to benefit from spirit release?

More important than diagnosis is the patient's attitude and openness to work in the spiritual dimension. Some people are too frightened, others totally reject the spiritual approach.

Most case reports have dealt with mild or moderate cases of emotional disturbance. Among the most dramatic have been cases of sexual dysphoria. Patients treated by spirit release, when on the brink of a sex change operation, have experienced a complete change of attitude and have cancelled the operation.

My experience, as a psychiatrist with access to patients in hospital, is that, no matter what the condition, anyone able to trust and to co-operate fully can benefit.

But spirit release is not a cure-all; it is only one aspect of treatment, albeit an important one. Self-harm is an area in which spirit release is particularly indicated, since such patients often have the spirits of suicides with them.

However, it is important also to treat the historical causes of the deep psychological pain which such patients experience.

Schizophrenia presents serious problems, since it is often impossible to establish the necessary trust, and the patient's connection to reality may be too tenuous for effective therapeutic contact. Modi (1997) describes a case, successfully treated, first by remote spirit release through a relative, then by direct release with the therapist.

Remote spirit release allows therapy from a distance. It is usually done with two therapists, one acting as scanner. The scanner projects part of her consciousness to the target subject. Any attached entities may use her voice to speak to the facilitator.

Remote work is only done with the patient's consent, or where this is not feasible, for instance with a young child, with the agreement of the patient's higher self. It is preferable to have the patient consciously involved in the procedure of spirit release, whenever possible.

It is rare to find one who can give good counsel. It is more rare to find one who listens to advice. It is difficult to find an expert physician. Fewer still will take his medicine.

Spiritualism

By M. Willcocks PhD

A number of eminent people have supported investigations in the field of Spiritualism, including the British writers Sir Arthur Conan Doyle and Sir Oliver Joseph Lodge.

Unlike many other religions, Spiritualism does not tie its adherents to a creed or dogma. Rather, the philosophy of Spiritualism is founded upon seven basic principles, which were developed and derived through the mediumship. These Seven Principles, which act as guidelines for the development of a personal philosophy of how to live one's life, are stated as follows:

The Fatherhood of God; The Brotherhood of Man; The Communion of Spirits and the Ministry of Angels; The continuous existence of the human soul; Personal responsibility; Compensation and retribution hereafter for all the good and evil deeds done on earth; Eternal progress open to every human soul. Although spiritualism, the belief that the dead manifest their presence to people, usually through a clairvoyant or medium, has been practised in one form or another since prehistoric times, modern spiritualism is the result of 19th-century occurrences and research.

In the 1840s, there was a child medium named Margaret Fox capable of quite incredible hypnotic results. Her sister and father aroused sensational news stories that spurred the creation of the cult of spiritualism. It was given impetus by the writings of another American medium, Andrew Jackson Davis, who asserted that he also was capable of performing certain intellectual feats in a trance that he could not perform normally.

At about the same time, British surgeon James Braid provided a scientific explanation of mesmerism and thus helped to establish the modern technique of hypnosis. In 1872 a former British clergyman, William Stainton Moses, became editor of the spiritualist paper Light and wrote several books on spiritualism. The movement was publicly discredited after the appearance of a number of charlatans, whose demonstrations were recognised as simple tricks of prestidigitation.

Margaret Fox herself, as a grown woman, claimed that she had used tricks to make her 'spirit rappings'. Nevertheless, serious investigators believed some truth lay behind the reports of other mediums. The Society for Psychical Research was founded and a fund was established to examine the claims of spiritualism. Easy and conventional comments made upon Spiritualism by journalists seem to be singularly lacking in logical sense, and there seems to be an underlying assumption by the media that the more often a dishonest medium or fraudulent seance is discovered, the more spiritualism is diminished.

As a matter of intellectual justice it is desirable to protest against this confused argument, which connects the proved falsity of knaves with the probable falsity of psychic phenomena. The two things have no logical connection. No conceivable number of false mediums affects the probability of the existence of real mediums one-way or the other. If anything, the argument might as well be turned the other way. It could be said, with rather more reason, that as all hypocrisies are the evil fruits of public virtue, so in the same way the more real spiritualism there is in the world the more false spiritualism there is likely to be.

Stress Management

By Derek Webster

Stress accounts for over 70 per cent of visits to your GPs surgery and for the loss of 6.7 million working days, costing society about £3.7 billion. Stress Management is thus important, not only to the individual, but to society as a whole.

The term stress, as applied by Hans Selye, the founding father of the movement, is used to imply effect, the causal factors being termed 'Stressors'. These stressors do not directly create stress but are mediated by the way we think about them – our self-talk, beliefs and attitudes. This we call cognitive appraisal. If the stress continues for long enough it creates distress and disease.

Thus: STRESSORS + COGNITIVE APPRAISAL = STRESS -> DISEASE

Although the same physical reaction can occur to positive triggers, producing eustress rather than distress, it usually doesn't last very long and therefore is unlikely to create disease. I prefer to call this positive arousal in order to simplify the equation.

How then do we manage stress?

We can deal with the stressor directly by trying to change it or get away from it. You could, for example, get a divorce, move, or give up your job, but it may not always be possible or advantageous to do this.

You can deal with the stress directly by learning relaxation skills. Stress and relaxation are defined as opposites. If you relax correctly, and for long enough periods, I can guarantee that your stress related illnesses will disappear for as long as you do it. But I suspect that when the next lot of stressors come along the first thing you will stop is your relaxation practice. And to some extent relaxation is closing the stable door after the horse has bolted. Theoretically if you didn't get stressed you wouldn't have to relax!

So maybe the thing to do is change the way you think about the stressors and there are many ways of doing this – REBT, NLP and TA for example, as well as by taking up particular philosophies or through life itself. Unfortunately, this isn't the whole answer either, although it can produce the most profound effects.

Much of the stress response is a bad habit and can occur even when there are no stressors for you to think about or react to. Therefore it is worth learning to relax in order to resolve this. Furthermore it has been found that in a deeply relaxed state you are more likely to change your thinking and behaviour by means of a visualisation process.

Likewise, if your partner is chasing you around the house with an axe, hell bent on mutilation, there is little point in relaxing and persuading yourself that they are lovely really, and if you think nice thoughts they will stop it. Get the hell out of there! So what am I saying? In essence I'm pointing out that working on all three elements is important.

Your key initial strategy is to learn relaxation skills – this will help you to get rid of the symptoms that may be making your life such a misery. Relaxation is something quite physiologically specific and is best learned with the help of at least temperature and muscle biofeedback where specific criteria can be reached. You can then be sure you are truly producing the opposite of stress.

Learn how to change your thinking, beliefs and attitudes in order to reduce your negative emotions and enhance the positive ones by learning one of the numerous cognitive restructuring techniques.

When you can relax and have changed your thinking you may only occasionally have to remove yourself from the stressor. Usually you will be able to adapt or resolve it by using the other key skills of assertion and problem solving.

Any stress management training, especially for specific disorders needs to take all of this into account and above all teach skills. Make sure that your trainer whether personal, group or within a corporate setting, does not merely allude to things you need to learn, suggest diversions, or strategies that intervene between stressor and disease, leaving the rest of the equation intact and allowing the stress to break out in some other way.

"You can either take action, or you can hang back and hope for a miracle… miracles are great but they are so unpredictable and learn from the mistakes of others, you can't live long enough to make them all yourself" – **Eleanor Roosevelt.**

Tantra

By Mark Maxwell, the Brighton School Of Tantra

The body, our sensations, emotions and thoughts, in fact the whole of existence, are a manifestation of subtle energy. Tantra concentrates on developing our awareness of this subtle energy (Chi, Chakras, meridian channels, the aura). Through this development we begin to realise the ultimate nature of reality.

We can learn to recognise, practice and stabilise our innate, enlightened perspective. This is not a path of detachment from the world but one of immersion in it. Many spiritual dogmas consider the body as an unnecessary, even evil accessory to spiritual life. Tantra sees it as a profound vehicle for transformation.

Tantra is amongst the oldest spiritual teachings from the east. It has its roots in the Hindu, Buddhist, Taoist, and Western Alchemical traditions and is essentially a path to enlightenment. What differentiates it from other spiritual philosophy is its use of the body as well as the mind as a tool for greater awareness.

The techniques involved are as numerous as the number of its teachers. However there are a few common themes that permeate their message.

Firstly that Tantra is essentially a path of the Heart. It is through the heart that we can reconcile the apparent separation between spirit and matter, and it is through the heart that we can experience the sublime love and compassion that lies behind the 'bliss' of enlightenment.

Secondly Tantric practice focuses on certain tools and techniques. Commonly a practitioner uses meditation, visualisation, ritual and physical exercises e.g. Yoga, Chi Kung and Mudra (hand and body postures) to increase awareness of the enlightened perspective. They may also use Yantras and Mandalas (art for meditation) and the chanting of Mantras. Ultimately, however, one simply aspires to be continually present, spontaneous and blissful in every aspect of life.

Sexual practices are a smaller part of more authentic teachings. Sexual Tantra uses the highly potent zing energy of arousal to stimulate and balance the subtle energy centres (Chakras) of the body/mind. Through sex we can more easily experience the reality of our unity with others and the world around us. We can also speed up the evolution of our awareness and creative potential and develop our understanding of the 'bliss' mentioned above.

Certain methods of enhancing and controlling orgasm are used to prolong intercourse and heighten our ecstatic feelings. These take time and patience to master but the end result is very rewarding. Psychotherapeutic methods are often used to overcome sexual neuroses and encourage greater levels of communication between partners. In essence Sexual Tantra enables us to walk the spiritual path, which can often be a rather lonely experience, hand in hand with our lover. These highly stylised

TANTRA

THE BRIGHTON SCHOOL OF TANTRA.
Meditation, Massage, Chi Kung and Sexual Tantra Classes. Develop awareness and ecstatic sensuality through the subtle energies of the body/mind. INFO: Flat1, 4 Adelaide Crescent, Hove, BN3 2JD. Tel: 01273 746928 e-mail: unwinding@easynet.co.uk

eastern traditions are continually being adapted for the western seeker. The modern world, with all its intensity and interest in ecstatic experience, resonates strongly with Tantra. It will undoubtedly be corrupted by some and tremendously healing for others. Beware of cheap imitations.

The aspirant should know that some techniques (especially energy channelling) could be very powerful. Practising without the reliable foundation and support of an experienced practitioner, during what is often an overwhelming journey, can be dangerous. My advice is to begin by searching within. Know first your intention and motivation. If these are clear then you will find what you are looking for.

The Father of Medicine
By M Willcocks PhD

There are many references to Hippocrates, the father of medicine, in this book. Hippocrates, circa 460-377BC, unlike many figures in the Ancient World, was not a product of mythology. As Greek civilisation developed and reading and writing became increasingly important, notable scientists, mathematicians and writers began to be identified.

Hippocrates was one of them, a doctor who worked on the Greek island of Cos. He is regarded as the 'father of medicine' because his followers wrote over 60 medical books covering a wide range of medical topics including gynaecology, head wounds and diseases. He also founded a medical school on Cos.

Hippocrates developed a new approach to medicine by refusing to use gods to explain illnesses and disease. This meant that medicine came to be seen as a science rather than a religion.

Hippocrates stressed the importance of observation, diagnosis and treatment and developed the theory that the body had four humours – black bile, yellow bile, phlegm and blood. Illness occurred, he believed, if one of these humours was out of balance and the body therefore contained too much or too little of it.

He stressed the importance of fresh air, a good diet and plenty of exercise to help the body heal itself. All of Hippocrates's students had to follow a strict ethical code which governed their behaviour as doctors.

Students swore that they would maintain patient confidentiality and never deliberately poison a patient. Even today, doctors entering the profession can choose to swear the Hippocratic oath. This oath was an attempt to place doctors on a higher footing than other healers and set them apart as specialists.

Hippocrates's ideas were a strange mixture of common sense and factual inaccuracies. His suggestions about diet and exercise are as valid today as they were 2,400 years ago, as was his use of observation.

However, his belief in the Four Humours was completely wrong. Strangely enough, this theory lasted until the 17th century, but the importance of exercise and diet was forgotten after the Romans!

Hippocrates's most important contributions were in the development of the medical profession and in a code of conduct for doctors.

Toe Reading

By Anthony Hampton

Toe reading is not a method of clairvoyance, it does not foretell the future for an individual but rather it can point the way that person may wish to take by their own free choice.

Feet are as individual as are the people that own them, no two pairs of feet are exactly the same they come in all shapes arid sizes. Similarly no two sets of toes on those feet will be an exact mirror image. They can be completely different in length, shape and direction. They may be crooked, cross over or under another toe, have flat, pointed or rounded ends. Some may appear to be clawing to get a grip whilst others appear to be floating in mid air.

Compare your own toes to those of a very young child, generally speaking they have beautifully straight toes, graduated in length and in perfect symmetry. It would appear that as we mature and become aware the toes become distorted and out of shape, some quite ugly in appearance. Why should this be so? What is it that causes the toes to change so dramatically.

Imre Somogyi found the study of feet and toes to be very interesting and after much research and many observations came to the realisation that the toes were in effect a mirror of a persons personality and soul.

Energy passes down through the body then outwards at the hands and feet and returns to the head in a continual cycle in a similar manner to the magnetic energy that flows through and out of a bar magnet. The energy that flows through the human body can be likened to magnetic energy in that it cannot be detected by our normal five senses, we only know it exists by what it does.

In the human body the flow of energy can be disturbed by illness or the condition of the internal organs causing a slowing or deflection from its normal route resulting in disharmony. Reflexologists for example can detect this and identify the area of the body where an imbalance is present.

In a similar way personality imbalances appear to be reflected in the toes causing them to become distorted in various ways. Mr Somogyi came to realise that each individual toe registered part of the human character and he gave a meaning and purpose to each.

Trager

What is Trager work? Think about softening, widening. Think about lengthening, expanding. Think about light, lighter, and lighter still. Think about a dancing cloud.

Now take a moment and notice how your body feels just thinking of these things. TRAGER movement education both creates and operates from a feeling state of pleasurable, effortless, easy movement.

Trager Psychophysical Therapy has been around since the 1930s and has gained popularity steadily in the UK over the last four years.

How long does it take?

A full Trager experience is 90 minutes, which includes an exploration into Mentastics.

Mentastics? Is that a related cult?

Very funny. Mentastics is the exercise, homework, side of Trager bodywork. Based on neuromuscular re education, integration and effortlessness it is a series of movements to use yourself to recreate the sensations you experienced while being treated by the practitioner.

How much does it cost?

About £60 in the comfort of your home or £55 – £75 at a studio.

How many sessions does it take to notice a difference?

Three in quick succession.

What are some DIY techniques?

Trager can be used in your everyday life with these easy to follow techniques: Let one arm drop softly by your side and gently waggle the fingers of your hand and think about feeling the bones.

How much does that hand weigh? Now do the same on the other side. You may find your arm visibly lengthens as you relax.

Sitting down, imagine that your head is attached to the ceiling by a large rubber band. Feel how that affects your posture- making you straighter but not bolt upright. Feel your shoulders softly come down as your head bobs on the elastic.

Now imagine that you have a paintbrush fixed to the top of your head and that you are gently painting the ceiling with it.

Allow your head to wobble from side to side with tiny little movements.

Couches and Treatment Equipment

By M. Willcocks Ph.D

There are many tools such as treatment couches used by therapists; this piece will help to describe the use of a selection of these tools/devices;

Postural Drainage Boards: A postural drainage board, couch or table is used to position the patient effectively for physiotherapy, deriving maximum benefit from gravity in helping to clear secretions.

Pep Mask: (positive expiratory pressure) mask is a breathing device, which causes resistance to expiration.

Percussors/Vibrators: A precursor or vibrator is a mechanical device that assists in the mobilisation of bronchial secretions by applying vibratory pressure to the chest wall during postural drainage.

Inhaled Medication Equipment: Inhaled medications can be an essential component of the therapist's equipment, for the purposes of inhalation.

Nebuliser: An inhalation set consists of a nebuliser, mask or mouthpiece, and tubing. It is used in conjunction with a compressor, which forces air through the nebuliser, aerosolising the medication and pushing it through the mouthpiece or mask for inhalation.

Puffer: A puffer is used to deliver aerosolised medication from a pressurised container. These devices are often used to deliver bronchodilators and inhaled steroids.

Aero Chamber: The Aero Chamber is attached to the metered dose inhaler (puffer), and holds a puff of medication until the patient is ready to inhale it deeply.

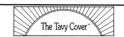
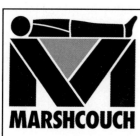

Tui-na

By Amanda Rogers

Tui-na, which literally means 'push - grasp', is an ancient system of healing dating back more than 4,000 years. An invigorating massage it is often accompanied with moxibustion – a herb of mutwort burnt close to the skin to heat the blood and improve energy flow.

Other techniques often used in conjunction are cupping- cups are applied with heat and placed systematically on the body to create a vacuum and draw out toxins. Chi nei tsang – a treatment in its own right – is often applied, the focus being directed more specifically to the organs. Chinese herbs and martial arts can play a part as well.

Tui-na's unique approach is in the varied strokes employed. It differs from Shiatsu which is a modified Japanese form which came into being much later. Shiatsu applies constant pressure with the pad of the thumb or the palm directed downward while one hand maintains a connection with the tantien – the bodies energy source just below the navel.

Tui-na interweaves connective tissue work with energy work. using rocking, gripping, applying traction, friction rubbing, rolling and even pounding! Needless to say' it is quite dynamic, and leaves one feeling invigorated and elated!

Tui-na for children is also very popular! In the womb, the umbilical cord is our life energy. When the cord is cut the new-born has to breathe, and fend, for itself with the first breath. the whole of the ribcage expands like an accordion. As we go from infancy to adulthood there is a tendency to use only the upper part of our chest when we breathe.

When working the navel, releasing the tissues surrounding the organs, and 'clearing space' we enable the breath to once more be drawn deeply into the abdomen, nourishing, oxygenating, and releasing trauma that we build up and store over time.

The dichotomy is that our protective armour is what hurts us. Protection is the result of injury... injury occurs because of compensation... compensation is protection. Therefore, the more we free up our bodies the stronger we become and the less likely to injure ourselves and our environment.

The Chinese philosophy is that everything in nature exists in the hot, energy becomes matter and matter dissolves into energy. We can breakdown energy' and matter into five elements. They are Wood, Fire, Earth, Metal and Water. Each element either feeds – as in the mother, or contains – as in the father the corresponding element.

For example, water feeds wood. If a tree is thirsty then we know the water energy is disturbed. In the case of a forest fire the water which controls the fire is depleted. So the emphasis would be on energising the water element. Similarly in the body if there were dehydration or inflammation the water element would need to be addressed. Inside the elements lie the energetic pathways – each associated with a particular organ.

The blood filled organs that lie deep in

TUI-NA

MS A RODGERS, Clapham Common Clinic, 151-153 Clapham High Street, London, SW4 7SS. 0956 210454 the body are yin in nature, i.e. kidneys, heart etc. while the organs that are more vacuous are 'yang' in nature i.e. the intestines. Yin and Yang are the opposing forces that exist in all things. Yin is the dark side of the mountain – the cool, deep, nurturing aspect of nature. While Yang, the light side of the mountain, is fiery, expressive and creative. The expression 'opposites attract' is a result of this phenomenon!

Tui-na has withstood the test of time. Where many western therapies come in and out of fashion, Tui-na's roots lie deep because they follow the laws of nature. Those that become extinct are those who cannot adapt to a changing environment. This is the power of Tui-na, the recognition that the earth and our bodies are the same.

Coming of age

By M Willcocks PhD

A popular misconception is that Chinese medicine is acupuncture alone. But it is a far broader concept that also embraces the use of herbs, moxibustion, massage, medicinal foods and therapeutic massage, known as Tuina.

While interest in Oriental medicine – and other 'alternative' therapies – has been increasing in this country for a number of years, there are still many who remain unconvinced of their effectiveness. Criticism is sometimes justified – though this is most likely due to the damaging actions of a minority of ill-trained and unscrupulous practitioners rather than a true indication of Oriental Medicine's potential.

A growing concern is the lack of an official regulatory body – at present anyone may establish a practice, whether or not they possess the relevant qualifications.

Although a national register has been proposed, many people still feel that not enough is being done to develop and maintain standards and keep out the quacks. This may all be about to change, with the intervention of the Government's CAM (Complementary Alternative Medicine) initiative. The CAM proposals will require all therapists to be registered with a regulatory body within the BMA.

More and more people are turning to Oriental medicine, despite Western medical advances, as they seek an effective cure without side effects. In the proper hands, traditional Chinese medicine can produce just this result. Nonetheless, the discipline is still viewed by much of the orthodox medical establishment as suspect.

In Vietnam the use of Chinese medicine has long been accepted. Yet even there it is undergoing a number of changes in a bid to survive into the next millennium.

Much of the herbal medicine available both in Asia and the UK is still produced on a relatively small scale and in the traditional manner. However, at the Thien Hung Medicine Company on the outskirts of booming Ho Chi Minh City, hi-tech, automated production lines are churning out herbal pills for the domestic and foreign markets by the million. Probably the most convincing argument in favour of Thien Hung Medicine is Mr. Thien Long himself who uses his own medicines regularly. For a man of 70 he is in remarkable condition and, if the rumours are true, the father of seven children to three different wives – the latest of which is said to be half his age.

When even your GP can offer you acupuncture for the treatment of certain conditions, you know Oriental medicine is gaining acceptance.

Vegetarianism

By M Willcocks PhD

Eating patterns have changed significantly over the past few decades. One trend has been towards a decreased intake of fat because of evidence linking fat consumption to increased risk of heart disease and other health problems.

In addition, recent evidence indicates that adding more fruits, vegetables and grains, sources of nutrients such as complex carbohydrates, anti-oxidants and fibre, may help decrease the risk of certain chronic diseases. Dietary changes which emphasise the inclusion of more vegetarian foods can help accomplish the goals essential to a weight control programme. The value of a completely vegetarian way of eating depends on careful meal planning and attention to nutritional balance – limiting fat, saturated fat and cholesterol; using sugars, salt and sodium in moderation; eating vegetables and fruits.

Including a variety of foods is important. Vegetarian diets which omit complete groups of foods without sufficient substitutes can have adverse effects. The more limited and restrictive the diet, the greater the likelihood of developing nutrient deficiencies. Selecting adequate foods from each major category (protein, carbohydrate and fat) will enhance a vegetarian diet.

Vegetarian foods are often so high in bulk that people get full before they can eat enough to meet their caloric requirements and may thus find it difficult to maintain a healthy weight. This can usually be remedied by adding more high calorie, nutrient-dense foods such as fruit juices, dried fruits, nut and seed butters, granola and cheese.

Protein is critically important for many body functions and it must be supplied from food. Unlike most animal foods, not all vegetarian foods are rich in protein. The best sources are beans, lentils, nuts and soy products. To improve the quality of protein, and enable it to be used effectively, these foods should be eaten daily and combined with pasta, bread, rice and other grains.

Important nutrients such as zinc, an essential component of the immune system; iron and vitamin B12, which prevent anaemia; and calcium and vitamin D, necessary for maintaining bone health are readily available in animal foods. Even modest portions of meat, poultry and fish can supply enough zinc, iron and B12 to satisfy daily requirements, therefore some people continue to include them, but less frequently, or in smaller amounts.

Without these foods, the selection of appropriate alternatives is important. Good sources of zinc are seafood, eggs, cheese, whole wheat and wheat germ. Iron is found in legumes (lentils, beans, peanuts and peanut butter), soy products and dried fruits.

The type of iron present in plant

foods, however, is less readily available to the body and this can increase the risk of iron deficiency when only plant sources are consumed. Milk, yoghurt, and cheese supply B12, as well as calcium and vitamin D. It should be noted that Vitamin B12 is present only in animal foods and strict vegetarians need to take a supplement to obtain this nutrient.

Contrary to popular belief, adequate dietary fat is essential. However, no more than 30 per cent of calories should be supplied as fat and no more than ten per cent of calories as saturated fat.

The best vegetarian sources are oils (olive, canola, peanut). Some vegetarian diets may contain increased amounts of fat, especially saturated fat, from cream, eggs, cheese and margarine. Individuals seeking to improve their diets may benefit from vegetarian food choices, but attention to nutrient adequacy is imperative. Strict limitations and a lack of variety may have serious adverse affects. People who have very specific health care needs, such as growing children, pregnant women and the elderly, will not necessarily thrive on a complete vegetarian programme.

Strict adherence to one specific pattern is not necessary; optimal nutrition can be achieved in many ways. Including a variety of foods, paying careful attention to nutritional balance and enjoying whatever you eat, together provide a basis for healthy eating habits. People choose a vegetarian diet for a variety of religious, philosophical, and ethical beliefs. Some people abstain from eating meat for religious reasons, for example Jains, and some Buddhists and Hindus, who believe that the killing and eating of animals violates the ethical precept of ahimsa, or nonviolence.

Ecological reasons motivate other people, because much less land and food outlay is required to raise vegetables and grain than livestock.

Some people avoid animal products for health reasons. Vegetarians may live longer and have much lower risks for heart disease, cancer, diabetes and other serious illnesses. They also tend to be thinner, to have lower blood pressure and have a lower risk of osteoporosis, a condition in which the bones get weaker as a person ages. These health effects are attributed to the fact that vegetarian diets tend to be lower in fat and cholesterol and higher in fibre and certain vitamins.

People may adopt a vegetarian diet due to concerns about the methods used for raising animals. Most chickens, pigs and veal calves are raised in close confinement and are given chemical additives in their feed and these practices offend many people on health and humane grounds.

In the past it was thought that vegetarians might develop protein deficiencies if they did not carefully combine their foods. It is now known that such careful planning is not necessary. Protein deficiencies do not occur if one eats a variety of plant foods and eats enough to maintain one's weight.

However, many nutritionists believe that vegans should eat vitamin-enriched cereals or take a vitamin supplement for vitamin B-12, which is needed in small amounts for healthy blood and nerves.

VEGETARIAN

THE FLOWER IN HAND guest house is a lovely listed building perched just above the South Bay harbour. Superb sea views, charming en-suite rooms, great breakfasts, including veggie and vegan. £19.50 pppn. Tel 01723 371471

HIGHER VENTON FARM, Widecombe-In-The-Moor, Newton Abbot, Devon, TQ13 7TF. 01364 621235

Vibrational Energy Alignment

By Jenny Hok

What is Vibrational Energy? I believe that it will be the medicine of the 20th Century. A magnetic field surrounds the Earth – and indeed each and every animate and inanimate being on and within the earth has its own magnetic field. A magnetic field is made up of energy.

Energy is found in all objects. An old stone or rock will have a vibration. Sometimes you can feel the vibration by holding your hand over it. People, animals and plants all have their own individual vibration, the rate of vibration changing under differing circumstances.

When a magnetic field goes out of balance, this can be due to an imbalance or blockage, in the energy field, and this in turn can result in disease for both the earth and for humans. Both our environment and our bodies can suffer due to many different factors. As humans, we try to look after our bodies and heal them, but we are not as aware of our homes and gardens.

A house may be built on or near an old burial ground, or an underground stream. Possibly some tragedy took place at the site in the past, leaving a disturbed energy behind, which in turn could affect the well being of the household today.

There are so many things within the invisible which we do not understand. For example, I know of a lady who moved into a new home, where everything was fine until she hung an old pair of curtains in one room; the vibrational energy of the room changed and she began to feel very uneasy. The house was subjected to Vibrational Energy Alignment. The curtains were thrown away, the house treated and within 24 hours everything was back to normal and harmony restored.

One use of VEA is where the energy of a house seems at a low ebb. It is possible there is blocked energy within the area. By rebalancing the vibrations to heal the area, the energies will be heightened, and an improvement in the health of a sick person may be noticed.

Animals, dogs and cats for example, have a greater sense of awareness than humans. It is interesting to note that after a building has been treated; the household pets tend to demonstrate their well being before the humans have sensed the change.

The Vibrational Energy Alignment treatment is carried out with sound, using Tuning Forks to clear any blockages, cleanse areas, and re-balance both buildings and the people (and pets) who live in them.

This can be achieved via 'distant treatment' with the practitioner working from a plan of the house area and a list of the inhabitants.

VIBRATIONAL ENERGY ALIGNMENT

Healing your environment

Please write to:
Mrs J Hok
Middle Old Park
Farnham
Surrey
GU10 5EA

Or telephone:
(00 44) (0) 1252 715092

Or send your e-mail to:
jennyhok@bizonline.co.uk

Vision Improvement
By Peter Mansfield

Bates Vision Education is a proven, successful and natural method for improving eyesight. Dr W H Bates of New York described his method for improving eyesight without glasses or surgery in 1920.

It is based on the elimination of strain from the visual system, and the development of 'central fixation' through relaxation and awareness of contrast and movement. The 'Bates Method' has been described in many books and taught, in various forms, worldwide for more than 80 years, with good results for millions of people.

The way we see reflects the behaviour of our eyes. The behaviour of our eyes in turn reflects the way we use them, as well as the way we relate to ourselves and to the world: eyesight problems can therefore express both misuse and the reasons for it. The fluid nature of the human system, including the visual system means that changes in the way we think and act can change the way the eyes work, for better as well as for worse.

While the 'Bates Method' concentrates on practical ways of improving the use of the eyes, Dr Bates, especially in his later writings, also showed great awareness and interest in the origins of the mental strain which leads to impaired vision, eg in emotional distress and physical misuse. 'Bates Vision Education' develops and amplifies these threads, exploring connections to many other branches of education and therapy, and always reaffirming the central importance of working in a practical way with the experience of seeing. In this way we can use the goal of clear sight to help

---

Where can I find a Bates Vision Teacher?

Karen Banks	London WC1 020 7831 7924 & Nottingham	**01159 608855**
Wendy Finch	Nantwich, Liverpool & Bolton	**01270 624303**
Julia Galvin	Brighton	**01273 554388**
Francesca Gilbert	Kingston, Surrey	**020 8549 9246**
Peter Mansfield	Brighton. *peterm@argonet.co.uk*	**01273 424752**
Margaret Montgomery	Herts, London W1, Essex, S.Devon & Hants *margaret.montgomery@btinternet.com*	**01442 862228**
Ajay Sehgal	London W5 and NW5	**020 8560 1844**
Aileen Whiteford	Edinburgh, Glasgow & Aberdeen.	**01875 819595**
Kevin Wooding	Oxford & London NW6. *kkwooding@breathe.co.uk*	**01865 514224**

Registered Members of the Bates Association for Vision Education
www.seeing.org
Bave PO Box 25 Shoreham by sea BN43 6ZF

us evolve as sensitive and expressive beings, in all our physical, emotional, mental and spiritual aspects, in relationship to ourselves and the world.

Members of the Bates Association have been trained in the authentic Bates tradition with the added benefit of modern insights and techniques. They are bound by the Association's rules and code of professional conduct. Bates Vision Teachers do not diagnose or treat disease, nor prescribe spectacles. The work is educational in nature: no guarantee of any particular degree of improvement can or will be given and all teachers accept pupils on that understanding. It is the responsibility of the pupil to seek the advice of medical or optical practitioners as appropriate.

Bates Vision teachers may also have other professional skills which may have application to a pupil's needs. The Bates Association has no knowledge of members' competence or qualifications in other fields and intending pupils are advised to make their own enquiries to ensure that they will receive the help they require. Although teachers give individual lessons to adults, most work with children. Some can also offer lectures and workshops, intensive residential courses or teacher training.

Case history

Name: Charlotte; Age: 7; Condition: Short-sighted.

It is now more than five years since Charlotte first experienced trouble with her eyesight. Now at the age of 12, it was gratifying to learn that she is having no trouble with her eyesight at home or at school and has truly learned the difference between using her eyes well and using them badly.

According to the optician's original prognosis she should have been bound to glasses long ago – thus giving further evidence for our observation that glasses reward us in using our eyes badly, lock the habits in place and truly create a need for themselves.

Charlotte's mother had heard about the Bates Method, and decided to investigate this treatment. On finding a Bates practitioner, an initial assessment of Charlotte was that she was indeed short sighted, but there were signs that her sight was still in a flexible state.

Lessons progressed weekly and fortnightly for about nine months. Charlotte absorbed every new technique and suggestion quite happily. Charlotte's sight improvement is now complete and she will have natural vision for the rest of her life.

Words of **Wisdom**

"*The great secret of doctors, known only to their wives but still hidden from the public, is that most things get better by themselves; most things, in fact, are better in the morning*"

LEWIS THOMAS

Voice Work

By Roz Comins at the Voice Care Network UK

There is greater awareness today of the availability and benefits of both voice therapy and voice training. Voice therapy and voice training have different purposes.

The wide range of exercises can be used to remedy disorders and problems with voice, as well as to develop skills for acting, singing, teaching, preaching, work that involves the use of voice, and for recreation and personal satisfaction.

As voice can be affected by posture, breathing, general flexibility of the muscles that produce voice, how confidently the voice is used in speaking, it is not surprising that the work includes relaxation, easy physical alignment, breathing, easy voice, sustained sounds and working on rhythms and words.

Voice is essential for words. They are made as the voice flows through the mouth. When we are born and take breath for our first cry, our voice sounds for the first time.

The growing infant listens and repeats the sounds and rhythms of the voices heard and learns to talk. This is an important part of being human. Voice is central to our lives and with words it is our most immediate way of expressing our thoughts and feelings and of understanding those of others.

A speech and language therapist completes basic training then adds specialist voice therapy skills to their qualifications.

They work with patients in medical setting. Most of them work in the health service, but some are in independent

They provide clinical treatment and remediation for patient's difficulties and disorders of voice. These may be presented as hoarseness, discomfort or pain felt in the throat, or serious loss of voice.

When a voice problem arises and persists, especially if it lasts over three weeks, and if it is not caused by cold or infection, an appointment needs to be made with a GP.

After diagnosis a prescription may be provided or a consultation arranged with a specialist in Ear, Nose and Throat (ENT). When the consultant has diagnosed the problem, referral may be made for clinical treatment with a voice therapist. It is essential that the consultant makes the diagnosis before the treatment begins.

A voice teacher works in the field of education and has professional training in teaching and in voice. Sometimes they are known as voice coaches or trainers.

Their work aims to strengthen the voice, and to develop skills in using it effectively and creatively. Basic exercises and techniques that are relevant and useful will aim to motivate and encourage both practice and application.

Results are achieved through personal involvement and motivation. It is satisfying to control your voice and know it will work as you wish, that you can get attention, hold interest and achieve the response needed from your listeners.

Voice workshops are a satisfying introduction to freeing the voice and developing skills. Group work with others involved is a natural and satisfying way of working and exercises can include talking and responding.

Individual voice coaching although it can focus on personal needs, lacks the support and rapport of a working group.

There needs to be easy communication between therapist and patient and between teacher and student. Those who try voice workshops for the first time are advised to try a taster session, and to check the providers' qualifications and experience.

A simple analogy with sport may clarify the difference between a voice therapist and a voice teacher. In very general terms a voice trainer increases muscular stamina and skills like a sports coach, while a voice therapist is like a physiotherapist whose work is to treat muscles that are strained or overused.

A number of voice therapists are deeply interested in the normal voice and train both therapists and teachers.

VOICE WORK THERAPY

LOUISA HARMER LRAM, ARCM. Find your natural intuitive guidance. Allow your story to unfold. Heal you psyche. No sound is wrong.(An invitation to work in this new way) Individual Sessions, Groups, Workshops for 'up to date' information. Tel: 020 7603 3602 Mobile: 07939 093 3640. e-mail: louisaharmer@yahoo.com. Applegarth Studio, Augustine Road, London, W14 OHZ. Sound & Voice.

Voice Care Network UK
Registered Charity No 1070980

Provides: **Information on voice care**
Voice awareness workshops
Voice coaching

A tutor list of: **Voice teachers & Speech and**
Language Therapists, professionally
trained and highly experienced

Contact: **Phone/fax: 01926 864000**
e.mail: **vcnuk@btconnect.com**
Website: **www.voicecare.org.uk**
Address: **VCN, 29 Southbank Road, Kenilworth CV8 1LA**

Water – a lifelong friend

By M Willcocks PhD

Hydrotherapy is the external application of water to the entire human body or a part of it for therapeutic purposes. It generally is available as part of spa therapy and has evolved into a separate form of treatment.

People have bathed in natural hot springs (and cold bodies of water) since the beginning of recorded history. Contemporary hydrotherapy pools are small, shallow, heated swimming pools. Some are circular and use jets to make the water swirl around; others are rectangular. The water is usually chlorinated, and the natural alkalinity of tap water is sometimes reduced until the water is neutral.

The main advantages of hydrotherapy relate to buoyancy and to heating or cooling. The human body immersed in water is buoyed up. Muscles need exert only a fraction of their normal effort to maintain a normal posture in the water.

A patient who is too weak to move an injured or convalescent limb without aid may be able to perform a full range of movements in a hydrotherapy pool. Polio victims and paraplegics may derive great benefit from this form of physical therapy.

The body may be warmed or cooled by using water that is relatively hot or cold. Hot water is initially stimulating, but then promotes muscular relaxation. It reduces pain and improves circulation. Cold water lowers body temperature, reduces blood circulation, increases muscle tone, reduces swelling after injury and reduces muscular pain. The use of baths for such purposes as well as for religious purification, personal cleanliness and private or social relaxation dates from at least the time of ancient Greece.

The use of spas in Europe became popular early in the 19th century. Little evidence exists that mineral waters supply anything specific that ordinary warm water or physiotherapy cannot.

Several kinds of therapeutic baths produce results through the selected temperature of the water, aided in some instances by the stimulation produced by a jet such as a needle shower or a whirlpool.

Baths at skin temperature are relaxing and sedative; those hotter or colder are stimulating. Baths may be given by submersion in water or, in the form of wet packs, by wrapping the body in wet sheets or towels.

All of the body may be submerged, or only a particular part may be bathed, as, for example, in the arm bath or footbath, or the sitz bath for the pelvic region.

The hot bath stimulates, relieves pain (particularly of cramps and sometimes of arthritis), controls convulsions, and induces sleep. Quickening the pulse and respiration, it also increases perspiration, thereby relieving the kidneys of part of their work and temporarily decreasing weight. Hot packs are helpful in muscular disorders. The cold bath is helpful in reducing high fever and limiting inflammation.

Stimulating baths are generally of short duration to avoid exhaustion; sedative warm baths may be continued for hours or, in the treatment of certain nervous diseases, for days. Kinotherapeutic baths, in which a routine of exercise is carried on while the patient is submerged, were successful in restoring the use of muscles damaged by poliomyelitis when that disease was still widespread. They are used today in the treatment of some bone diseases and fractures. When any substance intended to effect, or assist in, the cure of disease is added to the bath medium, the bath is called medicated. Soap, bath salts, bath oil and similar detergents are so common that they are not usually considered medicines.

Alcohol sponge baths are cooling and are useful in the prevention of bedsores. A hot bath with mustard added was a traditional remedy for infant convulsions, and alkaline baths have been used extensively in the treatment of rheumatic conditions.

Medicated vapours, both natural and artificial, are used in steam baths; the vapours often are allowed to fill a closed room in which the patient can walk about, exposing both skin and lungs to their effects.

Steam cabinets, which enclose the body from the neck down, are also used to give vapour baths. Carbonated waters are sometimes used, as are brines, although their value is uncertain.

Among the most popular medicated baths are those in which the waters of natural warm mineral springs are used. Thousands of people suffering from a wide variety of ailments frequent mineral baths in search of the cures attributed to local waters and muds, although their medical value is generally doubted.

Bathing has been part of religious practice as ritual purification since early times. It is still important among Hindus and Muslims. The mikvah in Orthodox Judaism and baptism in Christianity are derived from ritual bathing.

Bathing has also been considered important to health and comfort in some societies, notably those of the ancient Greeks and Romans and those of the West in modern times. Bathing may also have a social function, as in ancient times and in Turkey, Iran, and Japan.

The early Christian church, which considered physical cleanliness less important than spiritual purity, did not encourage private bathing and it censured the licentiousness of Roman public baths.

Bathing, especially in chilly northern Europe, came to be regarded as unhealthy and was frowned upon as an indulgence. Medieval builders paid more attention to fortifications and fireplaces than to water supply and drains.

Although many late medieval cities had public baths, which offered refreshment and entertainment to mixed company, such facilities were generally considered extremely disreputable.

Bathing, for most of the population, was rare. In northeastern Europe, where Roman influence had not penetrated and the church took longer to become established, the Finns and Russians developed steam baths, derived from the steam baths of the ancient Scythian nomads on the Eurasian steppe.

Finnish and Russian families built small wooden rooms or huts (sauna) with benches around the walls. Water thrown on heated rocks created dense clouds of steam, in which the bathers sweated.

They were then soaped, rubbed, flogged with softened birch twigs, and washed with tepid water. Finally they were splashed with cold water or plunged into snow or an icy stream.

Islamic societies, in southern Europe and the Middle East, which valued baths for religious, hygienic and social purposes, developed sophisticated bathing facilities. The rich built splendid baths in their homes. Public baths were built in every town that had a mosque. Some large cities, such as Cordoba in Spain, had hundreds of baths, which men and women visited separately.

In Constantinople and other Turkish cities, public baths served the same functions as Roman baths. They consisted of a large, domed, steam-heated central room surrounded by smaller rooms, the whole decorated with marble or mosaics. One could spend the day at the baths, enjoying refreshments and meeting friends. Turkish baths, like Roman baths, in time degenerated into resorts of idleness and indulgence.

The Japanese also set great store by social bathing. Almost every house had a bath, which was an indoor wooden tub or a garden pool. Washing was done first in private, but a whole family enjoyed soaking in a hot tub. In addition many large public baths were at mineral or hot springs where many families bathed together. These customs continue in modern Japan.

The puritanical spirit of the 16th-century Reformation further discouraged bathing in Europe and similarly affected the American colonies. In the 18th and 19th centuries, more secular in outlook, the wealthy adopted the habit of visiting natural medicinal or hot springs for their health.

It became fashionable to spend a few weeks each year taking the waters at such resorts as Bath in England, Vichy in France, Baden-Baden in Germany, or Saratoga Springs, New York, in the U.S.

Luxury hotels, fine shops, concert halls and casinos grew up around the baths. In 19th century cities, however, dirt and disease increased as a result of the Industrial Revolution. Cities were begrimed by factory smoke and overcrowded with people seeking factory work.

After an outbreak of cholera in London, demand gradually arose for improved bathing facilities. By the late 19th century, private houses of the upper classes were being built with separate bathrooms supplied with running water in fixtures of wood, copper, or iron. Municipal and private corporations built public baths for the general populace.

By the late 20th century, cleanliness was generally recognised as desirable, and as a result of mass production, most city dwellings had their own indoor baths. New housing was usually provided with one or more bathrooms, equipped with hot and cold running water in fixtures usually of gleaming porcelain enamel. Showers became commonplace.

Water Retention

Expanding waistline? It may not be what you eat

By M Willcocks PhD

Water retention can be a regular little demon that makes waistbands tighten, bras leave tram lines, rings wedge and ankles and feet swell.

With what seems like the flash of a devil's wand anything up to 8lbs can appear on the scales as if from nowhere. The why and how can be a mystery, but there's one thing all sufferers agree on – water retention is not a pretty sight!

The good news is we don't have to put up with it. There are ways forward and they are pretty painless.

Water retention is caused by a malfunctioning of the kidneys. In most cases it is not a signal that you have kidney problems – although if you are over 45 and find yourself suddenly suffering with bloating and swelling, especially of the ankles, then it would be a good idea to see your GP and ask for a general check.

Water retention can be a sign of renal hypertension, high blood pressure or heart problems so a GP check would eliminate worries and allow you to take on board the self-help cures we are discussing here.

In the vast majority of cases, water retention is the result of the kidneys not being allowed to do their job properly. And what a job it is! They are the lynch pin of an elaborate system designed by evolution to deal with everything we take in by mouth, air and through our skin. They can identify the good things our body needs, like vitamins and minerals, which they send back into the bloodstream. And they detect the nasties, like unwanted pollutants, which along with general waste they send into the body's reject and eject system. Without them we would be dead!

They work 24 hours a day and are also responsible for making sure that all parts of the body get water as and when they need it. And this is where we hit the nub of the water retention problem.

The kidneys take water from wherever they can find it within the body; if there isn't enough then they perform sluggishly. If water doesn't arrive where it's needed, the body thinks a drought-emergency is imminent and goes into panic mode. Instead of using and eventually shedding the water it has at its disposal in our cells and tissues it holds on to it and stores it in all those familiar places!

The cure is simple, so long as you don't fall into a common trap. Water retention doesn't mean you are holding too much water and therefore should drink less! Quite the contrary.

The answer is to drink more, try and drink at least one litre, preferably two, water naturally, every day. And that's on top of other drinks like tea or coffee. Bottled water is best, but tap water will do. Avoid salt on and in food, it only encourages the body to cling on to its water. Eat more fruit and vegetables, both are full of water as well as nutrition.

Keep the water flowing in and the kidneys will make sure it keeps on flowing out!

Yoga

By M. Willcocks PhD

This ancient practice is usually linked with many misconceptions. People tend to visualise bodies curled in pretzels, standing on your head or chanting while sitting in the lotus position. While meditation can be combined with yoga, and yoga does consist of many positions, it is as easy to learn as any new sport.

The benefits are unlimited. Yoga builds strength, composure and energy and can be practised in your own home. One of the main focuses of yoga is breath control. As you read this article you are more than likely breathing incorrectly. The majority of people do not breathe the right way and do not even realise it, whether they are working out or simply doing their day-to-day activities.

All athletes know breathing correctly is essential to a good workout. So why not apply this to all activities in your life? The notion of taking a class to learn to breathe may sound amusing, but breathing is the main component in the foundation of yoga. Learning to do this correctly will increase your stamina and precision in a sport and in your daily energy.

The first basic lesson you will learn in yoga class is deep, rhythmic breathing. This method actually feeds oxygen to your body's organs. Providing this oxygen to your body helps fight fatigue. Lungs that are well exercised by these breathing methods lower the chances of respiratory illness and colds. Just as you work out other parts of your body, the lungs too need a workout!

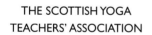
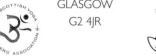

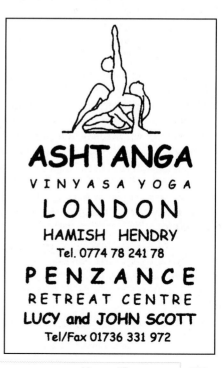

Breathing exercises also work the diaphragm and help to improve the form of the body. It is believed that through yoga you can prolong life and slow down ageing. Slow and rhythmic breathing through proper yoga can slow the heart rate down. This is restful to the heart. Since breathing is the key to life, full use of your lungs provides your body with more oxygen, without it organs and cells deteriorate faster. These exercises also relax the mind and ease tension. Yoga emphasises emotional balance for a healthy body and mind. This system of breath control in yoga is known as Pranayama. There are many breathing techniques, and it is always recommended to learn with a teacher.

A key to proper breathing lies in your posture. People who suffer from tension know that tight muscles in the shoulder area can affect the way you stand. This can throw the entire back out of alignment. Yoga can relieve this and by learning exercises poor posture can be eliminated, along with teaching relaxation of the neck, shoulders and upper back.

Some of the benefits which have been mentioned are energy, stamina, posture and flexibility. Yoga is an excellent way to improve your performance in sports. One of the elements yoga focuses on is the body's movement. Some athletes through training their body, suppress their natural ability. They train to build muscle and neglect the idea of natural movement. In yoga you will learn to become fully aware of body.

As mentioned before, breathing is the cornerstone of yoga. Learning to breathe properly alone will increase your athletic ability. Yoga helps with flexibility. Stretching through yoga you will have less of a chance of injury, than you do with regular stretching exercises. You will learn your body's limitations. It is surprising to know that most athletes know little about their own body and how it works. This will be learned through yoga classes.

Yoga also teaches the athlete balance. Runners can greatly benefit from this. Most runners display a certain position while jogging. They tend to lean forward and look as though they are falling! This is not only a strain on the body, but a waste of energy. The runner is off balance and the body is out of alignment. Yoga will teach you to align your body fully: head, neck and shoulders, aligned with the spine. It will teach a relaxed position of the arms and natural position of the pelvis. Arms hang loose and all of the work is done by the legs. Bad running habits leave muscles tense, improving your position will actually build stamina and speed.

There are many other great benefits of yoga, especially for women. This is not to say men will not benefit through yoga, it is for everyone. Yoga can help with backache,

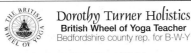

weakness and swelling. Yoga exercises aids natural childbirth by strengthening the pelvic muscles. As stated before, always consult your physician first.

Yoga also helps with the toning of the body after pregnancy. Women tend to gather excess fat in the lower body. Yoga firms this area along with the pelvic muscles after delivery.

Before commencing Yoga exercises you are advised to consult a professional in the art, there are several in this directory and on the: naturalhealthdirect.com website.

Getting started.

The best way to get started in Yoga is to either find a qualified teacher or buy a good book or tape, if you're not sure where to start looking, you will find a variety of practitioners advertising in this directory.

Types of Yoga

There are over a hundred different schools of Yoga. Some of the most well known are described below:

Hatha Yoga: The physical movements and postures, plus breathing techniques. This is what most people associate with Yoga practice.

Raja Yoga: Called the "royal road," because it incorporates exercise and breathing practice with meditation and study, producing a well-rounded individual.

Jnana Yoga: The path of wisdom; considered the most difficult path.

Bhakti Yoga: The practice of extreme devotion in one-pointed concentration upon one's concept of God.

Karma Yoga: All movement, all work of any kind is done with the mind centred on God.

Tantra Yoga: A way of showing the unseen consciousness in form through specific words, diagrams, and movements. One of the diagrams that are used to show the joining of the physical and spiritual bodies is two triangles superimposed upon one another. The downward-pointing triangle represents the physical body, or the female aspect having to do with work, action, and movement; the upward-pointing triangle represents the spiritual body of support, energy, and vastness.

Kashmir Shaivism: Everything in the universe, according to this thought, has both male and female qualities. Although it is impossible to describe these qualities exactly, some words that could be associated with the male principle are consciousness, energy, mind, and potentiality.

The female principle could be described in terms such as manifestation, movement, and form. Many other Yogic philosophies, such as Vedanta, recognise only the male principle, saying that the female aspect — that is, the manifest world — is unreal; that is why you often see pictures of ascetics attempting to negate their body through suffering and self-denial. They are attempting to prove to themselves that the world, or the female aspect, is not important.

Kashmir Shaivism, on the other hand, recognises that these male and female principles are an equal partnership; they are so interdependent that they cannot be separated; they are, in fact, one thing. The feeling of attraction between them creates the immense complexity of the universe that we enjoy and celebrate.

Also unlike other philosophies, Kashmir Shaivism is based in emotion rather than intellect. In fact, Shaivism says that intellectual understanding by itself will never lead us to 'realisation' — the summit of Yoga — because it blocks our ability to experience the full power of that male/female consciousness in ourselves.

Who Can Practice Yoga?

Yoga is suitable for most adults of any age or physical condition. Because of the non-strenuous nature of our approach to exercise, even those with physical limitations can find a beneficial routine of Yoga.

Yoga exercises are not recommended for children (those under 16) because their bodies' systems are still growing, and the effect of Yoga exercises on the glandular and other systems may interfere with those natural changes. Children may, however, safely practice meditation and simple breathing exercise (as long as the breath is never held); these techniques can greatly help children with emotional upset, anger and fear management, and stress coping.

Yoga exercises for women during menstruation is not recommend, regular practice of breathing and meditation, however, is encouraged

History of Yoga

No one knows exactly when Yoga began, but it certainly predates written history. Stone carvings depicting figures in Yoga positions have been found in archaeological sites in the Indus Valley dating back 5,000 years or more.

There is a common misconception that Yoga is rooted in Hinduism; on the contrary, Hinduism's religious structures evolved much later and incorporated some of the practices of Yoga. Other religions throughout the world have also incorporated practices and ideas related to Yoga.

The tradition of Yoga has always been passed on individually from teacher to student through oral teaching and practical demonstration. The formal techniques that are now known as Yoga are, therefore, based on the collective experiences of many individuals over many thousands of years.

The particular manner in which the techniques are taught and practised today depends on the approach passed down in the line of teachers supporting the individual practitioner.

One of the earliest texts having to do with Yoga was compiled by a scholar named Patanjali, who set down the most prevalent Yoga theories and practices of his time in a book he called Yoga Sutras ('Yoga Aphorisms') as early as the first or second century B.C. or as late as the fifth century A.D. Exact dates are unknown.

The system that he wrote about is known as 'Ashtanga Yoga', or the eight limbs of Yoga, and this is what is generally referred to today as Classical Yoga. Most current adherents practice some variation of Patanjali's system.

The eight steps of Classical Yoga are 1) yama, meaning 'restraint' – refraining from violence, lying, stealing, casual sex, and hoarding; 2) niyama, meaning 'observance' – purity, contentment, tolerance, study, and remembrance; 3) asana, physical exercises; 4) pranayama, breathing techniques; 5) pratyahara, preparation for meditation, described as 'withdrawal of the mind from the senses'; 6) dharana, concentration, being able to hold the mind on one object for a specified time; 7) dhyana, meditation, the ability to focus on one thing (or nothing) indefinitely; 8) samadhi, absorption, or realisation of the essential nature of the self. Modern Western Yoga classes generally focus on the third, fourth, and fifth steps.

Yoga probably arrived in Europe in the late 1800s, but it did not become widely known until the 1960s, as part of the youth culture's growing interest in anything Eastern. As more became known about the beneficial effects of Yoga, it gained acceptance and respect as a valuable method for helping in the management of stress and improving health and well-being.

Many doctors now recommend Yoga practice to patients with back pain, heart conditions, arthritis, depression, and other chronic conditions.

Yoga and Religion

The common belief that Yoga derives from Hinduism is a misconception. Yoga actually predates Hinduism. The techniques of Yoga have been adopted by Hinduism as well as by many other world religions.

Yoga is a system of techniques that you can use for a number of goals, from simply reducing stress or increasing limberness all the way to becoming more self-aware.

There can be a 'spiritual' dimension to Yoga practice if you practice meditation and start to become aware that there is more to you than just your physical body. This is sometimes called mystical awareness, because it puts you in touch with intuition, creativity, and other aspects of yourself that you may not have known about before.

This is not the same as organised religion, which involves a set of teachings that everyone in that religion believes in.

Religion also usually demands that you have faith without any experience in what you are supposed to have faith in.

The spiritual aspects of Yoga are strictly individual; no one tells you what you will experience or what is inside your own mind, because naturally it is different for everyone!

This type of individual practice will not interfere with your own religion — in fact, many of our students who have practiced for many years continue to follow the religious traditions they have grown up in without feeling any conflict.

YOGA

SOUTH LONDON VINIYOGA: Small group classes and group tuition in South London. For details ring Geoff Farrer 0171 703 1495 or send stamped addressed envelope to 88b Talfourd Road, London, SE15 5NZ.

EXPERIENCE YOGA. Allows gentle movement, breathing techniques and relaxation to help you balance your daily life. Classes also given for pregnancy. Individual classes available. Beginners welcome. Telephone. 0208 958 7515 e-mail h.marlow@yoga56freeserve.co.uk

YOGA IN IRELAND-Dingle -West Kerry. Classes, day/weekend workshops, HOLIDAYS, individual tuition also BOWEN technique. Highly acclaimed Deep RELAXATION C.D. available. Ilonka Miclos Tel: 0353[0]669151765 Fax: 00353[0]66152242. E-mail eoin@duigo.com

YOGA PLACE E2 – Yoga classes, courses , workshops. All levels catered for. Programme includes different styles ranging from the slower to the more dynamic -Iyengar & Scaravelli inspired yoga and Astanga Vinyasa and pregnancy yoga. Tel: 020 7739 5195. www.yogaplace.co.uk e-mail: info@yogaplace.co.uk

ELAINE SHILLITOE B.W.Y Yoga Teacher. West Yorkshire. A sensitive approach Asana,Pranayama,Relaxation.Concentration and Meditation. To create inner peace and well being. Also Aromatherapy, Kinesiology, Acupressure, Massage, Bach Flower Remedies and Reiki. More information please call 01274 870372

Zero Balancing

By M Willcocks PhD

Zero Balancing (ZB) is a gentle, yet powerful hands on method of balancing body energy with body structure. With the client fully clothed and lying down, finger pressure and held stretches are used to invite the release of tension accumulated in the deep structure of the body.

It provides a point of stillness around which the body can relax, giving the person the opportunity to let go of unease and pain and experience a new level of integration.

And so the great question in holistic bodywork is – how can a therapist get his/her hands on both a person's energy and on the physical structure? How can health practitioners precisely and simultaneously balance the physical and energetic aspects of their clients?

Today this question is being addressed elegantly by what may be the most revolutionary development in bodywork of the last quarter century. As a hands on skill it is an eminently teachable and a non-invasive means to restore and maintain well being. From thousands of reports its therapeutic impact is so profound as to evoke spiritual metaphors. For massage and body workers, movement therapists, acupuncturists, psychotherapists and all manner of medical professionals, ZB can provide practical access to both sides of the body/energy equation.

The tool developed by ZB to effect energetic and structural domains are the fulcrums. Fulcrum is defined in the dictionary as 'a position, element or agency through, around or by means of which vital powers are exercised'.

The ZB fulcrum is built by the therapist in such a manner that his or her energy and structure is brought into contact with the energy and structure of a client. In addition to this structural/energetic interface at least two other dimensions are added to the fulcrum, resulting in a complicated geometric form.

Because the proper function of the skeletal system is one of the theoretical bases for ZB and the literal basis underlying the muscles and fascia of the body, soft tissue pain and dysfunction are often relieved through ZB.

Headaches, neck and shoulder pain, low back dysfunction and many other physical symptoms may be dramatically affected by the application of the various fulcrums. Similarly, alignment will be improved through the attention paid to the foundation joints. Clients report the experience of a new uprightness and enhanced relationship of their body to gravity.

Feelings of being taller and lighter with a greater fluidity to everyday movements are commonly reported. Although more difficult to prove, it is hoped that ZB, as it brings the deepest structures and energetic domains of the body into graceful balance, has an ameliorative impact on disease and

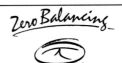

For a current list of Certified Zero Balancers or information about Zero Balancing Workshops please send a large SAE to:

ZBA UK, 10 Victoria Grove, Bridport, Dorset, DT6 3AA
Tel: **01308 420007**

degenerative processes in the body. Psychologically, sustained or acute trauma can imprint on the background field, impede or destabilise the internal energy flows and may, ultimately, affect the vertical energy flow. By emphasising fulcrums into the key energetic and structural domains crucial to the individual, ZB helps balance the psyche. Clients report a heightened sense of calmness and a lessening of needless anxiety.

The ZB client may experience the release of emotions as old stress patterns held within the various energetic domains are relieved. A restored sense of hope and power is commonly reported. This likely stems from sustained experiences within the working state. Living in a sustained manner within this expanded state of consciousness allows a more flexible, expansive perspective on problems which in an everyday state of mind may seem insuperable or overwhelming.

For many clients the most intriguing and revolutionary aspect of ZB is its spiritual impact. Intriguing because it is at once exciting and difficult to believe, given our materialistic culture and upbringing, that hands can touch another person's spirit directly and hold, amplify or balance it.

In our culture today, many people are engaged in a search for a more sustainable and harmonious way to live. There is a hunger for deeper feelings of clarity and connectedness. Revolutionary in that it provides a dramatic and body-felt amplification of this experiential realm, ZB provides a much needed and direct experience in sustained harmony, clarity and connectedness. Its theory and practice has some essential contributions to make toward the urge and need for wisdom.

The dense energy domain which ZB primarily focuses on is experienced as deep within us but not as ego. It has more in common with the 'elan vital', that vital energy or spirit which infuses us and enables us to live. ZB has discovered that this domain is accessible through the skeletal system, particularly the foundation joints.

To have identified an anatomical locus for spirit fruitfully challenges the conceptual monopoly which religion has had on spiritual experience. Spirit, from this perspective, is directly accessible through an enlightened approach to anatomy. It does not require the subscription to any particular belief system. This allows for the spread and democratisation of spiritual experience which is essential to our age if we are to move beyond ego-based lifestyles and the politics of disintegration.

Freedom is a word that not used much since the 1960s – those incredibly inspiring times in which, to paraphrase a song, many groups of people were walking and talking with their minds and hearts set on a higher level of integration for mankind.

Perhaps freedom fell into disuse because we simply lacked the deeper technologies for its achievement. This is really the science of samadhi! Samadhi means enlightenment or freedom from illusion. ZB frees the background field from past vibrations which linger in time beyond their usefulness; frees the internal energy flows from past and present stressors which needlessly impede our life function; and balances the skeletal system, thus freeing the core/source energy of our lives.

All this work heightens the perception that the source of our happiness lies not in the (in any case impossible) satisfaction of the ego, but rather in the appreciation and honouring and re-creation of this life we share on this earth at higher and higher levels of structural and energetic integrity. Through its energy model, simplicity of transmission and practice, and powerful therapeutic impact, ZB represents a qualitative step in this integrative process.

Charitable Organisation and Associations

A.C.R.E ....Gloucestershire 01285 653477

Albany Trust ....London 020 8767 1827

Association for Professional Healers ....Preston 01772 316726

Association of Professional Sugaring ....Oxfordshire 07957 587606

Bioregional Developoment Group ....Surrey 020 8773 2322

British College of Naturopathy & Osteopathy ...London 020 7592 3100

C.L.E.S ....Manchester 0161 236 1891

Craniosacral Therapy Education Trust ....London 07000 785 778

D.E.M.O'S ....London 020 7321 2200

Friends of the Earth ....London 020 7490 1555

Good Gardeners Association ....Gloucestershire 01452 750402

The Greenhouse Trust ....Norfolk 01603 631007

The International College of Oriental Medicine ..Sussex 01342 313106

Lapis Fellowship ....Essex 01206 572205

National Urban Forestry Unit ....Wolverhampton 01902 828600

Neals Yard Agency for Personal Developement .London 0870 444 2702

Permaculture Association ....London 01654 712188

The Raptor Foundation ....Cambridgeshire 01487 741140

The Soil Association ....Bristol 0117 929 0661

The Trinity Centre ....Essex 01206 561150

Unstone Grange Trust ....Derbyshire 01246 412344

Directory

ACUPUNCTURE

AIKIDO

ALCHEMY

ALEXANDER TECHNIQUE

ALLERGY TESTING

ALOE VERA

ALTERNATIVE DENTISTRY

AMATSU

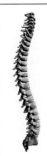
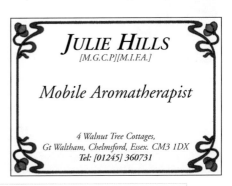

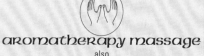

AROMATHERAPY (CONT)

Kent	Madden, L 36
	Natural Balance 44
Kent	Ryan, N 37
Lanarkshire	Bankier, F 40
	Muller, V 45
Lancashire	Chadwick, E 37
	Sandra Day School of Health . . .45
	Total Care Therapy 37
Leicestershire	Duhy, C 42
London	Aromatherapy
	Organisations Council 44
	Morris, M 45
	Roques – O'Neil, R 43
	The Relaxation Place 39
Merseyside	The Health & Beauty Centre . . .45
Middlesex	Darling, J 27
Oxfordshire	Jenny Wren Remedies 39
	Mann, B 38
Perthshire	McPherson, N 40
Roxburghshire	Natures Touch 45
Staffordshire	Barr, H 45
	Williscroft, B 45
Surrey	Seymour, L 45
West Midlands	Davies, E 40

AROMATHERAPY (CONT)

West Midlands	Victoria Aromatherapy 38
Wiltshire	Bodysense Aromatherapy 40
Worcestershire	Penrice, C 45
Yorkshire	Atkinson, E & Wood, C 42
	Choice Aromas 39
	Hinchliffe, J 329
	Hodkin, A 45
	P A Aromatherapy 45
	Parry, K 45
	Shackleton, R 45
	White, A 39

AROMATHERAPY PRODUCTS & ESSENTIAL OILS

Cambridgeshire	Eve Taylor (London) Ltd 52
Cheshire	Aquarius Aromatherapy 46
	Cameo Essential Oils 52
Cornwall	Plantain 49
Denbighshire	Celestial Design 47
Devon	Essence Serene 48
Hampshire	New Horizon Aromatics 50
Ireland	Unicorn Products (Eire) Ltd 48
Leicestershire	Quinessence Aromatherapy 48
	Scentimental 51
London	Alexander Essentials Ltd 50

AROMATHERAPY PRODUCTS & ESSENTIAL OILS (CONT)

London	Aromacushion Ltd	.46
Oxfordshire	New Seasons	.52
Somerset	Harmony Oils Ltd	.49
Sussex	Aromadot	.46
Sussex	Good Scents	.47
Tyne & Wear	Feel Good Aromatherapy	.47
Warwickshire	Purple Flame	.49

ART, DRAMA & DANCE THERAPY

Bristol	Dominique Pahud & David Thorogood	.60
Cambridgeshire	Holliday, C	.60
Dorset	Doorway To Power	.147
Gloucestershire	Scenario	.59
Kent	Wilson, V	.60
London	Black, K	.55
	Eeabe	.56
	Institute for Arts in Therapy & Education	.57, 60
	Mendoza, H	.60
	Pomegranite	.60
	Riley, F	.60
Middlesex	Rose, H	.60
Powys	The Aquarian Studio	.54

ART, DRAMA & DANCE THERAPY (CONT)

Surrey	Kemp, I	.60
Sussex	Branscombe, J	.60
	Cruthers, H	.60

ASTROLOGY

Cambridgeshire	Jones, P	.253
Nottinghamshire	Faculty of Astrological Studies	.61
Surrey	Brooker, J	.172
West Lothian	Saunders, J	.61

AURA SOMA

Bedfordshire	Goodwin, C	.63
	Grace, K	.350
Buckinghamshire	Rainbow Studio	.62
Cambridgeshire	Hurst, S	.64
Cheshire	Irving, R	.64
	Tilston, A	.64
Co Durham	Taylor, R	.64
Hampshire	Bull, I	.64
Kent	Lennard, J	.64
Lincolnshire	Asiact	.62
London	Graham, L	.64
Middlesex	Open Door Therapies	.64
Suffolk	White, M	.62
Surrey	Rosenberg, S	.63

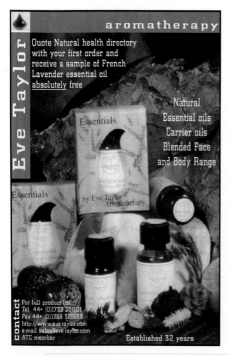
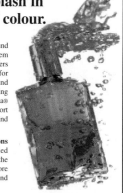

AURA SOMA (CONT)
Sussex Aura Soma Direct 63
 Castle, P 187

AYURVEDIC MEDICINE
London Depala, R 65

BACH FLOWER REMEDIES
Cheshire Gill, S 319
Co Durham Midgley, C 68
Devon Hollingsworth, E 68
Dorset Turner, H M 318
Hampshire Shiner, S 68
Leicestershire Snuggs, M 68
London Baird, J 68
 Lewis, I 68
 Lomas, C 68
Oxfordshire The Bach Centre 66
 Gins, F 67
 Ritchie, N 68
Pembrokeshire Going For Health 68
Somerset Taylor, C 68
Sussex Haywards Heath
 Natural Therapy Rooms 66
 Rawlings, M 329
 Vaines, E 67
West Midlands Miller, V 68
Yorkshire Smith, Y 68
 Thurlow, N 335

BODY ELECTRONICS
Devon Bodyelectronics 69

BOOKS MAGAZINES & PUBLISHERS
London Moksha Press 70
Sussex Mayfair Publishing 70

BOWEN TECHNIQUE
Ayrshire Health, Stress & Injuries Clinic .73
Berkshire Lidiard, L 337
 Norris, T 297
Cheshire Emery, S 71
 Evans, D & Mee, B 71
Devon Berry, R 80
Dorset The Bowen Association (UK) ...76
 Jenkins, R 71, 78
Fifeshire Caldwell, S 72
 The Complementary
 Therapy Clinic 75
Ireland Bowen Therapists Ireland 74
Kent Austin, N 74

BOWEN TECHNIQUE (CONT)
Lanarkshire Doherty, R 72
 Healthy Backs 73
 Kenilworth Medical Centre 75
Lancashire The Reiki Way 220
Lincolnshire Barton, M 78
London Rahs, E 80
Merseyside Beer, P 74
Middlesex Mills, J 192
Norfolk Jones, G 71
Northamptonshire Wild Wood
 Complementary Therapies 239
Nottinghamshire Hughes, P 73
Oxfordshire Feary, H 78
Perthshire Smith, I 72
 Macdonald, A 79
Shropshire Wilkinson, S 76
Somerset European College of
 Bowen Studies 77
 Underwood, M 76
Stirlingshire Martin, L 72
Surrey Milton, R 79
 Rigby, C 80
Warwickshire Gentilli, A 80
 The Physical Therapy Clinic 75
West Lothian Ward, E 344
Yorkshire Slack, D 75

BREATHWORK
Cumbria Rhouvier, S 373

BUQI
London Leong, T 81

BUSINESS OPPORTUNITIES
Essex Magnetic World 83
Gloucestershire Nutrition For Life 82
Warwickshire Natural Health Options 270

BUTEYKO

CANCER CARE

CHILDREN & BABY PRODUCTS

CHINESE HERBAL MEDICINE

CHIROPRACTIC

COLLOIDAL SILVER

COLONIC HYDROTHERAPY

COLOUR PUNCTURE

COLOUR THERAPY

COMPLEMENTARY HEALTH CARE CLINICS & CENTRES

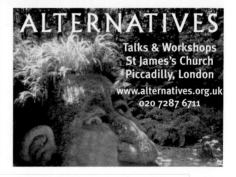

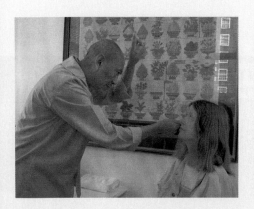 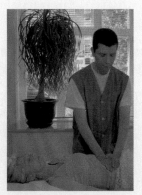

COUNSELLING & PSYCHOTHERAPY (CONT)

CRANIOSACRAL THERAPY

CRYSTAL HEALING

CRYSTAL HEALING (CONT)

CRYSTALS

DANCE, SOUND & HEART MEDITATION

DETOXIFICATION

DOWSING

EARTH HEALING

EDUCATION, TRAINING & WORKSHOPS

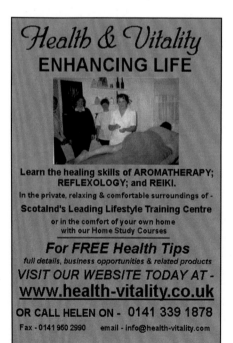

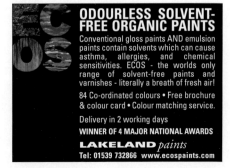

NO OTHER ENVIRONMENTALLY FRIENDLY WASHING PRODUCTS ARE MORE EFFECTIVE & 'DOWN TO EARTH'.

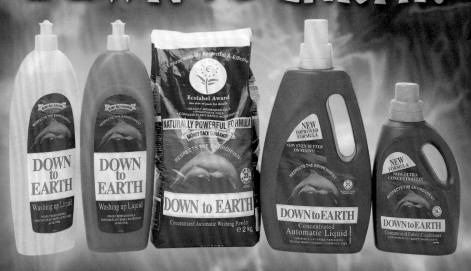

Phosphate-free and readily biodegradable, Down to Earth contains plant derived ingredients that help protect the environment, while optimising performance. It's therefore no surprise that we are the only washing powder to be independently judged and awarded the Eco label by the European Union. If you would like to find out more about how to help your environment, call the DOWN TO EARTH GREENLINE, FREEPHONE 0500 646645 (UK only)

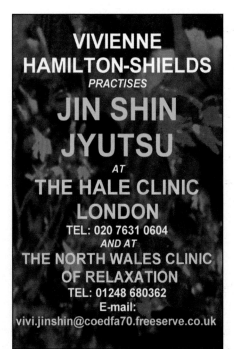

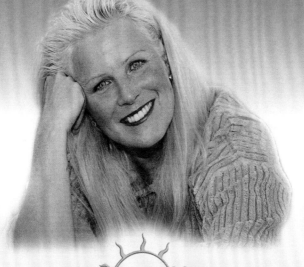

NUTRITION (CONT)

NUTRITIONAL PRODUCTS

NUTRITIONAL THERAPY

ORGANIC FOOD & DRINK

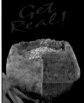

We understand
that you care about what you eat
Organic

With over 700 products in some of our largest stores, you can trust Tesco to provide you with a fantastic range of quality Organic food at low prices.

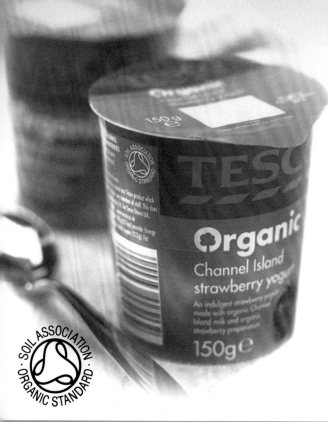

If you've ever thought that choosing organics meant limiting your choice, think again. We've re-launched our organic range to ensure we offer yo an organic alternative for all your everyday products. But that's not all we also offer a selection of more exotic organic lines so you can find organic products to suit every occasion.

You can trust us to provide you with the highest quality organic food at low prices. All our organic products are grown and produced to regulations laid down by the United Kingdom Register of Organic Food Standards. And all our products are certified by approval bodies such as the Soil Association who ensure that these strict standards are adhered to

TESCO
'The UK's favourite Organic Retailer'
as voted in Mintel Survey published in Supermarketing Magazine 30/6/00

ORGANIC PRODUCTS & SERVICES
Devon — Golden Fleeces 284
Suttons 284
Herefordshire — Sunnybank Vine Nursery .282, 284
Willy Winkle 283
Ireland — Natural Instincts 284
Surrey — Clearly Natural 283

OSTEOPATHY
Bedfordshire — Leighton Buzzard Centre 285
Co Durham — Teesdale Osteopathic Clinic ...285
London — The Replingham Clinic 119

PAST LIFE WORK
London — Cheetham, A 205
Derbyshire — Pheonix Healing Centre 287
Suffolk — Wallace, G 286

PERSONAL CARE
Cheshire — Clover Leaf Centre 289

PERSONAL DEVELOPMENT
Cumbria — Rhouvier, S 373
Inverness-Shire — Herbert, M 290

PHYSIOTHERAPY
Bedfordshire — Leighton Buzzard Centre 293
London — Hobar Therapeutic Services ...293
Vanbrugh Physiotherapy Clinic 292

PILATES
Bedfordshire — Boyle, K 299
Leighton Buzzard Centre 296
Berkshire — Norris, T 297
Wakefield, F..............297
Buckinghamshire — Eales, C 299

PILATES (CONT)
Devon — The Pure Pilates Studio 299
Hertfordshire — Locher, K 299
Lanarkshire — Stearn, L 299
Nottinghamshire — Burnett, P 299
Shropshire — Hatch, L 299
Surrey — Garrett, O 297
West Lothian — Brigid McCarthy Pilates Studio .299
Edinburgh Pilates Centre 299

PRANIC HEALING
Hampshire — Humby, H 302
London — Nelson, C 303

PRECONCEPTUAL CARE
Surrey — Barnes, B 305
Foresight 304

PSYCHONEURO IMMUNOLOGY
London — Healthworks 308

QI GONG
Surrey — Gerchi, D 310
Sussex — Brighton School of Tantra 361

RADIONICS
Gloucestershire — Stewart, C A 313
London — Keys College of Radionics 149
Oxfordshire — The Radionic Association 312
Yorkshire — Temple, J 313

REBIRTHING
Cambridgeshire — Wilkins, P 316
Dorset — Artemis, C (Doorway to Power) .147
Dumfries & Galloway — Lewis, F 316
Greater Manchester — McCallum, C 316
London — Breathworks 314
British Rebirth Society 315
Cheetham, A 205
Gabriel, C 316
Lange, G 316
The London College of Holistic Breath Therapy 316

REFLEXOLOGY
Berkshire — Edmonds, A 332
Grey, P.................325
Buckinghamshire — Helen Elizabeth 317
Cambridgeshire — Evans, J 332
Taylor, R 326

HOBAR THERAPEUTIC SEVICES

PHYSIOTHERAPY, REMEDIAL
SPORTS INJURIES
AROMATHERAPY TREATMENTS
MUSICIANS CLINIC

London SW and Surrey North
Tel: 020 8405 4707

REFLEXOLOGY (CONT)

REFLEXOLOGY (CONT)

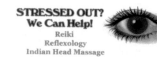
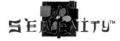

REGRESSION THERAPY
Yorkshire   Thurlow, N 335

REIKI
Berkshire   Lidiard, L 337
                   The Reiki School 337
Cambridgeshire   Hurst, S 64
                   Mason, M 333
Cheshire   Gill, S 319
                   Marston, S 334
Cumbria   Murphy, I, RGN 45
Derbyshire   Peak School of Reiki 336
Dyfed   Perfect Scents 328
Hampshire   The Wellbeing Consultancy . . .336
Herefordshire   Pinches, J E 328
Ireland   Solanus Garden 43
Kent   Pellatt, G J Y 337
Lancashire   The Reiki Way 220
London   Bailey, S 213
                   Cross, M and Knight, K 252
                   Topham, S 333
                   Zenined, L 336
Merseyside   Reiki Dawn 333
Norfolk   Gilmour, M 334
Oxfordshire   Gins, F 67
Somerset   Cariad West 335
Surrey   Cowieson, M 330
                   Raworth, J 334
Sussex   Durham, Y 226
                   Spiers, B 334
                   Tera-Mai Association 336
                   Wildor, C 335
Warwickshire   Hitchco, J 333
                   Patricia Owen &
                   Barbara Thompson 222
West Lothian   Heaven Scent 337
Worcestershire   Kordas, A 137
Yorkshire   Stratton, K 339
                   Thurlow, N 335

SEKHEM
Berkshire   Hodgson, A 340
Cambridgeshire   Cornell, J 340
Fifeshire   Buyers, J M 339
Lancashire   Guest, G 340
Lincolnshire   Green, G 340
London   Busaan Warham, G 339
                   Cochin – De Billy, S 340
West Lothian   Trubridge, F 339
Yorkshire   Stratton, K 339

SHAMANIC REIKI
Sussex   Castle, P 187

SHAMANISM
London   Alvardo, S 132
                   Amoda 342
Yorkshire   The Shamanic
                   Research Foundation 341

SHEN THERAPY
Dorset   Collins, D 342
Fifeshire   McCathie, M 344
Lanarkshire   McClennan, J & Phillips, I 346
                   Morton, F 344
Perthshire   Shen Therapy Centre 345
Perthshire   Campbell, D and R 346
Tyne & Wear   McLane, I 346
West Lothian   Barlow, C 344
                   Ward, E 344
Worcestershire   Heart of England Centre 346

SHIATSU
Fifeshire   Lamont, M 347
Kent   Lucy Moorhead Shiatsu &
                   Counselling 347
Northumberland   Robinson-Begg, C 347
Surrey   Wallace, S 347
Sussex   The Art of Unwinding 360

SKENAR
Wiltshire   Life Energies Ltd 348

SOUND THERAPY
Bedfordshire   Grace, K 340
Bristol   Thompson, E 349
London   D'angelo, J 350
Surrey   Sound Works 150

Kingsley Media Ltd
Kingsley House
College Road
Keyham
PLYMOUTH
PL2 1NT

Dear Reader,

We hope that you have found this directory useful and that you will use the therapies, services and products contained it its pages. We have been as careful as possible to ensure that all advertisers are bona fide, and would appreciate your comments, good or indifferent. All such comments will be passed to the appropriate advertiser.

The next edition in this series will be available in January 2002. If you use a therapist, service or product you feel should be included in the next edition, please write to us or E-mail: editor@naturalhealthdirect.com.

Freepost address: **KINGSLEY MEDIA (FREEPOST PY2100) PLYMOUTH PL2 1ZZ** (No stamp required).

Wishing you good health and peace.

Louise O'Neill

Louise O'Neill
Editor

The Editor wishes to say a special thank you to all the contributing authors whose knowledge and hard work has been invaluable to the compilation of this edition of the Natural Health Directory.

Adrian Tindale at the
British Aikido Association

Alan Sanderson

Ali Northcott

Amanda Rogers

Andina Seers

Angela Bradbury at the
Guild of Naturopathic Iridologists

Angelica Hochadel

Belinda Barnes

Brian Gibbons

Brian H Butler at the
Association of Systematic Kinesiology

Bridgitte Scott

British Chiropractic Association

Chris Retzler

Chrissie Hardisty and Silvia Hartman-Kent at the
Association for Meridian Therapies

Christine Green

Claire Maxwell-Hudson

Dario Gerchi

Darren Higgins

Debbie Thomas

Dennis Altram at Amatsu UK

Derek Webster

Dominic Yeoman

Don Harrison at
the British Institute for Allergy Testing

Dr N. Sathiymoorthy at
the Ayurvedic Medical Association

Dr. Liesbeth Ash and David Ash

Editha Campbell, David Burmeister and
Michou Landon

Eileen Fairbane

Ellen Collinson

Feng Shui Society

Geraldine Sherborne

Gerd Lang

Helen Belot

Janie Godfrey at the
European College for Bowen Studies

Jayne Williams

Jenny Hok

Joan Diamond

John Fuller at the
British Complementary Medical Association

John Vernon

John Wilkes at the
Bowen Association

Kamini Alena Hola

Kate and Simon Kirkwood

Lauren Harrington

Linda Fellows

Lorrane Myers

Louise Smart

Marcus West

Margaret Barnes

Margaret Brooks

Margot Sunderland at the
Institute for Arts in Therapy and Education

Mark Maxwell at the
Brighton School of Tantra

Michael Grevis

Michael Kern

Michael Rust at the
British Society of Dowsers

Milo Seiwert

Narendra Mehta

Nicola Dunn

Nina Gallagher

Patrick Holford

Pauline Allen

Peter Atherton

Peter Aziz

Peter Mansfield

Pratibha Castle

Richard Morgan

Robert I. White & Professor Yilan Shen

Ron Bowles

Roz Comins at the Voice Care Network

Sheila Gill

Simon Duncan at the
British Reflexology Association

Stefan Ball at the Bach Centre

Sue Martin at the
Faculty of Astrological Studies

Sue Richter

Suzie Chiazzari

Teresa Leong

The British Acupuncture Council

The British Bio-Magnetic Association

The College of Past Life Regression

The Federation of Holistic Therapists

The High Touch Network

The Holographic Repatterning Association

The Journey

The McTimoney Chiropractic Association

The Metamorphic Association

The Munro Hall Clinic

The National Register of
Hypnotherapists and Psychotherapists

The Osteopathic Information Service

The Reiki College

The Rev Professor Andrew Lindzey

The School of Spinal Touch Therapy

The Shamanic Research Foundation

The Shen Therapy Institute

The Society of Homeopaths

The team at New Approaches

The World Federation of Healing

Tina Ricketts

Tony Hampton

Trudy Norris at the
National Institute for Medical Herbalists

Vida Butcher

Banish the hype
Have your detector ready

Thousands of vulnerable people are duped into spending millions of pounds on useless remedies and devices every year. Worse still, many with serious medical problems waste valuable time before getting proper treatment. As this delay may endanger lives, please seek professional advice before buying any 'cure' products.

There are ways to evaluate the genuineness of products, for instance:

Does the label claim that there are precious oils or essences in the product? Check the percentage claimed and do your research on the cost/availability of these additives. You will probably discover that the cost of the item cannot justify the high cost of the additive, hence the claim would be misleading and at worst utterly false.

Does the advertisement promise 'a quick and easy cure?' There is no such thing.

Is the product advertised as effective for a wide range of ailments or for an undiagnosed pain? Be careful.

Does the manufacturer use key words such as 'miraculous,' 'exclusive,' 'secret,' or 'ancient?' This is probably pure hype.

Is the product advertised as available from only one source, requiring payment in advance? Walk away.

Does the manufacturer use undocumented case histories that sound too good to be true? Ask for proof.

In addition, don't rely on promises of a 'money-back guarantee.' Be aware that many fly-by-night operators may never be there to respond to a refund request.

Being well informed enables you to spot fraud. Learn to recognise products by the above typical phrases that are often used to promote them. Have your hype detector switched on and don't buy when it bleeps.

Why is fraud successful

Fraud, or quackery, is a business that sells false hope. It preys on vulnerable people who are victims of conditions that have no complete medical cures, such as arthritis, multiple sclerosis and certain forms of cancer. It also thrives on the wishful thinking of those who want short-cuts to their personal appearance. Such vanity enables the 'cowboy element' of an essentially legitimate trade to make quick profits.

Those who wish to deceive the public have always been quick to exploit trends. Whilst legitimate medical science, natural and orthodox, is continually advancing, unscrupulous dealers are quick to market useless concoctions as medical 'breakthroughs.'

Whilst fraudulent selling of 'copycat' or bogus products invariably causes irreparable harm to bona fide products, the most damaging frauds of all are the ones that turn people away from proper medical diagnosis and treatment of serious illnesses.

How to spot the fraud.

Consumers can avoid problems and save money by learning some basic facts about fraud. The following sections discuss five conditions that can be susceptible to cure misrepresentations. This is not an exhaustive list, but it is representative and may help you become better informed and spend your money more effectively.

Arthritis

If you or a family member is one of the estimated millions of people who suffer from one of the many forms of arthritis, be aware that this condition invites a flood of useless products. This is because, so far, medical science has found no cure for arthritis. Thousands of dietary and natural 'cures' have been sold for arthritis like mussel extract, vitamin pills, desiccated liver pills, and honey and vinegar mixtures. In fact it has been proven that no herb, either by itself or in combination with other ingredients, is a cure for any form of arthritis. In addition, there is no medical evidence to suggest that a lack of vitamins or minerals causes arthritis or that taking vitamin or mineral supplements will give relief.

If you have arthritis and in search of a cure, you should know that arthritis is a serious condition that should be treated by a qualified health professional. Miracle 'cures,' copper bracelets, and even self-prescribed over-the-counter pain-relieving products cannot take the place of appropriate medical advice and treatment.

Cancer

Because the diagnosis of cancer can bring feelings of fear and hopelessness, many people who have been diagnosed as having a form of cancer may be tempted to turn to unproven remedies or clinics that promise a cure. As an aid to evaluating cancer-cure claims, keep in mind that there is no one device or remedy capable of diagnosing or treating all types of cancer. Cancer is a name given to a wide range of conditions requiring different forms of treatment determined by a qualified health professional. Medical science has been able to help many cancer patients, but use of a bogus remedy can delay proper diagnosis and treatment.

Weight Loss

If you, or others you know, are attempting to lose weight, consider these basic facts:

If you want to lose weight you must lower your calorie intake or increase your calorie use by exercise. Claims that you can eat all you want and lose weight effortlessly defy the rules of nature and thus belong to the annals of mythology. Any weight loss product can only be effective and sustain weight loss as part of a fitness programme. Any dietary product or programme will not be effective and long lasting without reducing your calorie intake or increasing your calorie use through exercise. If you want to lose weight and tone up as well, you must exercise. If you want to look good and be fit, particularly as you grow older, you must exercise.

Fat deposits

'Cellulite' is a name advertisers sometimes use for the fat that some people accumulate around their thighs, buttocks, and stomachs. Before you buy products advertised to dissolve 'cellulite,' here are some important things to keep in mind:

No amount of rubbing, wrapping, massaging or scrubbing will get rid of fat deposits. The best way to reduce fat deposits is by dieting to lose weight and exercising to improve muscle tone. No special vitamin or mineral supplement can dissolve fat deposits. Again, the best way to lose weight, including fat on thighs, buttocks, and stomach, is to follow a sensible diet and exercise programme.

Baldness

If you are bald or your hair is thinning, you may be a target for fraud. You should know that: no over-the-counter cream, lotion, or device can prevent baldness, induce new hair to grow, or cause hair to become thicker. Over-the-counter (non-prescription), do-it-yourself 'remedies' are ineffective because most baldness is hereditary. Ninety per cent of all baldness is due to the inherited trait known as 'male pattern baldness'; also, no over-the-counter cream, lotion, or device can treat other types of baldness, including those caused by ringworm, systemic disease, glandular defects or local infection.

For a proper diagnosis of the cause of baldness and to discuss possible treatment, consult a professional Trichologist. Artificial hair implants are dangerous and will not stimulate natural hair growth. The implanting of polyester or modacrylic fibres into the scalp can cause serious infections, bleeding and loss of natural hair. Such implants are generally recognised by doctors as unsafe and ineffective, and have a high probability of discomfort and pain, together with a high risk of infection, skin disease and scarring.

What you can do to help

Although the Government requires that over-the-counter health products to be subjected to stringent controls, many unscrupulous companies find loopholes in the law and sell products without meeting these requirements. Indeed, the Internet is the perfect vehicle for this because it can operate outside national laws.

Laws that prohibit fraud can be enforced against retailers and advertisers of bogus products or services. There are several agencies available to the public, Trading Standards being the most accessible; then there are Government, advertising and television watchdogs. By being aware of the fraud problem and by reporting suspicious products to the appropriate agency, you can help get dangerous or worthless products and services off the market.

Remember, if you are thinking of taking any health promoting or ailment cure supplements, consult your GP if you are taking other prescribed medicines to make sure they don't clash with the medication you are already taking.

Don't be afraid to complain, you are very important to the retailer, be it a small shop, supermarket, or multi national conglomerate, without you they have no business, so it is in their interest to investigate your complaint.

There is an old saying:

The highwayman demands 'your money OR your life,' but quacks demand 'your money AND your life!'

This statement is particularly true when it comes to dubious over-the-counter health products. Please take care and have a healthy 'natural' life.

M. Willcocks PhD

The Green Life Directory
Patron: Richard Briers OBE

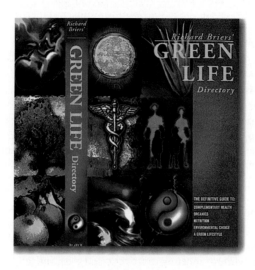

U **ntil now It has been difficult for the consumer to make natural choices, when being overwhelmed with product advertising and the lack of meaningful definitions as to what constitutes a natural product or service. The Green Life Directory does, for the first time, provide a single and targeted source of relevant information, enabling the public to choose a cleaner, healthier, more fulfiling life style.**

The Green Life Directory is the ultimate compendium, providing a way forward to a healthier lifestyle. It incorporates a comprehensive A–Z directory of manufacturers, producers, suppliers, shops, natural beauty and health farms/retreats, products and services, where to stay, eat and ecological attractions, plus authoritative articles by leading experts and generic descriptions of all facets of the rapidly growing GREEN industry.

A powerful presence in a heavy weight directory, to give this project substance we have enlisted the support of many widely recognised experts and professionals. The following is a specimen list of people assisting with this project, Patrick Holford–Nutrition. The University of Durham–Green Chemistry. Tom Flood–Conservation. The University of Exeter–Environmental studies. The Soil Association–Organic. Nature Watch–Company product. Professor Andrew Linzey–Animal care and many more.

Available at £7.95 from all branches of Waterstones, selected branches of WH Smith, and other retail outlets. If your local book shop does not have it in stock please ask them to order from: ABA Book Distribution, 59 College Road, Keyham, Plymouth PL2 1NT; Tel: 01752 519735; Email: aba@naturalhealthdirect.com.

Great titles from Kingsley Media Ltd

The Four Seasons Bed & Breakfast Guide
An extremely useful guide of 1200 pages packed with information on all parts of Britain with descriptions, potted history, places to go and things to do, also a selection of quality places to stay from hotels to guest houses.
PRICE: £12.50 (DISCOUNTED TO £7.95) + £4. POST & PACKING

The Bed & Breakfast Magazine
A magazine for the whole of Britain featuring thousands of places to go and things to do, with stories from celebrities, breakfast at 10.000 ft. etc. Also personally selected places to stay or eat. Great Value.
PRICE: £3.95 + £1.50 POST & PACKING

The Selected Bed & Breakfast Guide (Millennium Edition)
Another fabulous guide to the whole of Britain, bristling with what Britain has to offer, and places to stay from castles to guest houses at prices to suit every pocket.
PRICE: £9.95 (DISCOUNTED TO £6.95) PLUS £2. POST & PACKING

Travellers Choice: Hotels – Inns – Restaurants (Millennium Edition)
A really useful guide for the traveller packed with venues selected for quality and service at the right price, also featuring what to do and where to go in an informative, easy to use format.
PRICE: £9.95 (DISCOUNTED TO £6.95) PLUS £2. POST & PACKING

Eat In/Eat Out in Great Britain
A book to entertain all lovers of good food. It provides an eclectic mix of places to eat from the top echelons to simple tea rooms, plus an array of recipes gathered from restaurateurs and an assortment of specialist shops, farms and fisheries where the unusual can be sourced.
PRICE: £9.95 (DISCOUNTED TO £6.95) PLUS £2. POST & PACKING

The Discerning Visitor to East Anglia
A guide especially prepared for those who visit out of season. What to see and do and places to stay. A fascinating guide for discovering East Anglia.
PRICE: £7.95 (DISCOUNTED TO £5.95) + £2. POST AND PACKING

The Discerning Visitor to Wessex and Exmoor
A guide especially prepared for those who visit out of season What to see and do, places to stay and a complete guide to Bristol, Wiltshire, Somerset and Dorset.
PRICE: £7.95 (DISCOUNTED TO £5.95) + £2. POST AND PACKING

A Day Out in Cornwall and Days Out in Devon
Two essential magazines for visitors and locals alike. Packed with ideas for a day out, with information grids containing all the information you need to enjoy your holiday, find that special place to eat or simply enjoy what these holiday counties have to offer.
PRICE: £2.95 (DISCOUNTED TO £1.95) + £1 POST AND PACKING

Grandfather Parkyn's Eclipse
A unique and delightfully descriptive story of a 1,300-mile round trip from Cornwall to Edinburgh undertaken by the Mayor of Par and three companions in a Fiat tourer in 1927.
PRICE: £4.95 (DISCOUNTED TO £2.95) + £2 POST AND PACKING

All of the above titles are available from Waterstones, WH Smith and other leading book shops, if they do not have stock of your choice please ask them to order from: ABA Book Distribution, 59 College Road, Keyham, Plymouth PL2 1NT. Tel: 01752 519735

To order direct from the publisher please complete the following:

Please send the following title(s) ....

Please debit my credit card (card type) .... *(American Express and Diners Cards not accepted)*

Card Number ☐☐☐☐ ☐☐☐☐ ☐☐☐☐ ☐☐☐☐

Name On Card ....

Card Expiry _____/_____ Card Issue Number (where applicable) ....

Enclosed cheque in sum of £ .... **SEND TO: KINGSLEY MEDIA LTD, FREEPOST (PY2100), PLYMOUTH PL2 1ZZ (NO STAMP REQUIRED)**

Name and address. ....

....

....

.... Post code ....

Daytime telephone number ....